RED BOOK®
ATLAS
OF PEDIATRIC INFECTIOUS DISEASES

Editor
Carol J. Baker, MD, FAAP

American Academy of Pediatrics

141 Northwest Point Blvd

Elk Grove Village, IL 60007-1098

Developmental Editor: Martha Cook

Photo Editor: Mark Ruthman

Marketing Manager: Linda Smessaert

Production Manager: Theresa Wiener

Designer: Dave Roberts

Production: Peg Mulcahy

Copyeditor: Kate Larson

Library of Congress Control Number 2006930574
ISBN-13: 978-1-58110-247-5
ISBN-10: 1-58110-247-X
MA0381

The recommendations in this publication do not indicate an exclusive course of treatment or serve as a standard of care. Variations, taking into account individual circumstances, may be appropriate.

Brand names are furnished for identification purposes only. No endorsement of the manufacturers or products listed is implied.

3-174/0407

1 2 3 4 5 6 7 8 9 10

Table of Contents

Acknowledgments vi

Introduction vii

Image Credits viii

1/Actinomycosis 1

2/Adenovirus Infections 3

3/Amebiasis 4

4/Amebic Meningoencephalitis and Keratitis (*Naegleria fowleri, Acanthamoeba* species, and *Balamuthia mandrillaris*) 6

5/Anthrax 9

6/Arboviruses 12

7/*Arcanobacterium haemolyticum* Infections 15

8/*Ascaris lumbricoides* Infections 17

9/Aspergillosis 19

10/Babesiosis 21

11/Bacterial Vaginosis 22

12/*Bacteroides* and *Prevotella* Infections 24

13/*Balantidium coli* Infections (Balantidiasis) 26

14/*Baylisascaris* Infections 27

15/Blastomycosis 29

16/Borrelia Infections (Relapsing Fever) 31

17/Brucellosis 33

18/*Campylobacter* Infections 35

19/Candidiasis (Moniliasis, Thrush) 37

20/Cat-Scratch Disease *(Bartonella henselae)* 40

21/Chancroid 43

22/*Chlamydia trachomatis* 44

23/*Clostridium botulinum* (Botulism and Infant Botulism) 46

24/*Clostridium difficile* 48

25/Clostridial Myonecrosis (Gas Gangrene) 50

26/Coccidioidomycosis 52

27/*Cryptococcus neoformans* Infections (Cryptococcosis) 55

28/Cutaneous Larva Migrans 57

29/Cytomegalovirus Infection 58

30/Diphtheria 61

31/*Ehrlichia* and *Anaplasma* Infections (Human Ehrlichioses) 63

32/Enterovirus (Nonpoliovirus) Infections (Group A and B Coxsackieviruses, Echoviruses, and Numbered Enteroviruses) 67

33/Epstein-Barr Virus Infections (Infectious Mononucleosis) 69

34/*Escherichia coli* (Nondiarrheal) and Other Gram-Negative Bacilli (Septicemia and Meningitis in Neonates) 72

35/*Escherichia coli* Diarrhea (Including Hemolytic-Uremic Syndrome) 75

36/*Giardia intestinalis* Infections (Giardiasis) 80

37/Gonococcal Infections 82

38/Granuloma Inguinale (Donovanosis) 86

39/*Haemophilus influenzae* Infections 88

40/Hantavirus Pulmonary Syndrome 91

41/*Helicobacter pylori* Infections 94
42/Hepatitis A 95
43/Hepatitis B 97
44/Hepatitis C 101
45/Herpes Simplex 103
46/Histoplasmosis 109
47/Hookworm Infections (*Ancylostoma duodenale* and *Necator americanus*) 112
48/Human Herpesvirus 6 (Including Roseola) and 7 114
49/Human Immunodeficiency Virus Infection 116
50/Influenza 124
51/Kawasaki Disease (Mucocutaneous Lymph Node Syndrome) 127
52/Leishmaniasis 131
53/Leprosy 133
54/Leptospirosis 136
55/*Listeria monocytogenes* Infections (Listeriosis) 138
56/Lyme Disease (Lyme borreliosis, *Borrelia burgdorferi* Infection) 140
57/Lymphatic Filariasis (Bancroftian, Malayan, and Timorian) 144
58/Lymphocytic Choriomeningitis 146
59/Malaria 147
60/Measles 150
61/Meningococcal Infections 153
62/Molluscum Contagiosum 157
63/Mumps 159
64/*Mycoplasma pneumoniae* Infections 161
65/Nocardiosis 163
66/Onchocerciasis (River Blindness, Filariasis) 166
67/Human Papillomaviruses 169
68/Paracoccidioidomycosis (South American Blastomycosis) 172
69/Paragonimiasis 174
70/Parainfluenza Viral Infections 176
71/Parvovirus B19 (Erythema Infectiosum, Fifth Disease) 178
72/*Pasteurella* Infections 181
73/Pediculosis Capitis (Head Lice) 182
74/Pediculosis Corporis (Body Lice) 184
75/Pediculosis Pubis (Pubic Lice) 185
76/Pertussis (Whooping Cough) 186
77/Pinworm Infection *(Enterobius vermicularis)* 190
78/Pityriasis Versicolor (Tinea Versicolor) 192
79/Plague 195
80/Pneumococcal Infections 198
81/*Pneumocystis jiroveci* Infections 204
82/Poliovirus Infections 207
83/Rabies 210
84/Rat-Bite Fever 213
85/Respiratory Syncytial Virus 215
86/Rickettsialpox 217
87/Rocky Mountain Spotted Fever 219

88/Rotavirus Infections 223
89/Rubella 225
90/Salmonella Infections 229
91/Scabies 233
92/Schistosomiasis 236
93/Shigella Infections 239
94/Smallpox (Variola) 241
95/Sporotrichosis 246
96/Staphylococcal Infections 248
97/Group A Streptococcal Infections 261
98/Group B Streptococcal Infections 269
99/Non–Group A or B Streptococcal and Enterococcal Infections 272
100/Strongyloidiasis (Strongyloides stercoralis) 275
101/Syphilis 278
102/Tapeworm Diseases (Taeniasis and Cysticercosis) 294
103/Other Tapeworm Infections (Including Hydatid Disease) 297
104/Tetanus (Lockjaw) 299
105/Tinea Capitis (Ringworm of the Scalp) 302
106/Tinea Corporis (Ringworm of the Body) 305
107/Tinea Cruris (Jock Itch) 307
108/Tinea Pedis and Tinea Unguium (Athlete's Foot, Ringworm of the Feet) 308
109/Toxic Shock Syndrome 310
110/Toxocariasis (Visceral Larva Migrans, Ocular Larva Migrans) 316
111/Toxoplasma gondii Infections (Toxoplasmosis) 318
112/Trichinellosis (Trichinella spiralis) 323
113/Trichomonas vaginalis Infections (Trichomoniasis) 326
114/Trichuriasis (Whipworm Infection) 328
115/African Trypanosomiasis (African Sleeping Sickness) 329
116/American Trypanosomiasis (Chagas Disease) 331
117/Tuberculosis 333
118/Diseases Caused by Nontuberculous Mycobacteria (Atypical Mycobacteria,
    Mycobacteria Other Than Mycobacterium tuberculosis) 345
119/Tularemia 350
120/Endemic Typhus (Flea-borne Typhus or Murine Typhus) 353
121/Epidemic Typhus (Louse-borne Typhus) 354
122/Varicella-Zoster Infections 356
123/Vibrio cholerae Infections 363
124/West Nile Virus 365
125/Yersinia enterocolitica and Yersinia pseudotuberculosis Infections
    (Enteritis and Other Illnesses) 368
Index 371

Acknowledgments

The editor wishes to thank the following people who made the book possible: Larry Pickering, MD, FAAP, the editor of the *Red Book* 2000, 2003, and 2006; the members of the American Academy of Pediatrics Committee on Infectious Diseases; Edgar Ledbetter, MD, FAAP, who gave birth to the idea of photographs to accompany the *Red Book;* Martha Cook for her enthusiasm, excellent assistance, and never-ending encouragement; and my mother, who tolerated my temporary disappearance while completing this task.

Introduction

The American Academy of Pediatrics (AAP) *Red Book® Atlas of Pediatric Infectious Diseases* is a summary of key disease information from the AAP *Red Book®: 2006 Report of the Committee on Infectious Diseases*. It is intended to be a study guide for students, residents, and practitioners.

The visual representations of common and atypical clinical manifestations of infectious diseases provide diagnostic information not found in the print version of the *Red Book*. The juxtaposition of these visuals with a summary of the clinical features, epidemiology, diagnostic methods, and treatment information serve as a training tool and a quick reference. The *Red Book Atlas* is not intended to provide detailed treatment and management information but rather a big-picture approach that can be refined by consulting reference texts or infectious diseases specialists. Complete disease and treatment information from the AAP can be found on *Red Book® Online* at www.aapredbook.org.

The *Red Book Atlas* could not have been conceived without the dedication and tireless efforts of Edgar Ledbetter, MD, who for many years photographed disease manifestations in children. Many of these photographs were used in testing physicians during American Board of Pediatrics examinations. Some diseases rarely are seen today because of improved preventive strategies, especially vaccines. While photographs can't replace hands-on experience, they have always helped me to increase the likelihood of a correct diagnosis.

The study of pediatric infectious diseases has been a challenging and changing professional life that has brought me great joy. To gather information with my ears and eyes (the history and physical examination) and to put the many pieces together to arrive at a diagnosis is akin to investigating a mystery. On many occasions, just seeing *the* clue (a characteristic rash, an asymmetry, a swelling) will solve the medical puzzle, lead to recovery, and bring the satisfaction almost nothing can replace. It is my hope that the readers of the *Red Book Atlas* might find a similar enthusiasm for the field.

Carol J. Baker, MD
Editor

Image Credits

All images not included in the following list are from the American Academy of Pediatrics (AAP) courtesy of Edgar O. Ledbetter, MD.

Chapter 3 Amebiasis
Image 3.1: Centers for Disease Control and Prevention
Image 3.2: AAP, courtesy of Dimitri Agamanolis, MD
Images 3.3 and 3.4: Centers for Disease Control and Prevention

Chapter 4 Amebic Meningoencephalitis and Keratitis
Images 4.1–4.4: Centers for Disease Control and Prevention

Chapter 5 Anthrax
Images 5.1 and 5.2: Centers for Disease Control and Prevention
Image 5.3: Centers for Disease Control and Prevention, courtesy of Marshall Fox, MD
Image 5.5: Centers for Disease Control and Prevention
Image 5.6: Centers for Disease Control and Prevention, courtesy of James H. Steele, MD

Chapter 6 Arboviruses
Images 6.1 and 6.2: Centers for Disease Control and Prevention

Chapter 7 *Arcanobacterium haemolyticum* Infections
Image 7.1: Noni E. MacDonald, MD
Images 7.2–7.4: Gary D. Williams, MD, and Peter S. Karofsky, MD

Chapter 8 *Ascaris lumbricoides*
Images 8.2 and 8.3: Centers for Disease Control and Prevention

Chapter 9 Aspergillosis
Image 9.1: Centers for Disease Control and Prevention
Image 9.3: AAP, courtesy of Dimitri Agamanolis, MD

Chapter 11 Bacterial Vaginosis
Image 11.1: Centers for Disease Control and Prevention, courtesy of M. Rein, MD

Chapter 12 *Bacteroides* and *Prevotella* Infections
Image 12.2: Centers for Disease Control and Prevention
Image 12.3: Centers for Disease Control and Prevention, courtesy of V. R. Dowell, Jr, MD

Chapter 13 *Balantidium coli* Infections
Images 13.1 and 13.2: Centers for Disease Control and Prevention

Chapter 14 *Baylisascaris* Infections
Image 14.1: Centers for Disease Control and Prevention, courtesy of Gavin Hart, MD
Image 14.2: Michigan Department of Health
Image 14.3: Centers for Disease Control and Prevention
Image 14.4: Centers for Disease Control and Prevention, courtesy of Gavin Hart, MD

Chapter 15 Blastomycosis
Image 15.1: Centers for Disease Control and Prevention, courtesy of Libero Ajello, MD
Image 15.3: Dermatlas.org, courtesy of Sugathan Paramoo, MD, with permission

Chapter 16 *Borrelia* Infections
Image 16.2: Centers for Disease Control and Prevention

Chapter 17 Brucellosis
Image 17.2: Centers for Disease Control and Prevention, courtesy of Larry Stauffer, MD

Chapter 18 *Campylobacter* Infections
Image 18.1: AAP, courtesy of Robert Jerris, PhD
Image 18.2: Centers for Disease Control and Prevention
Image 18.3: Centers for Disease Control and Prevention, courtesy of W. A. Clark, MD

Chapter 19 Candidiasis
Image 19.3: James H. Brien, DO
Image 19.4: David Clark, MD
Image 19.6: AAP, courtesy of George A. Nankervis, MD, PhD

Chapter 20 Cat-Scratch Disease
Images 20.4–20.7: Michael Rajnik, MD

Chapter 21 Chancroid
Image 21.1: Centers for Disease Control and Prevention, courtesy of J. Pledger, MD
Image 21.2: AAP, courtesy of Hugh L. Moffet, MD

Chapter 22 *Chlamydia trachomatis*
Image 22.1: Noni McDonald, MD

Chapter 23 *Clostridium botulinum*
Image 23.1: Charles G. Prober, MD
Image 23.2: AAP, courtesy of Hugh L. Moffet, MD
Image 23.3: Centers for Disease Control and Prevention

Chapter 24 *Clostridium difficile*
Image 24.2: Centers for Disease Control and Prevention
Image 24.3: Carol J. Baker, MD

Chapter 26 Coccidioidomycosis
Image 26.1: Centers for Disease Control and Prevention

Chapter 27 *Cryptococcus neoformans* Infections
Image 27.2: Centers for Disease Control and Prevention, courtesy of Edwin P. Ewing, Jr, MD

Chapter 28 Cutaneous Larva Migrans
Image 28.2: AAP, courtesy of George A. Nankervis, MD, PhD

Chapter 29 Cytomegalovirus Infection
Image 29.2: AAP, courtesy of George A. Nankervis, MD, PhD
Image 29.3: AAP, courtesy of Stacey W. Hedlund, DO
Image 29.4: Centers for Disease Control and Prevention, courtesy of Edwin P. Ewing, Jr, MD

Chapter 30 Diphtheria
Image 30.3: AAP, courtesy of George A. Nankervis, MD, PhD

Chapter 31 *Ehrlichia* and *Anaplasma* Infections
Image 31.1: Centers for Disease Control and Prevention
Images 31.2–31.4: Richard F. Jacobs, MD

Chapter 32 Enterovirus (Nonpoliovirus) Infections
Image 32.4: Michael Rajnik, MD

Chapter 33 Epstein-Barr Virus Infections
Images 33.2 and 33.3: James H. Brien, DO
Image 33.5: Centers for Disease Control and Prevention

Chapter 34 *Escherichia coli* (Nondiarrheal) and Other Gram-Negative Bacilli
Image 34.1: Carol J. Baker, MD

Chapter 36 *Giardia intestinalis* Infections
Image 36.1: Centers for Disease Control and Prevention

Chapter 37 Gonococcal Infections
Image 37.1: Centers for Disease Control and Prevention, courtesy of Norman M. Jacobs, MD
Image 37.2: Centers for Disease Control and Prevention, courtesy of J. Pledger, MD
Image 37.3: Centers for Disease Control and Prevention
Image 37.5: Centers for Disease Control and Prevention, courtesy of Joe B. Miller, MD

Chapter 38 Granuloma Inguinale
Image 38.1: AAP, courtesy of Robert Jerris, PhD
Images 38.2 and 38.3: Centers for Disease Control and Prevention, courtesy of Cornelio Arevalo, MD

Chapter 39 *Haemophilus influenzae* Infections
Images 39.1 and 39.6: Martin G. Myers, MD
Image 39.2: AAP, courtesy of George A. Nankervis, MD, PhD

Chapter 40 Hantavirus Pulmonary Syndrome
Image 40.1: Centers for Disease Control and Prevention
Image 40.2: Centers for Disease Control and Prevention, courtesy of James Gathany, MD
Image 40.3: Centers for Disease Control and Prevention
Image 40.4: David C. Waagner, MD
Image 40.5: Centers for Disease Control and Prevention, courtesy of Sherif R. Zaki, MD

Chapter 43 Hepatitis B
Image 43.1: Centers for Disease Control and Prevention
Image 43.2: Centers for Disease Control and Prevention, courtesy of Patricia Walker, MD

Chapter 44 Hepatitis C
Image 44.1: Centers of Disease Control and Prevention, courtesy of Susan Linsley

Chapter 45 Herpes Simplex
Image 45.1: Centers for Disease Control and Prevention
Image 45.3: Martha L. Lepow, MD
Images 45.4–45.6: Jerri Ann Jenista, MD
Image 45.7: AAP, courtesy of George A. Nankervis, MD, PhD
Image 45.8: Centers for Disease Control and Prevention, courtesy of N. J. Flumara, MD, and Gavin Hart, MD

Chapter 46 Histoplasmosis
Image 46.1: Centers for Disease Control and Prevention, courtesy of Edwin P. Ewing, Jr, MD
Image 46.3: Centers for Disease Control and Prevention

Chapter 47 Hookworm Infections
Images 47.2–47.4: Centers for Disease Control and Prevention

Chapter 48 Human Herpesvirus 6 (Including Roseola) and 7
Image 48.1: AAP, courtesy of George A. Nankervis, MD, PhD
Image 48.2: Stanley L. Block, Jr, MD

Chapter 49 Human Immunodeficiency Virus Infection
Images 49.1, 49.2, and 49.4–49.7: Baylor International Pediatric AIDS Initiative at Baylor College of Medicine, submitted by Mark W. Kline, MD
Image 49.3: Centers for Disease Control and Prevention, courtesy of Sol Silverman, Jr, DDS

Chapter 50 Influenza
Image 50.1: Immunization Action Coalition
Images 50.2 and 50.3: Carol J. Baker, MD

Chapter 51 Kawasaki Disease
Image 51.5: AAP, courtesy of George A. Nankervis, MD, PhD
Image 51.6: Charles G. Prober, MD
Image 51.7: Michael Rajnik, MD

Chapter 52 Leishmaniasis
Image 52.1: Jerri Ann Jenista, MD
Image 52.3: AAP, courtesy of Hugh L. Moffet, MD

Chapter 53 Leprosy
Image 53.1: Barbara A. Jantausch, MD
Images 53.2 and 53.3: Gary D. Williams, MD
Images 53.4 and 53.5: AAP, courtesy of Hugh L. Moffet, MD

Chapter 54 Leptospirosis
Image 54.2: Centers for Disease Control and Prevention

Chapter 55 *Listeria monocytogenes* Infections
Image 55.1: Martha L. Lepow, MD

Chapter 56 Lyme Disease
Image 56.3: AAP, George A. Nankervis, MD, PhD
Image 56.4: Michael Rajnik, MD

Chapter 57 Lymphatic Filariasis
Images 57.1–57.3: Centers for Disease Control and Prevention

Chapter 58 Lymphocytic Choriomeningitis
Image 58.1: Leslie L. Barton, MD

Chapter 59 Malaria
Images 59.1 and 59.2: Centers for Disease Control and Prevention

Chapter 60 Measles
Images 60.4 and 60.5: Centers for Disease Control and Prevention
Image 60.6: Stacey W. Hedlund, DO

Chapter 61 Meningococcal Infections
Image 61.1: Centers for Disease Control and Prevention
Image 61.2: Martin G. Myers, MD
Images 61.8 and 61.9: AAP, courtesy of Dimitri
Agamanolis, MD
Image 61.10: AAP, courtesy of Neal A. Halsey, MD

Chapter 62 Molluscum Contagiosum
Image 62.1: Edgar K. Marcuse, MD, MPH
Image 62.5: Centers for Disease Control and Prevention,
courtesy of Edwin P. Ewing, Jr, MD

Chapter 63 Mumps
Image 63.1: Centers for Disease Control and Prevention,
courtesy of Heinz F. Eichenwald, MD
Image 63.3: AAP, courtesy of Paul F. Wehrle, MD

Chapter 64 *Mycoplasma pneumoniae* Infections
Image 64.2: AAP, courtesy of Neal A. Halsey, MD

Chapter 65 Nocardiosis
Image 65.1: Charles G. Prober, MD

Chapter 66 Onchocerciasis
Image 66.1: Centers for Disease Control and Prevention,
courtesy of the World Health Organization
Image 66.3–66.5: Logical Images, with permission

Chapter 67 Human Papillomaviruses
Image 67.1: Gary Williams, MD
Image 67.3: Martin G. Myers, MD

Chapter 68 Paracoccidioidomycosis
Images 68.1–68.3: Centers for Disease Control
and Prevention

Chapter 70 Parainfluenza Viral Infections
Image 70.2: AAP, courtesy of Dimitri Agamanolis, MD

Chapter 71 Parvovirus B19
Image 71.3: AAP, courtesy of George A. Nankervis, MD,
PhD
Image 71.4: AAP, courtesy of Dimitri Agamanolis, MD

Chapter 72 *Pasteurella* Infections
Image 72.1: AAP, courtesy of Larry I. Corman, MD

Chapter 73 Pediculosis Capitis
Image 73.1: Edgar K. Marcuse, MD, MPH
Image 73.2: Centers for Disease Control and Prevention

Chapter 74 Pediculosis Corporis
Image 74.1: Denise Metry, MD, Texas Children's
Hospital, with permission

Chapter 75 Pediculosis Pubis
Image 75.1: Gary D. Williams, MD

Chapter 76 Pertussis
Images 76.5–76.7: Carol J. Baker MD

Chapter 77 Pinworm Infection
Image 77.1: Centers for Disease Control and Prevention
Image 77.2: Gary D. Williams, MD

Chapter 79 Plague
Images 79.1, 79.2, 79.4, and 79.5: Centers for Disease
Control and Prevention
Images 79.6 and 79.7: Centers for Disease Control and
Prevention, courtesy of Marshall Fox, MD

Chapter 80 Pneumococcal Infections
Image 80.2: AAP, courtesy of George A. Nankervis,
MD, PhD
Image 80.8: Immunization Action Coalition

Chapter 81 *Pneumocystis jiroveci* Infections
Image 81.1: Courtesy of Russell Byrnes, MD

Chapter 82 Poliovirus Infections
Image 82.1: Centers for Disease Control and Prevention,
courtesy of Stafford Smith, MD
Images 82.2 and 82.3: Centers for Disease Control
and Prevention
Image 82.4: Martin G. Myers, MD
Image 82.5: Centers for Disease Control and Prevention,
courtesy of Ivan Karp, PhD

Chapter 83 Rabies
Images 83.1–83.5: Centers for Disease Control
and Prevention

Chapter 84 Rat-Bite Fever
Images 84.1 and 84.2: AAP, courtesy of George A. Nankervis, MD, PhD

Chapter 85 Respiratory Syncytial Virus
Image 85.1: Centers for Disease Control and Prevention
Image 85.2: Martha L. Lepow, MD

Chapter 86 Rickettsialpox
Images 86.1 and 86.2: Centers for Disease Control and
Prevention

Chapter 87 Rocky Mountain Spotted Fever
Image 87.1: Centers for Disease Control and Prevention,
courtesy of Michael L. Levin
Image 87.7: Martin G. Myers, MD
Image 87.9: Centers for Disease Control and Prevention

Chapter 88 Rotavirus Infections
Image 88.1: Centers for Disease Control and Prevention,
courtesy of Erskine Palmer, MD

Chapter 89 Rubella
Image 89.2: Centers for Disease Control and Prevention
Image 89.3: AAP, courtesy of George A. Nankervis, MD,
PhD
Image 89.4: Charles G. Prober, MD
Image 89.5: Mary Rimsza, MD
Image 89.6: Centers for Disease Control and Prevention

Chapter 90 *Salmonella* Infections
Images 90.1 and 90.2: Martin G. Myers, MD
Images 90.3 and 90.6: Centers for Disease Control
and Prevention

Chapter 91 Scabies
Images 91.2 and 91.3: James H. Brien, DO

Chapter 92 Schistosomiasis
Image 92.1: Immunization Action Coalition
Images 92.2–92.4: Centers for Disease Control
and Prevention
Image 92.5: Dermatlas.org, courtesy of Douglas
Hoffman, MD, with permission

Chapter 94 Smallpox
Images 94.1, 94.2, and 94.5: AAP, courtesy of Paul F.
Wehrle, MD
Image 94.3: Centers for Disease Control and Prevention,
courtesy of Lyle Conrad, MD
Image 94.6: Centers for Disease Control and Prevention,
courtesy of John Noble, Jr, MD
Images 94.7–94.9: Centers for Disease Control
and Prevention
Image 94.10: Centers for Disease Control and
Prevention, courtesy of Moses Grossman, MD

Chapter 95 Sporotrichosis
Image 95.1: Centers for Disease Control and Prevention

Chapter 96 Staphylococcal Infections
Image 96.2: AAP, courtesy of George A. Nankervis,
MD, PhD
Images 96.4, 96.11, and 96.12: Martin G. Myers, MD
Image 96.16: AAP, courtesy of Dimitri Agamanolis, MD
Image 96.19: AAP, courtesy of George A. Nankervis,
MD, PhD

Chapter 97 Group A Streptococcal Infections
Image 97.1: Centers for Disease Control and Prevention
Image 97.6: Martin G. Myers, MD
Image 97.7: Michael Rajnik, MD
Image 97.8: AAP, courtesy of George A. Nankervis,
MD, PhD
Image 97.9: Michael Rajnik, MD
Images 97.10 and 97.11: AAP, courtesy of
Paul F. Wehrle, MD
Image 97.12: Martin G. Myers, MD
Image 97.13: Michael Rajnik, MD

Chapter 98 Group B Streptococcal Infections
Image 98.1: David Clark, MD

**Chapter 99 Non–Group A or B Streptoccocal and
Enterococcal Infections**
Image 99.1: Martin G. Myers, MD
Images 99.3–99.5: AAP, courtesy of George A.
Nankervis, MD, PhD

Chapter 100 Strongyloidiasis
Image 100.1: James H. Brien, DO
Image 100.3: Neal A. Halsey, MD

Chapter 101 Syphilis
Image 101.1: Centers for Disease Control and
Prevention, courtesy of Joyce Ayers, MD
Image 101.2: Neal A. Halsey, MD
Image 101.4: Centers for Disease Control and
Prevention, courtesy of Norman Cole, MD
Image 101.9: Charles G. Prober, MD
Image 101.12: James H. Brien, DO
Images 101.14, 101.16, and 101.17: Centers for
Disease Control and Prevention, courtesy
of Susan Lindsley, MD

Chapter 102 Tapeworm Diseases
Image 102.2: James H. Brien, DO
Image 102.4: David Waagner, MD

Chapter 103 Other Tapeworm Infections
Images 103.1 and 103.3: Centers for Disease Control
and Prevention

Chapter 104 Tetanus
Image 104.1: Immunization Action Coalition
Image 104.3: Martin G. Myers, MD
Image 104.4: Immunization Action Coalition
Image 104.5: Centers for Disease Control and Prevention
Image 104.6: Immunization Action Coalition

Chapter 105 Tinea Capitis
Image 105.2: Larry I. Corman, MD
Images 105.3 and 105.4: Stanley L. Block, Jr, MD
Image 105.5: Martin G. Myers, MD
Image 105.6: Charles G. Prober, MD

Chapter 106 Tinea Corporis
Image 106.1: Centers for Disease Control and
Prevention, courtesy of Arvind A. Padhye, MD
Image 106.3: Charles G. Prober, MD
Images 106.4 and 106.5: Larry I. Corman, MD

Chapter 107 Tinea Cruris
Image 107.1: Dermatlas.org, with permission

Chapter 108 Tinea Pedis and Tinea Unguium
Image 108.1: Centers for Disease Control and
Prevention, courtesy of Lucille K. George, MD
Image 108.3: Gary D. Williams, MD

Chapter 109 Toxic Shock Syndrome
Image 109.5: Centers for Disease Control and Prevention
Image 109.6: Michael Rajnik, MD

Chapter 110 Toxocariasis
Image 110.2: AAP, courtesy of Hugh L. Moffet, MD

Chapter 111 *Toxoplasma gondii* Infections
Image 111.2: AAP, courtesy of George A. Nankervis,
MD, PhD
Image 111.4: Charles G. Prober, MD
Images 111.5 and 111.6: Jerri Ann Jenista, MD
Images 111.7 and 111.8: Centers for Disease Control and
Prevention, courtesy of Edwin P. Ewing, Jr, MD

Chapter 112 Trichinellosis
Images 112.4 and 112.5: Centers for Disease Control
and Prevention

Chapter 113 *Trichomonas vaginalis* Infections
Images 113.1–113.3: Centers for Disease Control
and Prevention

Chapter 114 Trichuriasis
Images 114.1 and 114.2: Centers for Disease Control
and Prevention

Chapter 115 African Trypanosomiasis
Image 115.1: Centers for Disease Control and Prevention,
courtesy of Myron G. Shultz, MD

Chapter 116 American Trypanosomiasis
Images 116.1 and 116.2: Centers for Disease Control
     and Prevention

Chapter 117 Tuberculosis
Image 117.1: Centers for Disease Control and
     Prevention, courtesy of George P. Kubica, MD
Image 117.2: David P. Ascher, MD, and Howard
     Johnson, MD
Image 117.5: Martin G. Myers, MD
Images 117.6 and 117.7: Barbara A. Jantausch, MD

**Chapter 118 Diseases Caused by Nontuberculous
Mycobacteria**
Image 118.4: Centers for Disease Control and Prevention

Chapter 119 Tularemia
Image 119.1: Centers for Disease Control and Preven-
     tion, courtesy of Thomas F. Sellers, MD
Image 119.6: Centers for Disease Control and Preven-
     tion, courtesy of J. M. Clinton, MD

Chapter 120 Endemic Typhus
Image 120.1: Centers for Disease Control and Prevention

Chapter 121 Epidemic Typhus
Image 121.1: Centers for Disease Control and Preven-
     tion, courtesy of the World Health Organization

Chapter 122 Varicella-Zoster Infections
Image 122.1: David Clark, MD
Image 122.6: AAP, courtesy of George A. Nankervis,
     MD, PhD
Image 122.8: Centers for Disease Control and Preven-
     tion, courtesy of Joel D. Meyers, MD
Image 122.10: Barbara A. Jantausch, MD

Chapter 123 *Vibrio cholerae* Infections
Images 123.1–123.3: Centers for Disease Control
     and Prevention

Chapter 124 West Nile Virus
Image 124.1: Centers for Disease Control and Prevention
Image 124.2: Centers for Disease Control and
     Prevention, courtesy of W. J. Shieh, MD,
     and S. Zaki MD
Images 124.3 and 124.4: Centers for Disease Control
     and Prevention

**Chapter 125 *Yersinia enterocolitica* and *Yersinia
pseudotuberculosis* Infections**
Image 125.1: AAP, courtesy of George A. Nankervis,
     MD, PhD

1

Actinomycosis

Clinical Manifestations

Cervicofacial infections can occur after tooth extraction, oral surgery, or facial trauma or are associated with carious teeth. **Thoracic** disease manifests as pneumonia, which can be complicated by abscesses, empyema and, rarely, pleurodermal sinuses. Focal or multifocal masses can be mistaken for tumors. The appendix and cecum are common sites of **abdominal** actinomycosis; chronic localized disease often forms draining sinus tracts. Other sites include the pelvis and brain.

Etiology

Actinomyces israelii is the usual cause.

Epidemiology

Disease results from penetrating (including human bite wounds) and nonpenetrating trauma.

Incubation Period

Several days to several years.

Diagnostic Tests

Gram stain showing beaded, branched, grampositive bacilli with or without "sulfur granules"; acid-fast staining is negative (unlike Nocardia); tissue specimens can be used for 16s rRNA sequencing and PCR assay. Culture specimens must be processed anaerobically.

Treatment

Intravenous penicillin G or ampicillin is recommended for 4 to 6 weeks followed by high doses of oral penicillin, amoxicillin, erythromycin, clindamycin, doxycycline, or tetracycline for a total of 6 to 12 months. Surgical drainage or excision may be necessary.

Image 1.1
A sulfur granule from an actinomycotic abscess (hematoxylin-eosin stain). While pathognomonic of actinomycosis, granules are not always present. They represent calcified colonies of the organism.

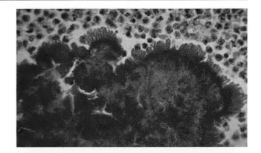

Image 1.2
Actinomycotic abscesses of the thigh of a 10-year-old child with chronic pulmonary, abdominal, and lower extremity abscesses. *Actinomyces* infections are often polymicrobial. *Actinobacillus actinomycetemcomitans* can accompany *Actinomyces israelii*.

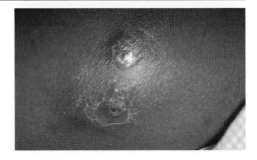

Image 1.3

Periosteal reaction along the left humeral shaft (diaphysis) in an 8-month-old boy with pulmonary actinomycosis. Clubbing in the presence of this chronic suppurative pulmonary infection and the absence of heart disease suggests that pulmonary fibrosis contributed to this infant's hypertrophic pulmonary osteoarthropathy.

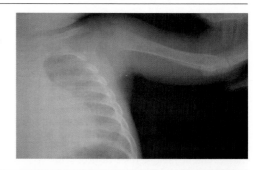

Image 1.4

Clubbing of the thumb and fingers of an 8-month-old boy with chronic pulmonary actinomycosis.

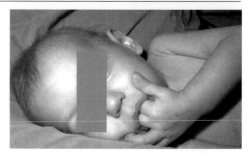

2

Adenovirus Infections

Clinical Manifestations

Upper **respiratory tract infection** manifestations include symptoms of the common cold, exudative pharyngitis, tonsillitis, otitis media, and pharyngoconjunctival fever. Life-threatening disseminated infection, severe pneumonia, meningitis, and encephalitis occasionally occur, especially among young infants or immunocompromised hosts. Adenoviruses are infrequent causes of acute hemorrhagic **conjunctivitis,** a pertussis-like syndrome, croup, bronchiolitis, and hemorrhagic cystitis. A few adenovirus serotypes cause **gastroenteritis.**

Etiology

DNA viruses comprising at least 51 distinct serotypes divided into 6 species (A–F). Some serotypes are associated primarily with respiratory tract disease (types 5 and 7), others with gastroenteritis (types 31, 40, and 41).

Epidemiology

Transmitted by respiratory tract secretions through person-to-person contact, aerosols, and fomites (adenoviruses are stable in the environment); epidemic keratoconjunctivitis often has been associated with nosocomial transmission in ophthalmologists' offices; enteric strains of adenoviruses are transmitted by the fecal-oral route and occur throughout the year, primarily affecting children younger than 4 years.

Incubation Period

2 to 14 days for respiratory tract infection; 3 to 10 days for gastroenteritis.

Diagnostic Tests

Cell culture of pharyngeal or eye secretions for respiratory tract disease. Immunoassay techniques are especially useful for diagnosis of diarrheal disease because enteric adenovirus types 40 and 41 usually cannot be isolated in standard cell cultures.

Treatment

Supportive.

Image 2.1
Adenoviral pneumonia in an 8-year-old girl with diffuse pulmonary infiltrates bilaterally. Most adenoviral infections in the healthy host are self-limited and require no specific treatment. Lobar consolidation is unusual.

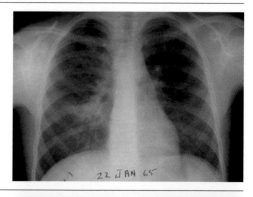

Image 2.2
Acute follicular adenovirus conjunctivitis. Adenoviruses are resistant to alcohol, detergents, and chlorhexidine and can contaminate ophthalmologic solutions and equipment. Instruments can be disinfected by steam autoclaving or immersion in 1% sodium hypochlorite for 10 minutes.

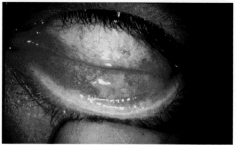

3

Amebiasis

Clinical Manifestations

Entamoeba histolytica infections include non-invasive intestinal infection, intestinal amebiasis, ameboma, and liver abscess. Patients with noninvasive intestinal infection can be asymptomatic or can have nonspecific intestinal tract complaints. People with intestinal amebiasis generally have 1 to 3 weeks of increasingly severe diarrhea progressing to grossly bloody dysenteric stools with lower abdominal pain and tenesmus. Weight loss and fever are common. Progressive colonic involvement can produce toxic megacolon, fulminant colitis, ulceration and, rarely, perforation, especially in patients inappropriately treated with corticosteroids or antimotility drugs. An ameboma can occur as an annular lesion of the cecum or ascending colon that can be mistaken for colonic carcinoma or a tender extrahepatic mass mimicking a pyogenic liver abscess.

Etiology

The pathogenic *E histolytica* and the nonpathogenic *Entamoeba dispar* are excreted as cysts or trophozoites in stools of infected people.

Epidemiology

Worldwide but more prevalent in developing countries; transmitted via amebic cysts by the fecal-oral route from contaminated food or water.

Incubation Period

Variable, typically 2 to 4 weeks.

Diagnostic Tests

Identification of trophozoites or cysts in stool specimens. Specimens of stool, endoscopy scrapings (not swabs), and biopsies should be examined by wet mount within 30 minutes of collection and fixed in formalin and polyvinyl alcohol.

Detecting serum antibody using indirect hemagglutination assay can be helpful, primarily for diagnosis of amebic colitis (approximately 85% sensitivity) and extra-intestinal amebiasis with liver involvement (up to 99% sensitivity).

Treatment

- **Asymptomatic cyst excreters (intraluminal infections):** Treat with a luminal amebicide such as iodoquinol, paromomycin, or diloxanide.
- **Patients with mild to moderate or severe intestinal symptoms or extraintestinal disease (including liver abscess):** Treat with metronidazole (or tinidazole), followed by a therapeutic course of a luminal amebicide (iodoquinol or paromomycin).

E dispar infection does not require treatment. Dehydroemetine followed by a therapeutic course of a luminal amebicide should be considered for patients for whom treatment of invasive disease has failed or cannot be tolerated. Corticosteroids and antimotility drugs administered to people with amebiasis can worsen the disease process.

Image 3.1
Trophozoite of *Entamoeba histolytica* (trichrome stain).

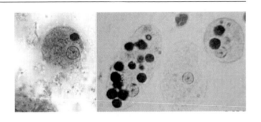

Image 3.2
Entamoeba histolytica. Amoebae in an intestinal ulcer.

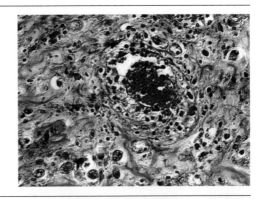

Image 3.3
Gross pathology of amebic *(Entamoeba histolytica)* abscess of liver. Tube of chocolate-like pus from abscess. Amebic liver abscesses usually are singular, large, and in the right lobe of the liver. Bacterial hepatic abscesses are more likely to be multiple.

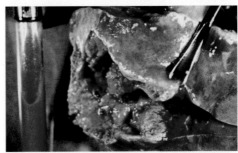

Image 3.4
This patient presented with invasive extraintestinal amebiasis affecting the cutaneous region of the right flank.

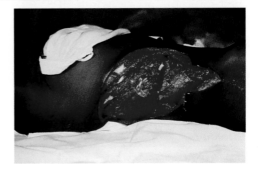

4

Amebic Meningoencephalitis and Keratitis
(Naegleria fowleri, Acanthamoeba species, and *Balamuthia mandrillaris)*

Clinical Manifestations

Naegleria fowleri can cause a rapidly progressive, almost always fatal, primary amebic meningoencephalitis. Early symptoms include fever and headache, quickly progressing to nuchal rigidity, lethargy, confusion, seizures, and altered consciousness.

Granulomatous amebic encephalitis caused by *Acanthamoeba* species and *Balamuthia mandrillaris* progresses slowly weeks to months after exposure. Signs and symptoms can include personality changes, seizures, headaches, nuchal rigidity, ataxia, cranial nerve palsies, hemiparesis, and other focal deficits. Fever often is low grade and intermittent. Skin lesions (pustules, nodules, ulcers) can be present without CNS involvement, particularly in patients with AIDS.

Amebic keratitis, usually attributable to *Acanthamoeba* species, occurs primarily in people who wear contact lenses and resembles keratitis caused by herpes simplex, bacteria, or fungi except for a more indolent course. Corneal inflammation, pain, photophobia, and secondary uveitis are predominant features.

Etiology

N fowleri, Acanthamoeba species, and *B mandrillaris* are free-living amebae that exist as motile, infective trophozoites and environmentally hardy cysts.

Epidemiology

N fowleri is found in warm freshwater and moist soil. Disease has been reported worldwide but is uncommon. In the United States, infection occurs primarily in the summer and usually affects children and young adults. *Acanthamoeba* species are distributed worldwide and are found in soil, freshwater and brackish water, dust, hot tubs, and sewage. The primary focus of infection most likely is skin or respiratory tract, followed by hematogenous spread to the brain.

Incubation Period

For *N fowleri*, several days to 1 week and for *Acanthamoeba* and *Balamuthia,* unknown.

Diagnostic Tests

N fowleri can be seen by microscopic demonstration of the motile trophozoites on a wet mount of centrifuged CSF or culture on 1.5% non-nutrient agar layered with enteric bacteria held in Page saline solution. The CSF shows polymorphonuclear pleocytosis, an increased protein concentration, a normal to very low glucose concentration, and no bacteria.

For *Acanthamoeba* species, the CSF typically shows a mononuclear pleocytosis and an increased protein concentration with normal or low glucose but no organisms. *Acanthamoeba* species, but not *Balamuthia* species, can be cultured by the same method used for *N fowleri*.

Treatment

Amphotericin B is the drug of choice for meningoencephalitis caused by *N fowleri*, although treatment often is unsuccessful.

Effective treatment for CNS infections caused by *Acanthamoeba* species and *B mandrillaris* has not been established. Patients with keratitis attributable to *Acanthamoeba* organisms have been treated successfully with prolonged courses of combinations of topical propamidine isethionate plus neomycin-polymyxin B sulfate-gramicidin ophthalmic solution, or topical polyhexamethylene biguanide, or chlorhexidine gluconate and various azoles (eg, miconazole, clotrimazole, fluconazole, or itraconazole) as well as topical corticosteroids. Early diagnosis is important for a good outcome.

Image 4.1

Naegleria fowleri trophozoite in CSF (trichrome stain). Note the typically large karyosome.

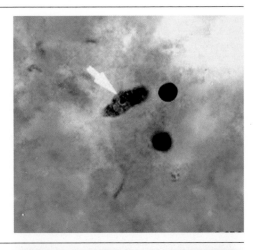

Image 4.2

Histopathologic features of amebic meningo-encephalitis due to *Naegleria fowleri* (direct fluorescent antibody stain).

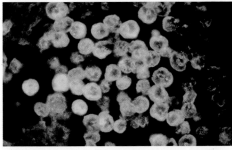

Image 4.3

Balamuthia mandrillaris trophozoites in brain tissue.

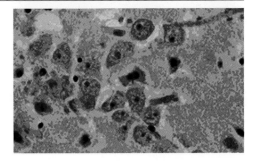

Image 4.4

A: CT scan. Note the right fronto-basal collection (arrow) with a midline shift right to left. B: Brain histology. Three large clusters of amebic vegetative forms are seen (hematoxylin-eosin stain, 250x). Inset: Positive indirect immunofluorescent stain on tissue section with anti-*Naegleria fowleri* serum.

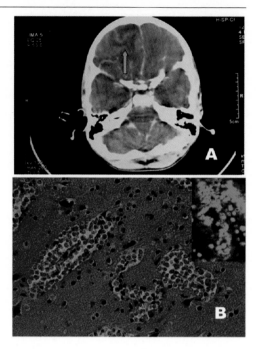

5

Anthrax

Clinical Manifestations

Cutaneous anthrax begins as a pruritic papule that enlarges and ulcerates forming a central black eschar. The lesion is painless, with surrounding edema, hyperemia, and regional lymphadenopathy. Patients can have fever, malaise, and headache. **Inhalational** anthrax is the most lethal form of disease. A prodrome of fever, sweats, nonproductive cough, chest pain, headache, myalgias, malaise, and nausea and vomiting may occur initially, followed by dyspnea, hypoxia, and fulminant shock resulting from hemorrhagic mediastinal lymphadenitis, hemorrhagic pleural effusions, bacteremia, and toxemia. A widened mediastinum is the classic finding on imaging of the chest.

Gastrointestinal tract disease can be intestinal or oropharyngeal. Patients with the intestinal form have symptoms of nausea, anorexia, vomiting, and fever progressing to severe abdominal pain, massive ascites, hematemesis, and bloody diarrhea. Oropharyngeal anthrax can include posterior oropharyngeal ulcers that typically are unilateral and associated with marked neck swelling, regional adenopathy, and sepsis. Hemorrhagic meningitis can result from hematogenous spread after acquiring any form of disease.

Etiology

Bacillus anthracis is an aerobic, gram-positive, encapsulated, spore-forming, nonmotile rod. *B anthracis* has 3 major virulence factors, an antiphagocytic capsule, and 2 exotoxins called lethal and edema toxins.

Epidemiology

B anthracis spores remain viable in the soil for decades. Natural infection of humans occurs through contact with infected animals or contaminated animal products, including carcasses, hides, hair, wool, meat, and bone meal. Internationally, outbreaks of gastrointestinal tract anthrax have occurred after ingestion of undercooked or raw meat. In the United States, the incidence of naturally occurring human anthrax decreased from an estimated 130 cases annually in the early 1900s to one case in 2006. Most cases (>95%) are cutaneous infections among animal handlers or mill workers.

Incubation Period

Generally less than 2 weeks for all forms of anthrax.

Diagnostic Tests

Depending on the clinical presentation, Gram stain and culture should be performed on specimens of blood, pleural fluid, CSF, and tissue biopsy or discharge from cutaneous lesions. Gram-positive bacilli seen on peripheral blood smears or in CSF can be an important initial diagnostic finding. Identification of suspect *B anthracis* isolates can be performed through the Laboratory Response Network in each state. Clinical evaluation of patients with suspected inhalational anthrax includes a chest radiograph to evaluate for widened mediastinum and pleural effusion.

Treatment

Naturally occurring cutaneous disease can be treated effectively with penicillins and/or tetracyclines; for bioterrorism-associated cutaneous disease, ciprofloxacin or doxycycline is recommended for initial treatment until antimicrobial susceptibility data are available. Because of the risk of concomitant inhalational exposure, consideration should be given to continuing an appropriate antimicrobial regimen for postexposure prophylaxis as well as administration of vaccine. Ciprofloxacin is recommended as part of an initial multidrug regimen for treating inhalational anthrax, anthrax meningitis, cutaneous anthrax with systemic signs, and gastrointestinal anthrax until results of antimicrobial susceptibility testing are known. Because of intrinsic resistance, cephalosporins and trimethoprim-sulfamethoxazole should not be used for therapy.

Image 5.1

A photomicrograph of *Bacillus anthracis* bacteria using Gram stain technique.

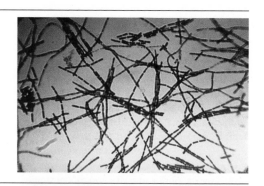

Image 5.2

Cutaneous anthrax. Vesicle development occurs from day 2 through day 10 of progression.

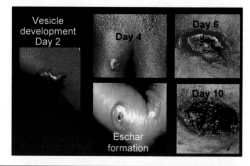

Image 5.3

This micrograph reveals submucosal hemorrhage in the small intestine in a case of fatal human anthrax (hematoxylin-eosin stain, 240x). Note the associated arteriolar degeneration.

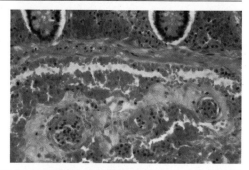

Image 5.4

Anthrax ulcers on the hand and wrist of an adult. The cutaneous eschar of anthrax had been misdiagnosed as a brown recluse spider bite. Edema is common and suppuration is absent.

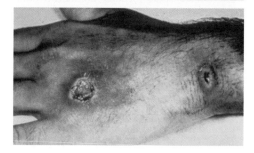

Image 5.5

Brain section revealing an intraventricular hemorrhage.

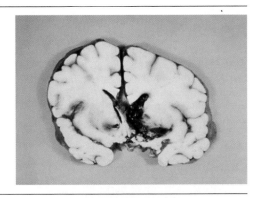

Image 5.6

Cutaneous anthrax lesion on the skin of the forearm.

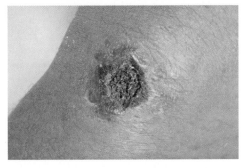

6

Arboviruses

(Also see West Nile Virus, p 365.)

(Including California Serogroup [Primarily La Crosse] Encephalitis, Eastern and Western Equine Encephalitis, Powassan Encephalitis, St Louis Encephalitis, Venezuelan Equine Encephalitis, Colorado Tick Fever, Dengue Fever, Japanese Encephalitis, and Yellow Fever)

Clinical Manifestations

Arboviruses (arthropod-borne viruses) are spread by mosquitoes, ticks, sandflies, or other arthropods and produce 4 principal clinical syndromes: (1) CNS disease (including encephalitis, aseptic meningitis, and flaccid paralysis); (2) an undifferentiated febrile illness, often with rash and headache; (3) acute polyarthropathy; and (4) acute hemorrhagic fever, sometimes accompanied by hepatitis. Some arboviruses can cause congenital infection.

Etiology

More than 550 arboviruses are classified in a variety of taxonomic groups, principally in the families Bunyaviridae, Togaviridae, and Flaviviridae, with more than 150 arboviruses known to cause human disease.

Epidemiology

Most arboviruses are maintained in nature through cycles of transmission among birds or small mammals by arthropod vectors. Humans and domestic animals are infected incidentally as "dead-end" hosts. Important exceptions are dengue fever, yellow fever, Oropouche, and chikungunya viruses because infected vectors spread disease from person to person. For the other arboviruses, person-to-person spread does not occur except through blood transfusion, intrauterine transmission, and possibly human milk. There also is evidence that Venezuelan encephalitis virus may be spread via respiratory tract secretions.

In the United States, mosquito-borne arboviral infections usually occur during summer and autumn, but in the South, cases occur throughout the year.

Incubation Period

Selected medically important arboviral infections are outlined in Table 6.1.

Diagnostic Tests

Detection of virus-specific IgM antibody in CSF is confirmatory, and presence of antibody in a serum specimen is presumptive evidence of recent infection in a patient with acute CNS infection. A greater than 4-fold change in serum IgM or IgG antibody titer in paired serum specimens obtained 2 to 4 weeks apart confirms a case. PCR assays to detect several arboviruses are available in reference laboratories. Serologic testing for dengue virus and arboviruses transmitted in the United States is available through several commercial, state, research, and reference laboratories. In patients with encephalitis, viral isolation should be attempted from a CSF specimen.

Treatment

Active clinical monitoring and supportive interventions can be lifesaving in patients with dengue hemorrhagic fever, yellow fever, and acute encephalitis.

Table 6.1

Disease Caused by Arboviruses in the Western Hemisphere

Disease[1]	Geographic Distribution of Virus	Clinical Syndrome	Incubation Period, Days
California serogroup viruses (primarily La Crosse)	Widespread in the US and Canada, including the Yukon and Northwest Territories; most prevalent in upper Midwest	Encephalitis; aseptic meningitis; coma	5–15
Colorado tick fever	Western US and Canada	Febrile illness—can be biphasic; can cause aseptic meningitis, leukopenia, and thrombocytopenia	1–14
Dengue fever and dengue hemorrhagic fever	Tropical areas worldwide: Caribbean, Central and South America, Asia, Australia, Oceania, Africa[2]	Febrile illness—can be biphasic with rash; hemorrhagic fever, shock	2–7
Eastern equine encephalitis virus	Eastern seaboard and Gulf states of the US (isolated inland foci); Canada; South and Central America	Encephalitis; coma; death; serious neurologic sequelae	3–10
Mayaro fever	Central and South America	Febrile influenza-like illness and polyarthralgia	1–12
Oropouche virus fever[2]	South America	Febrile illness	2–6
Powassan encephalitis virus	Canada; northeastern, north central, and western US, Russian Federation	Encephalitis; neurologic sequelae	4–18
St Louis encephalitis virus	Widespread: central, southern, northeastern, and western US; Manitoba and southern Ontario; Caribbean area; South America	Encephalitis with slow disease progression including fever, headache, confusion, weakness, tremor	4–14
Venezuelan equine encephalitis virus	Central and South America and southern US	Encephalitis	1–4
West Nile encephalitis virus	Asia; Africa; Europe; US	Febrile illness; aseptic meningitis; encephalitis; flaccid paralysis	5–15
Western equine encephalitis virus	Central and western US; Canada; Argentina, Uruguay, Brazil	Encephalitis; neurologic impairment in infected infants; congenital infection	2–10
Yellow fever	Tropical areas of South America and Africa[2]	Febrile illness, hepatitis, hemorrhagic fever, organ dysfunction	3–6

1 All are mosquito-borne except Colorado tick fever and Powassan, which are tick-borne, and Oropouche virus fever, which is midge-borne.
2 Mosquito vectors *Aedes aegypti* (yellow fever, dengue) and *Aedes albopictus* (dengue) are found in the United States and could transmit introduced virus.

Image 6.1

An electron micrograph of yellow fever virus virions.

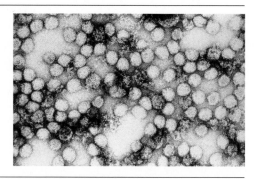

Image 6.2

Staining of West Nile virus antigen in the cytoplasm of a Purkinje cell in the cerebellum (immunohistochemistry, 40x).

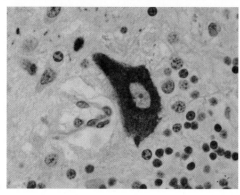

7

Arcanobacterium haemolyticum Infections

Clinical Manifestations

Acute pharyngitis often is indistinguishable from that caused by group A streptococci. Fever, pharyngeal exudate, lymphadenopathy, rash, and pruritus are common, but palatal petechiae and strawberry tongue are absent. A maculopapular or scarlatiniform exanthem is present in 50% of cases, beginning on the extensor surfaces of the distal extremities, spreading centripetally to the chest and back and sparing the face, palms, and soles. Respiratory tract infections that mimic diphtheria, including membranous pharyngitis, sinusitis, and pneumonia, and skin and soft tissue infections, including chronic ulceration, cellulitis, paronychia, and wound infection, also occur. Invasive infections, including septicemia, peritonsillar abscess, Lemierre syndrome, brain abscess, orbital cellulitis, meningitis, endocarditis, osteomyelitis, and pneumonia, are rare.

Etiology

Arcanobacterium haemolyticum is a facultative anaerobic gram-positive bacillus formerly classified as *Corynebacterium haemolyticum*.

Epidemiology

Pharyngitis occurs primarily in adolescents and young adults. Long-term pharyngeal carriage is rare. An estimated 0.5% to 3% of acute pharyngitis is attributable to *A haemolyticum*.

Incubation Period

Unknown.

Diagnostic Tests

A haemolyticum grows best in 5% CO_2 on rabbit or human blood–enriched agar, but colonies are small and have narrow bands of hemolysis not visible for 48 to 72 hours.

Treatment

Erythromycin is the drug of choice for treating tonsillopharyngitis. Trimethoprim-sulfamethoxazole should not be used. In rare cases of disseminated infection, parenteral penicillin plus an aminoglycoside is used until susceptibility testing can be performed.

Image 7.1
Arcanobacterium haemolyticum (Gram stain). *A haemolyticum* appears strongly gram-positive but becomes more gram-variable after 24 hours of incubation.

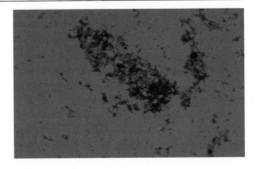

Image 7.2

Arcanobacterium was isolated from pharyngeal culture of this 12-year-old boy with a rash that was followed by mild desquamation.

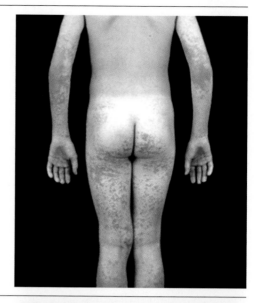

Image 7.3

Arcanobacterium-associated rash on dorsal surface of hand in the 12-year-old boy in Image 7.2.

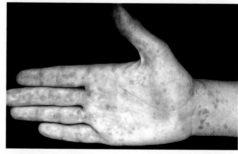

Image 7.4

Although not present in this patient with facial skin lesions associated with *Arcanobacterium haemolyticum* pharyngitis, a pharyngeal membrane similar to that of diphtheria may occur.

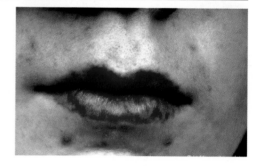

8

Ascaris lumbricoides Infections

Clinical Manifestations

Most infections are asymptomatic. Moderate to heavy infections can lead to malnutrition, nonspecific gastrointestinal tract symptoms, or acute intestinal obstruction. During the larval migratory phase, an acute transient pneumonitis (Löffler syndrome) associated with fever and marked eosinophilia can occur. Worm migration can cause peritonitis after intestinal wall penetration, and common bile duct obstruction resulting in biliary colic, cholangitis, or pancreatitis. Adult worms can be stimulated to migrate by stressful conditions (eg, fever, illness, or anesthesia) and by some anthelmintic drugs.

Etiology

Ascaris lumbricoides is the most widespread of all human intestinal roundworms.

Epidemiology

Infection with *A lumbricoides* is widespread but is most common in the tropics, in areas of poor sanitation, and where human feces are used as fertilizer. If infection is untreated, adult worms can live for 12 to 18 months, resulting in daily excretion of large numbers of ova.

Incubation Period

Interval between ingestion of the egg and development of egg-laying adults is approximately 8 weeks.

Diagnostic Tests

Ova can be detected by microscopic examination of stool. Occasionally, patients pass adult worms from the rectum, from the nose after migration through the nares, and from the mouth in vomitus.

Treatment

Albendazole, mebendazole, or ivermectin is recommended for treatment of asymptomatic and symptomatic infections. Although limited data suggest that these drugs are safe in children younger than 2 years, the risks and benefits of therapy should be considered before administration.

In cases of partial or complete intestinal obstruction, piperazine solution can be given through a gastrointestinal tube; however, it is not available in the United States. If piperazine is not available, conservative management (nasogastric suction, intravenous fluids) can result in resolution of obstruction, at which point albendazole, mebendazole, or ivermectin may be given. Surgical intervention occasionally is necessary to relieve intestinal or biliary tract obstruction. If surgery is performed, massaging the bowel to eliminate the obstruction is preferable to incision into the intestine. Endoscopic retrograde cholangiopancreatography can be used for extraction of worms from the biliary tree.

Image 8.1
Ascaris lumbricoides ovum.

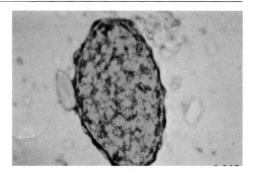

Image 8.2
A fertilized ascaris egg, still at the unicellular stage, the usual stage when the eggs are passed in the stool (complete development of the larva requires 18 days under favorable conditions).

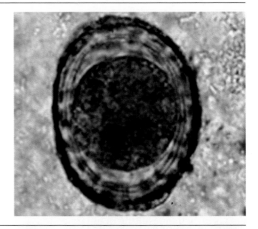

Image 8.3
An adult ascaris. Diagnostic characteristics are tapered ends and length of 15 cm to 35 cm.

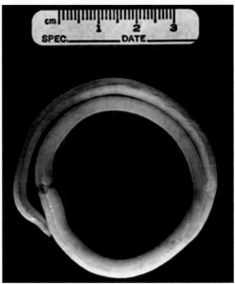

Image 8.4
A mass of large roundworms from a human infestation of ascaris.

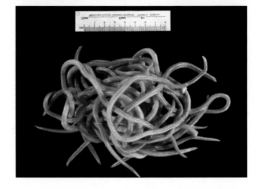

9

Aspergillosis

Clinical Manifestations

- **Invasive aspergillosis** occurs in immuno-compromised patients with prolonged neutropenia (eg, cytotoxic chemotherapy), graft-versus-host disease, or impaired phagocyte function (eg, chronic granulomatous disease, immunosuppressive therapy, corticosteroids). Invasive infection usually involves pulmonary, sinus, cerebral, or cutaneous sites. Rarely, endocarditis, osteomyelitis, meningitis, infection of the eye or orbit, and esophagitis occur. The hallmark of invasive aspergillosis is angio-invasion with resulting thrombosis. Patients with chronic granulomatous disease rarely display angioinvasion.
- **Aspergillomas** and **otomycosis** are 2 syndromes of nonallergic colonization by *Aspergillus* species in immunocompetent children. Aspergillomas ("fungal balls") grow in pre-existing pulmonary cavities or bronchogenic cysts without invading pulmonary tissue; almost all patients have underlying lung disease, such as cystic fibrosis or tuberculosis. Patients with otomycosis have chronic otitis media with colonization of the external auditory canal by a fungal mat that produces a dark discharge.
- **Allergic bronchopulmonary aspergillosis** is a hypersensitivity lung disease that manifests as episodic wheezing, expectoration of brown mucus plugs, low-grade fever, eosinophilia, and transient pulmonary infiltrates, and occurs most commonly in children with asthma or cystic fibrosis.
- **Allergic sinusitis** is characterized by symptoms of chronic sinusitis with dark plugs of nasal discharge.

Etiology

Aspergillus species are ubiquitous molds that grow on decaying vegetation and in soil. *Aspergillus fumigatus* is the usual cause of invasive aspergillosis.

Epidemiology

The principal route of transmission is inhalation of conidia (spores), but contaminated aerosolized water supply (eg, shower heads) can cause disease. Nosocomial outbreaks of invasive pulmonary aspergillosis have occurred in which the probable source of the fungus was a nearby construction site or faulty ventilation system.

Incubation Period

Unknown.

Diagnostic Tests

Dichotomously branched and septate hyphae, identified by microscopic examination of 10% potassium hydroxide wet preparations or of Gomori methenamine-silver nitrate stain of tissue or bronchoalveolar lavage specimens, are suggestive of the diagnosis. Isolation of *Aspergillus* species in culture is required for definitive diagnosis. A serologic assay for detection of galactomannan, a molecule found in the cell wall of *Aspergillus* species, is available commercially, but false-positive results occur frequently in children. A negative galactomannan test result does not exclude the diagnosis of invasive aspergillosis. This test should not be used in patients with chronic granulomatous disease. In **allergic aspergillosis,** diagnosis is suggested by a typical clinical syndrome with elevated total concentrations of IgE (>1000 ng/mL) and *Aspergillus*-specific serum IgE, eosinophilia, and a positive result of a skin test for *Aspergillus* antigens. In people with cystic fibrosis, the diagnosis is more difficult because wheezing, eosinophilia, and a positive skin test result not associated with allergic bronchopulmonary aspergillosis often are present.

Treatment

Voriconazole or amphotericin B in high doses is the drug of choice for invasive aspergillosis. Treatment duration should be individualized for each patient.

Surgical excision of a localized invasive lesion (eg, sinus debris, accessible pulmonary or cerebral lesions) often is warranted.

Image 9.1

This micrograph depicts the histologic features of aspergillosis including the presence of conidial heads.

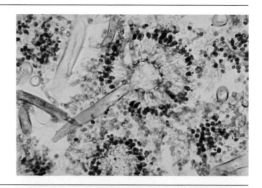

Image 9.2

Aspergilloma at intravenous line site in a 9-year-old boy with acute lymphocytic leukemia.

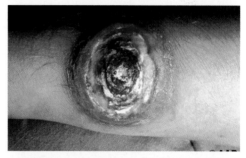

Image 9.3

Pulmonary aspergillosis in a patient with acute lymphocytic leukemia (fungus ball).

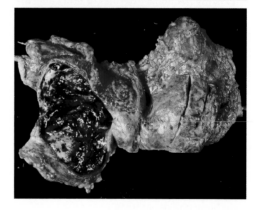

10

Babesiosis

Clinical Manifestations

In people who are symptomatic, gradual onset of malaise, anorexia, and fatigue typically occur, followed by intermittent fever with temperatures as high as 40°C (104°F) and signs and symptoms including chills, sweats, myalgias, arthralgias, headache, nausea, and vomiting. Less common findings are hyperesthesia, sore throat, abdominal pain, conjunctival injection, photophobia, weight loss, and nonproductive cough. Clinical signs generally are minimal, often consisting only of fever, although mild splenomegaly, hepatomegaly, or both are noted occasionally. If untreated, illness can last for a few weeks to several months, with a prolonged recovery. Severe illness is most likely to occur in people older than 40 years, people with asplenia, and people who are immunocompromised. It often presents with fever and hemolytic anemia. Many clinical features are similar to those of malaria.

Etiology

Babesia species are intraerythrocytic protozoa; *Babesia microti* has caused most cases in the United States.

Epidemiology

In the United States, the primary reservoir host for *B microti* is the white-footed mouse *(Peromyscus leucopus)*, and the primary vector is the tick *(Ixodes scapularis)*. Babesiosis also can be acquired through blood transfusions. Human cases of babesiosis have been acquired in the Northeast, Midwest, and West Coast of the United States (especially California, Connecticut, Kentucky, Massachusetts, Minnesota, Missouri, New Jersey, New York, Rhode Island, Washington, and Wisconsin). Most vector-borne human cases of babesiosis occur during late spring, summer, or autumn.

Incubation Period

1 week to several months.

Diagnostic Tests

Microscopic identification of the organism on Giemsa- or Wright-stained thick or thin blood smears. People with babesiosis may have concurrent Lyme disease, so diagnostic tests for *Borrelia burgdorferi* should be considered.

Treatment

Clindamycin plus oral quinine or atovaquone plus azithromycin. Exchange blood transfusions should be considered for severely ill people, especially but not exclusively for people with parasitemia levels of 10% or greater.

Image 10.1
Babesia microti in a peripheral blood smear. Note the typical intraerythrocytic location of the organisms. Babesiosis is usually a mild infection except in patients with asplenia.

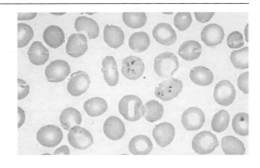

11

Bacterial Vaginosis

Clinical Manifestations

Bacterial vaginosis (BV), a syndrome primarily occurring in sexually active adolescent and adult females, is characterized by changes in vaginal flora. Symptoms can include a thin white or gray, homogenous vaginal discharge with a fishy odor. Bacterial vaginosis is asymptomatic in up to 50% of cases and usually is not associated with abdominal pain, pruritus, or dysuria.

Vaginitis and vulvitis in prepubertal girls usually have a nonspecific cause and rarely are manifestations of BV. In prepubertal girls, other predisposing causes of vaginal discharge include foreign bodies or infections attributable to group A streptococci, herpes simplex virus, *Neisseria gonorrhoeae, Chlamydia trachomatis, Trichomonas vaginalis,* or *Shigella* species or other enteric bacteria.

Etiology

The cause of BV is not clear. Typical microbiologic findings include an increase in concentrations of *Gardnerella vaginalis, Mycoplasma hominis, Ureaplasma* species, and anaerobic bacteria and a marked decrease in the concentration of *Lactobacillus* species.

Epidemiology

BV is the most prevalent vaginal infection in sexually active adolescents and adult females. Although the evidence of sexual transmission of BV is inconclusive, the condition is uncommon in sexually inexperienced females.

Incubation Period

Unknown.

Diagnostic Tests

The clinical diagnosis of BV requires the presence of 3 of the following symptoms or signs:

- Homogenous, gray or white, noninflammatory vaginal discharge that smoothly coats the vaginal walls
- Vaginal fluid pH greater than 4.5
- A fishy odor of vaginal discharge before or after addition of 10% potassium hydroxide
- Presence of "clue cells" (squamous vaginal epithelial cells covered with bacteria, which cause a stippled or granular appearance and ragged "moth-eaten" borders) on microscopic examination. Clue cells usually constitute at least 20% of vaginal epithelial cells.

A Gram stain of vaginal secretions is an alternative means of establishing a diagnosis. Cocci and a paucity of large gram-positive bacilli consistent with lactobacilli are characteristic. Culture for *G vaginalis* is not recommended because the organism may be found in females without BV, including females who are not sexually active.

Treatment

All nonpregnant patients who are symptomatic require treatment with metronidazole or clindamycin topically.

Pregnant women with symptoms of BV should be treated. Topical intravaginal clindamycin cream is not recommended during pregnancy because it can result in preterm labor. Metronidazole is the preferred treatment during pregnancy. Routine treatment of male sexual partners is not recommended because treatment has no influence on relapse or recurrence rates.

Image 11.1

This photomicrograph reveals bacteria adhering to vaginal epithelial cells known as clue cells. Clue cells are epithelial cells that have had bacteria adhere to their surface, obscuring their borders and imparting a stippled appearance.

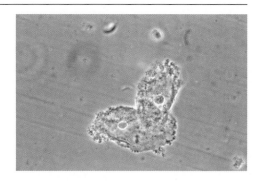

12

Bacteroides and *Prevotella* Infections

Clinical Manifestations

Bacteroides and *Prevotella* species from the **oral cavity** can cause chronic sinusitis, chronic otitis media, dental infection, peritonsillar abscess, cervical adenitis, retropharyngeal space infection, aspiration pneumonia, lung abscess, empyema, or necrotizing pneumonia. Species from the **gastrointestinal tract** are recovered in patients with peritonitis, intra-abdominal abscess, pelvic inflammatory disease, postoperative wound infection, or vulvovaginal and perianal infections. Soft tissue infections include synergistic bacterial gangrene and necrotizing fasciitis. Invasion of the bloodstream from the oral cavity or intestinal tract can lead to brain abscess, meningitis, endocarditis, arthritis, or osteomyelitis. **Skin involvement** includes omphalitis in newborn infants, cellulitis at the site of fetal monitors, human bite wounds, infection of burns adjacent to the mouth or rectum, and decubitus ulcers. Most infections are polymicrobial.

Etiology

Most *Bacteroides* and *Prevotella* organisms associated with human disease are pleomorphic, nonspore-forming, facultatively anaerobic, gram-negative bacilli.

Epidemiology

Bacteroides and *Prevotella* species are part of the normal flora of the mouth, gastrointestinal tract, or female genital tract. Members of the *Bacteroides fragilis* group predominate in the gastrointestinal tract flora; members of the *Prevotella melaninogenica* (formerly *Bacteroides melaninogenicus*) and *Prevotella oralis* (formerly *Bacteroides oralis*) groups are more common in the oral cavity. These species cause infections usually after alteration of a physical barrier after trauma, surgery, or chemotherapy. Except in infections resulting from human bites, no evidence of person-to-person transmission exists.

Incubation Period

Usually 1 to 5 days.

Diagnostic Tests

Anaerobic culture media are necessary for recovery of *Bacteroides* or *Prevotella* species. Because infections usually are polymicrobial, aerobic cultures also should be obtained. A putrid odor suggests anaerobic infection. Use of an anaerobic transport tube or sealed syringe is recommended for collection of clinical specimens.

Treatment

Abscesses should be drained when feasible. Clindamycin is active against virtually all mouth and respiratory tract *Bacteroides* and *Prevotella* isolates and is recommended by some experts as the drug of choice for anaerobic infections of the oral cavity and lungs. Some species of *Bacteroides* and almost 50% of *Prevotella* produce beta-lactamase. A beta-lactam penicillin active against *Bacteroides* combined with a beta-lactamase inhibitor can be useful to treat these infections. *Bacteroides* species of the gastrointestinal tract usually are resistant to penicillin G but are predictably susceptible to metronidazole and, sometimes, clindamycin.

Image 12.1

Prevotella melaninogenica (previously *Bacteroides melaninogenica*) and group A beta-hemolytic streptococcus were cultured from a submandibular subcutaneous abscess aspirate from this 12-year-old boy. There was no apparent dental, pharyngeal, or middle ear infection.

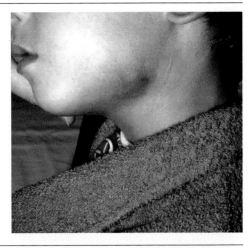

Image 12.2

Prevotella melaninogenica, pigmented colonies.

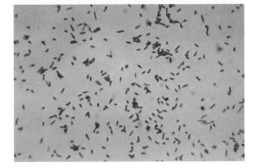

Image 12.3

This photomicrograph shows *Bacteroides fragilis* after being cultured in a thioglycollate medium for 48 hours. *B fragilis* is a gram-negative rod that constitutes 1% to 2% of the normal colonic bacterial microflora in humans. It is associated with extraintestinal infections such as abscesses and soft tissue infections, as well as diarrheal diseases.

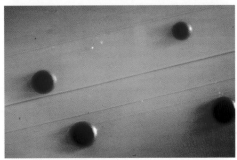

13

Balantidium coli Infections

(Balantidiasis)

Clinical Manifestations

Most human infections are asymptomatic. Acute infection is characterized by rapid onset of nausea, vomiting, abdominal discomfort or pain, and bloody or watery mucoid diarrhea. Infected patients can develop chronic intermittent episodes of diarrhea. Rarely, organisms spread to mesenteric nodes, pleura, or liver. Inflammation of the gastrointestinal tract and local lymphatic vessels can result in bowel dilation, ulceration, and secondary bacterial invasion.

Etiology

Balantidium coli, a ciliated protozoan, is the largest pathogenic protozoan known to infect humans.

Epidemiology

Pigs are believed to be the primary host reservoir of *B coli*. Cysts excreted in feces can be transmitted directly from hand to mouth or indirectly through fecally contaminated water or food. The excysted trophozoites infect the colon. A person is infectious as long as cysts are excreted in stool. The cysts can remain viable in the environment for months.

Incubation Period

Unknown but may be several days.

Diagnostic Tests

Diagnosis of infection is established by scraping lesions via sigmoidoscopy, histologic examination of intestinal biopsy specimens, or ova and parasite examination of stool. Stool examination is less sensitive, and repeated stool examination may be necessary to diagnose infection because shedding of organisms can be intermittent and trophozoites quickly degenerate.

Treatment

The drug of choice is tetracycline. Tetracycline should not be given to children younger than 8 years unless the benefits of therapy are greater than the risks of dental staining. Alternative drugs are metronidazole and iodoquinol.

Image 13.1
Balantidium coli trophozoites are characterized by their large size (40 µm–>70 µm); the presence of cilia on the cell surface, which are particularly visible in B; a cytostome (arrows); a bean-shaped macronucleus that is often visible (A); and a smaller, less conspicuous micronucleus.

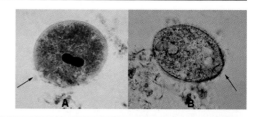

Image 13.2
Balantidium coli cyst in stool preparation.

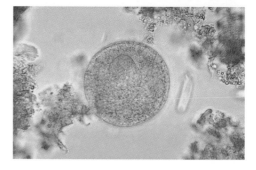

14

Baylisascaris Infections

Clinical Manifestations

Baylisascaris procyonis, a raccoon roundworm, is a rare cause of human eosinophilic meningoencephalitis. In a young child, presentation is acute CNS disease (eg, altered mental status and seizures) accompanied by peripheral and CSF eosinophilia. Severe neurologic sequelae or death is a typical outcome. *B procyonis* is a rare cause of predominantly extraneural disease in older children and adults. Ocular larva migrans can result in unilateral or bilateral neuroretinitis; direct visualization of worms in the retina sometimes is possible.

Etiology

B procyonis is a 10- to 25-cm roundworm (nematode) with a life cycle usually limited to its asymptomatic definitive host, the raccoon, and to soil.

Epidemiology

B procyonis is found throughout the United States; an estimated 22% to 80% of raccoons harbor the organism in the intestines. Embryonated eggs containing infective larvae are ingested from the soil by raccoons and grow to maturity in the small intestine, from which adult female worms shed millions of eggs per day. The eggs are 60 to 80 μm in size and have an outer shell, which permits long-term viability in soil.

Geophagia/pica is the most important risk factor for *Baylisascaris* infection, especially for neural larva migrans. Groups at highest risk include children 1 to 4 years of age and children with developmental delay.

Diagnostic Tests

Baylisascaris infection may be confirmed by specific serologic assays (serum, CSF) available only in research laboratories or by pathologic examination of tissue in which larvae with characteristic morphologic features sometimes may be visualized.

Treatment

Albendazole, in conjunction with high-dose corticosteroids, has been advocated most widely. However, treatment with anthelmintic agents and/or anti-inflammatory therapies (eg, corticosteroids) may not affect clinical outcome once CNS disease manifestations are evident. Some experts advocate the use of additional anthelmintic agents.

Image 14.1
Infective *Baylisascaris procyonis* egg (diameter, 70 μm) containing coiled second-stage larva that was recovered from soil and debris at a raccoon latrine (40x).

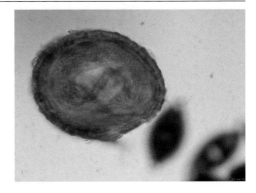

Image 14.2

Baylisascaris is raccoon roundworm, which may cause ocular and neural larval migrans and encephalitis in humans.

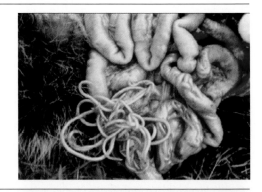

Image 14.3

Biopsy-proven *Baylisascaris procyonis* encephalitis in a 13-month-old boy. Axial T2-weighted MRIs obtained 12 days after symptom onset show abnormal high signal throughout most of the central white matter (arrows) compared with the dark signal expected at this age (broken arrows).

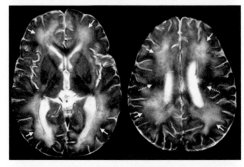

Image 14.4

Neuroimaging of human *Baylisascaris procyonis* neural larval migrans (NLM). In acute NLM, axial flair MR image (at the level of the posterior fossa) demonstrates abnormal hyperintense signal of cerebellar white matter.

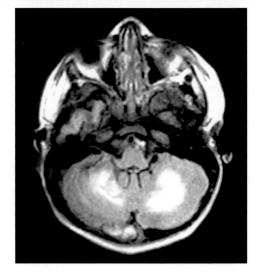

15

Blastomycosis

Clinical Manifestations

The major clinical manifestations of blastomycosis are pulmonary, cutaneous, and disseminated disease. Children commonly have pulmonary disease with a variety of flu-like symptoms and radiographic appearances. Skin lesions can be nodular, verrucous, or ulcerative, often with minimal inflammation. Abscesses generally are subcutaneous but can involve any organ. Disseminated blastomycosis usually begins with pulmonary infection and can involve skin, bones, CNS, abdominal viscera, and kidneys.

Etiology

Blastomycosis is caused by *Blastomyces dermatitidis*, a dimorphic fungus existing in infected tissues as the yeast form and in soil as the mycelial form, and is infectious for humans.

Epidemiology

Infection is acquired through inhalation of conidia produced from hyphae of the mycelial form from soil. Person-to-person transmission does not occur. Areas with endemic infection in the United States are the southeastern and central states and the midwestern states bordering the Great Lakes. Blastomycosis can occur in immunocompromised persons, but is rare in people infected with HIV.

Incubation Period

Approximately 30 to 45 days.

Diagnostic Tests

Thick-walled, figure-of-eight shaped, broad-based, single-budding yeast forms may be seen in sputum, tracheal aspirates, CSF, urine, or material from lesions processed with 10% potassium hydroxide or a silver stain. Children with pneumonia who are unable to produce sputum may require an invasive procedure to establish the diagnosis. Because serologic tests lack adequate sensitivity, every effort should be made to obtain appropriate specimens for culture.

Treatment

Amphotericin B is the treatment of choice for severe or life-threatening infection. Oral itraconazole or fluconazole has been used for mild or moderately severe infections. Data regarding the efficacy of itraconazole and fluconazole therapy in children are limited.

Image 15.1
Histopathology of blastomycosis (methenamine silver stain). Yeast cell of *Blastomyces dermatitidis* undergoing broad-base budding.

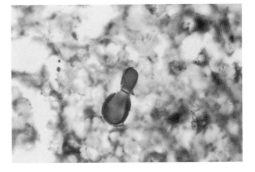

Image 15.2

Cutaneous blastomycosis (face). Most lesions are caused by hematogenous spread from a pulmonary infection.

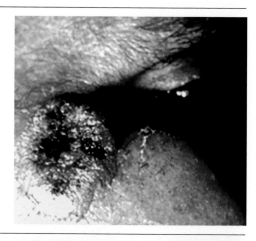

Image 15.3

An adult, whose pemphigus was under control following parenteral pulse steroid treatment and 2 years of oral steroid maintenance, developed a fungating growth on his right shin following a minor injury to his leg. Culture of tissue obtained from a skin biopsy revealed chromoblastomycosis.

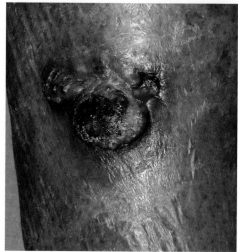

16

Borrelia Infections
(Relapsing Fever)

Clinical Manifestations

Relapsing fever is characterized by the sudden onset of high fever, shaking chills, sweats, headache, muscle and joint pains, and nausea. A fleeting macular rash of the trunk and petechiae of the skin and mucous membranes sometimes occur. Complications include hepatosplenomegaly, jaundice, thrombocytopenia, iridocyclitis, cough with pleuritic pain, pneumonitis, meningitis, and myocarditis. Untreated, an initial febrile period of 2 to 7 days terminates spontaneously by crisis. The initial febrile episode is followed by an afebrile period of several days to weeks, then by one or more relapses. Relapses typically become progressively shorter and milder as afebrile periods lengthen. Infection during pregnancy often is severe and can result in preterm birth, abortion, stillbirth, or neonatal infection.

Etiology

Borrelia recurrentis is the only spirochetal species that causes louse-borne (epidemic) relapsing fever. Worldwide, at least 14 *Borrelia* species cause tick-borne (endemic) relapsing fever, including *Borrelia hermsii, Borrelia turicatae,* and *Borrelia parkeri* in North America.

Epidemiology

Most tick-borne relapsing fever in the United States is caused by *B hermsii,* typically from tick exposures in rodent-infested cabins in western mountainous areas. *B turicatae* infections occur less frequently; most cases have been reported from Texas and often are associated with tick exposures in rodent-infested caves. *B parkeri* causes the lowest number of infections and is associated with burrows, rodent nests, and caves in arid areas or grasslands in the western United States.

Infected body lice and ticks remain alive and infectious for several years without feeding. Relapsing fever is not transmitted person to person.

Incubation Period

2 to 18 days, with a mean of 7 days.

Diagnostic Tests

Spirochetes can be observed by darkfield microscopy and in Wright-, Giemsa-, or acridine orange-stained preparations of thin or dehemoglobinized thick smears of peripheral blood or in stained buffy coat preparations. Serum antibodies to *Borrelia* species can be detected by enzyme immunoassay and Western immunoblot analysis at some laboratories, but these tests are not standardized and are affected by cross-reactions with other spirochetes.

Treatment

Treatment with doxycycline produces prompt clearance of spirochetes and remission of symptoms. For children younger than 8 years and for pregnant women, penicillin and erythromycin are the preferred drugs. A Jarisch-Herxheimer reaction (an acute febrile reaction accompanied by headache, myalgia, and an aggravated clinical picture lasting <24 hours) commonly is observed during the first few hours after initiating antimicrobial therapy. However, the Jarisch-Herxheimer reaction in children typically is mild and usually can be managed with antipyretic agents alone.

Single-dose treatment using a tetracycline, penicillin, or erythromycin is effective for curing louse-borne relapsing fever.

Image 16.1
Borrelia in peripheral blood smear. The spirochetes can be seen with darkfield microscopy and in Wright-, Giemsa-, or acridine orange-stained smears.

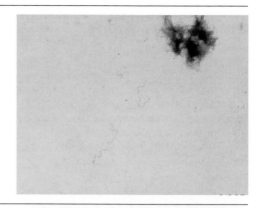

Image 16.2
Ornithodoros hermsii nymph. The length of the soft-bodied tick is 3.0 μm, excluding the legs. It is responsible for transmitting endemic relapsing fever.

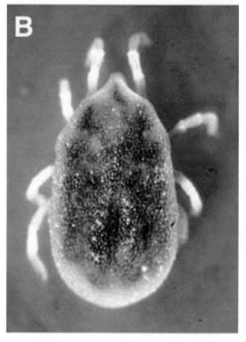

17

Brucellosis

Clinical Manifestations

Manifestations are acute or insidious and include fever, night sweats, weakness, malaise, anorexia, weight loss, arthralgia, myalgia, abdominal pain, and headache. Physical findings include lymphadenopathy, hepatosplenomegaly and, occasionally, arthritis. Serious complications include meningitis, endocarditis, and osteomyelitis.

Etiology

Brucella species are small, nonmotile, gram-negative coccobacilli. The species that infect humans are *Brucella abortus, Brucella melitensis, Brucella suis* and, rarely, *Brucella canis.*

Epidemiology

Brucellosis is a zoonotic disease of wild and domestic animals. Humans contract the disease by contact with infected animals or their secretions or by ingesting unpasteurized milk or milk products. Infection can be transmitted by inoculation through cuts and abrasions in the skin, inhalation of contaminated aerosols, contact with the conjunctival mucosa, or oral ingestion. Most cases occur in immigrants or travelers returned from areas with endemic infection and can result from ingestion of unpasteurized dairy products.

Incubation Period

Most people become ill within 3 to 4 weeks of exposure.

Diagnostic Tests

A definitive diagnosis is established by recovery of *Brucella* species from blood, bone marrow, or other tissue. Serologic testing can confirm a diagnosis with a 4-fold or greater increase in antibody titers in serum specimens collected at least 2 weeks apart. Increased concentrations of IgG agglutinins are found in acute infection, chronic infection, and relapse. Cross-reactions can occur with *Yersinia enterocolitica* serotype 09, *Francisella tularensis,* and *Vibrio cholerae.*

Treatment

Prolonged antimicrobial therapy is imperative for achieving a cure. Relapses generally are associated with premature discontinuation of therapy. Combination therapy is recommended with tetracycline (or trimethoprim-sulfamethoxazole if tetracyclines are contraindicated) and rifampin. For treatment of serious infections or complications, including endocarditis, meningitis, and osteomyelitis, streptomycin or gentamicin for the first 14 days of therapy in addition to a tetracycline (or trimethoprim-sulfamethoxazole if tetracyclines are contraindicated) is recommended. For life-threatening complications, such as meningitis or endocarditis, the duration of therapy with combination drugs often is extended for several months. Surgical intervention should be considered in patients with deep tissue abscesses.

Image 17.1
A calcified *Brucella* granuloma in the spleen of a man with fever of several years' duration.

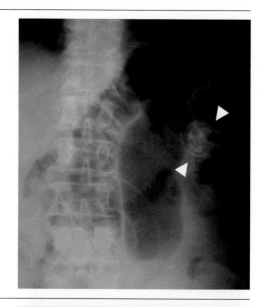

Image 17.2
Brucella melitensis colonies. *Brucella* species colony characteristics: fastidious, usually not visible at 24 hours; grows slowly on most standard laboratory media (eg, sheep blood, chocolate and trypticase soy agars); pinpoint, smooth, entire translucent, nonhemolytic colonies at 48 hours.

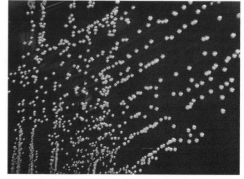

18

Campylobacter Infections

Clinical Manifestations

Predominant symptoms of *Campylobacter* infections include diarrhea, abdominal pain, malaise, and fever. Stools may contain visible or occult blood. In neonates and young infants, bloody diarrhea without fever may be the only manifestation of infection. Abdominal pain can mimic pain produced by appendicitis or intussusception. Mild infection lasts 1 or 2 days and resembles viral gastroenteritis. Most patients recover in less than 1 week, but 20% have a relapse or a prolonged or severe illness. Severe or persistent infection can mimic acute inflammatory bowel disease. Bacteremia is uncommon but can occur in neonates, in people with HIV infection, and in healthy and malnourished children. Immunocompromised hosts may have prolonged, relapsing, or extra-intestinal infections, especially with *Campylobacter fetus* and other "atypical" species. Immunoreactive complications, such as acute idiopathic polyneuritis (Guillain-Barré syndrome), Miller Fisher syndrome (ophthalmoplegia, areflexia, ataxia), reactive arthritis, Reiter syndrome (arthritis, urethritis, and bilateral conjunctivitis), and erythema nodosum, can occur during convalescence.

Etiology

Campylobacter species are motile, comma-shaped, gram-negative bacilli that cause gastroenteritis. *Campylobacter jejuni* and *Campylobacter coli* are the most common species isolated from patients with diarrhea. *C fetus* predominantly causes systemic illness in neonates and debilitated hosts.

Epidemiology

The gastrointestinal tract of domestic and wild birds and animals is the reservoir of infection. *C jejuni* and *C coli* have been isolated from feces of chickens, turkeys, and water fowl.

Many farm animals and meat sources can harbor the organism, and pets (especially young animals), including dogs, cats, hamsters, and birds, are potential sources of infection. Transmission of *C jejuni* and *C coli* occurs by ingestion of contaminated food or by direct contact with fecal material from infected animals or people. Improperly cooked poultry, untreated water, and unpasteurized milk have been the main vehicles of transmission. Person-to-person spread occurs occasionally, particularly among very young children. Enteritis occurs in people of all ages. Excretion of *Campylobacter* organisms typically lasts 2 to 3 weeks without treatment.

Incubation Period

Usually 1 to 7 days.

Diagnostic Tests

C jejuni and *C coli* can be cultured from feces, and *Campylobacter* species, including *C fetus,* can be cultured from blood. Laboratory identification of *C jejuni* and *C coli* in stool specimens requires selective media, microaerophilic conditions, and an incubation temperature of 42°C. The presence of motile, curved, spiral, or S-shaped rods resembling *Vibrio cholerae* by stool phase contrast or darkfield microscopy can provide rapid, presumptive evidence for *Campylobacter* species infection.

Treatment

Rehydration is the mainstay for all children with diarrhea. Erythromycin and azithromycin shorten the duration of illness and prevent relapse when given early during gastrointestinal tract infection. Treatment with erythromycin or azithromycin usually eradicates the organism from stool within 2 or 3 days. *C fetus* generally is susceptible to aminoglycosides, meropenem, imipenem, and extended-spectrum cephalosporins.

Image 18.1

Campylobacter jejuni. Gram stain faintly staining short, curved, or spiral-shaped gram-negative rods from a culture of the organism.

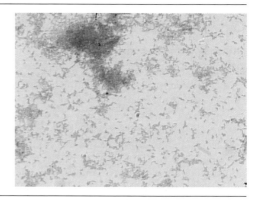

Image 18.2

This Gram-stained image shows the spiral rods of *Campylobacter fetus* subsp *fetus* taken from an 18-hour brain-heart infusion, and a 7% addition of rabbit blood agar plate culture.

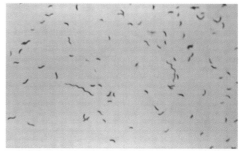

Image 18.3

Blood agar plate culture of *Campylobacter fetus* subsp *intestinalis*. *C fetus* causes prolonged, relapsing, or extraintestinal illness in immuno-compromised hosts. During convalescence *C fetus* infections had been associated with Guillain-Barré syndrome, reactive arthritis, and erythema nodosum.

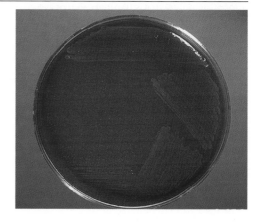

19

Candidiasis

(Moniliasis, Thrush)

Clinical Manifestations

Mucocutaneous infection results in oral-pharyngeal (thrush) or vaginal candidiasis; intertriginous lesions of the gluteal folds, neck, groin, and axilla; paronychia; and onychia. Dysfunction of T-lymphocytes, other immunologic disorders, and endocrinologic diseases are associated with chronic mucocutaneous candidiasis. Oral candidiasis can be the presenting sign of HIV infection or primary immunodeficiency. Esophageal and laryngeal candidiasis can occur in immunocompromised patients. Disseminated or **invasive candidiasis** occurs in very low birth weight newborn infants and in immunocompromised or debilitated hosts, can involve virtually any organ or anatomical site, and can be rapidly fatal. Candidemia or candiduria, respectively, can occur with or without systemic disease in patients with indwelling vascular or urinary catheters.

Etiology

Candida albicans causes most infections. Other species, including *Candida tropicalis, Candida parapsilosis, Candida glabrata, Candida krusei, Candida guilliermondii, Candida lusitaniae,* and *Candida dubliniensis,* also can cause serious infections in immunocompromised hosts.

Epidemiology

Candida species are present on skin and in the mouth, intestinal tract, and vagina of immunocompetent people. Vulvovaginal candidiasis is associated with pregnancy, and newborn infants can acquire the organism in utero, during passage through the vagina, or postnatally. Person-to-person transmission occurs rarely. Patients with neutrophil defects are at increased risk. Patients undergoing intravenous alimentation or receiving broad-spectrum antimicrobial agents, especially extended-spectrum cephalosporins, carbapenems, and vancomycin, or requiring long-term indwelling central venous catheters, have increased susceptibility. Postsurgical patients can be at risk, particularly after cardiothoracic or abdominal procedures.

Incubation Period

Unknown.

Diagnostic Tests

The presumptive diagnosis usually can be made clinically, but other organisms or trauma also can cause similar mucosal lesions. Yeast cells and pseudohyphae can be found in *C albicans*–infected tissue and are identifiable by microscopic examination of scrapings suspended in 10% to 20% potassium hydroxide. Endoscopy is useful for diagnosis of esophagitis. Ophthalmologic examination can reveal typical retinal lesions that can arise from candidemia. Lesions in the brain, kidney, liver, or spleen may be detected by ultrasonography or CT; however, these lesions may not appear by imaging until late in the course of disease or after neutropenia has resolved. A definitive diagnosis of invasive candidiasis requires isolation of the organism from a usually sterile site or demonstration of organisms in a tissue biopsy specimen.

Treatment

Mucous Membrane and Skin Infections. Oral candidiasis in immunocompetent hosts is treated with oral nystatin suspension or clotrimazole troches applied to lesions. Fluconazole can be beneficial for immunocompromised patients with oropharyngeal candidiasis or esophagitis. Skin infections are treated with topical nystatin, miconazole, clotrimazole, naftifine, ketoconazole, econazole, or ciclopirox. Vulvovaginal candidiasis is treated with topical azoles. Oral azole agents should be considered for recurrent or refractory cases.

For chronic mucocutaneous candidiasis, fluconazole and itraconazole are effective drugs. Low-dose amphotericin B given intravenously is effective in severe cases. Relapses are common and treatment should be viewed as a lifelong process. Keratomycosis is treated with corneal baths of amphotericin B in conjunction with systemic therapy. Patients with candiduria, especially patients with neutropenia, renal allographs, undergoing urologic manipulation, and infants with low birth weight, should be treated with fluconazole or a short course of low-dose amphotericin B intravenously.

Systemic Infections. Amphotericin B, fluconazole, caspofungin, micafungin, or anidulafungin is the drug of choice for treating people with invasive candidiasis, but data for caspofungin, micafungin, and anidulafungin in children and neonates are limited. Nearly all *Candida* species are susceptible to amphotericin B. Short-course therapy can be used for intravenous catheter-associated infections, provided the catheter is removed promptly and there is no evidence of systemic disease. Lipid-associated preparations of amphotericin B can be used if significant nephrotoxicity or clinical failure is observed with conventional amphotericin B therapy. However, lipid-associated preparations should not be used as first-line drugs. Flucytosine can be given with amphotericin B for *C albicans* infection involving the CNS if enteral administration is feasible. Fluconazole also has been used successfully for treatment of invasive candidiasis. Fluconazole is not an appropriate choice for therapy before the infecting *Candida* species is known because *C krusei* is resistant to fluconazole, and up to 50% of *C glabrata* also can be resistant. Treatment of disseminated candidiasis always should include removal of infected central vascular catheters and avoidance or reduction of systemic steroid therapy.

Image 19.1
Candida albicans (thrush) infection of the tonsils and uvula of an otherwise healthy 6-month-old infant. The white exudate resembles curds of milk.

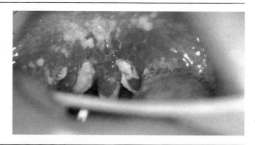

Image 19.2
Cutaneous candidiasis with typical satellite lesions in an infant boy.

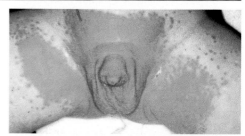

Image 19.3
Candidiasis, congenital, in an infant boy.

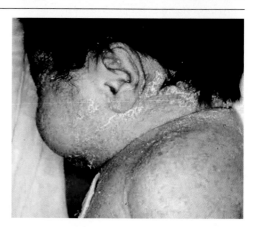

Image 19.4
Chronic mucocutaneous candidiasis in a
15-year-old immunodeficient boy. Impaired T-cell
function predisposes patients to this infection.

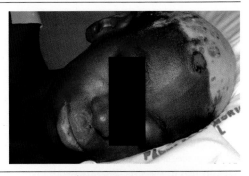

Image 19.5
Chronic mucocutaneous candidiasis.

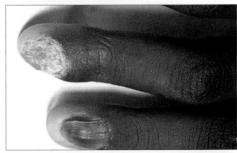

Image 19.6
An immunocompromised 5-year-old black male
with multiple candida granulomatous lesions, a
rare response to an invasive cutaneous infection.
These crusted, verrucous plaques and horn-like
projections require systemic antifungal therapy.

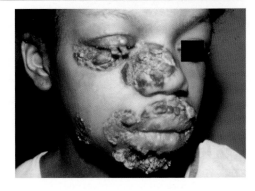

20

Cat-Scratch Disease

(Bartonella henselae)

Clinical Manifestations

Fever and mild systemic symptoms occur in approximately 30% of patients, but the predominant manifestation is regional lymphadenopathy. A skin papule often is found at the presumed site of bacterial inoculation and usually precedes development of lymphadenopathy by 1 to 2 weeks. The skin overlying affected lymph nodes typically is tender, warm, erythematous, and indurated, and nodes may suppurate spontaneously. Occasionally, infection can produce Parinaud oculoglandular syndrome, in which inoculation of the eyelid conjunctiva results in conjunctivitis and ipsilateral preauricular lymphadenopathy. Less common manifestations of cat-scratch disease (CSD) include encephalopathy, aseptic meningitis, fever of unknown origin, neuroretinitis, osteolytic lesions, granulomata in the liver and spleen, pneumonia, thrombocytopenic purpura, erythema nodosum, relapsing bacteremia, and endocarditis.

Etiology

Bartonella henselae is a fastidious, slow-growing, gram-negative bacillus.

Epidemiology

CSD incidence is unknown. Most cases occur in people younger than 20 years. Cats are the common reservoir. More than 90% of patients with CSD have a history of recent contact with apparently healthy cats, often kittens. No evidence of person-to-person transmission exists.

Incubation Period

From scratch to appearance of the primary cutaneous lesion is 7 to 12 days; from appearance of the primary lesion to lymphadenopathy is 5 to 50 days.

Diagnostic Tests

The indirect immunofluorescent antibody assay for detection of serum antibodies to antigens of *Bartonella* species is useful for diagnosis of CSD. Early histologic changes in lymph node specimens consist of lymphocytic infiltration with epithelioid granuloma formation. Later changes consist of polymorphonuclear leukocyte infiltration with granulomas that become necrotic.

Treatment

Management of localized CSD is aimed primarily at relief of symptoms because the disease can be self-limited. Painful suppurative nodes can be treated with needle aspiration for relief of symptoms; incision and drainage should be avoided, and surgical excision generally is unnecessary. Several oral antimicrobial agents (azithromycin, erythromycin, ciprofloxacin, trimethoprim-sulfamethoxazole, rifampin) and parenteral gentamicin are effective in the treatment of CSD.

Complicated cases in immunocompromised people should be evaluated in consultation with an infectious diseases specialist to determine the most appropriate therapy.

Image 20.1
Cat-scratch granuloma of the wrist with anterior axillary lymphadenitis in a 4-year-old boy. Cat-scratch disease is a common cause of chronic lymphadenopathy in children.

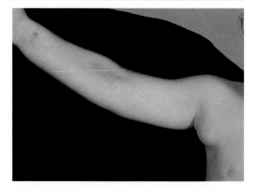

Image 20.2
Parinaud oculoglandular syndrome (inoculation of the conjunctivae with ipsilateral preauricular adenopathy) in a 6-year-old boy.

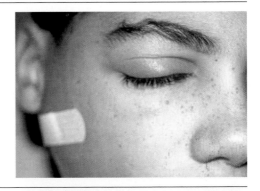

Image 20.3
A papule at each of 2 inoculation sites on the arm of a patient with cat-scratch disease.

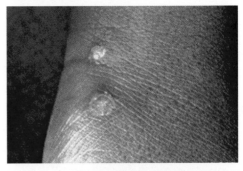

Image 20.4
A 2-year-old child with suppurative right axillary lymphadenopathy secondary to cat-scratch disease.

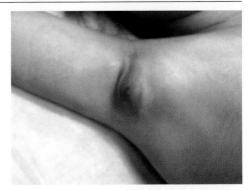

Image 20.5
Sanguinopurulent exudate aspirated from the axillary node of the patient in Image 20.4 with cat-scratch disease.

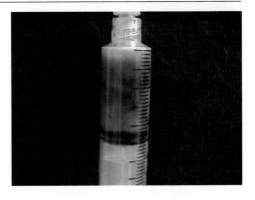

Image 20.6

Cat-scratch disease granuloma of the finger in a 12-year-old boy with epitrochlear node involvement.

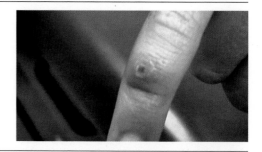

Image 20.7

Epitrochlear suppurative adenitis of cat-scratch disease in the child in Image 20.6 with a cat-scratch granuloma of the finger.

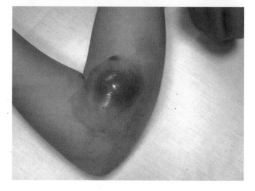

21

Chancroid

Clinical Manifestations

The genital ulcer begins as a tender erythematous papule, becomes pustular, and erodes over several days, forming a sharply demarcated, somewhat superficial lesion with a serpiginous border. The base of the ulcer is friable and can be covered with a gray or yellow, necrotic, and purulent exudate. Unlike a syphilitic chancre, which is painless, the chancroidal ulcer often is painful, tender, and nonindurated. The ulcer can be associated with a painful, unilateral inguinal adenitis (bubo), which often is fluctuant.

Many females are asymptomatic but can, depending on the site of the ulcer, have less obvious symptoms, including dysuria, dyspareunia, vaginal discharge, pain on defecation, or rectal bleeding.

Etiology

Haemophilus ducreyi, a gram-negative coccobacillus.

Epidemiology

Chancroid is an STI that is associated with poverty, urban prostitution, and illicit drug use. Chancroid is endemic in some areas of the United States. Coinfection with syphilis or HSV occurs in as many as 10% of patients. Chancroid is a well-established cofactor for transmission of HIV.

Incubation Period

3 to 10 days.

Diagnostic Tests

The diagnosis is made on the basis of clinical findings and exclusion of other infections associated with genital ulcer disease. Confirmation can be made by recovery of *H ducreyi* from a genital ulcer or lymph node aspirate. If chancroid is suspected, the laboratory should be informed.

Treatment

Recommended regimens include azithromycin or ceftriaxone (in a single dose). Adenitis often is slow to resolve and may require needle aspiration or surgical incision. Patients should be reexamined 3 to 7 days after starting therapy to verify that healing is occurring.

Image 21.1
Adolescent male with chancroid lesions of the groin and penis affecting the ipsilateral inguinal lymph nodes.

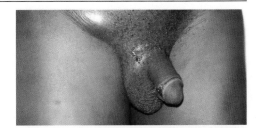

Image 21.2
Ulcerative chancroid lesions with inflammation of the shaft and glans penis caused by *Haemophilus ducreyi.* Chancroid lesions are irregular in shape, painful, and soft (non-indurated) to touch.

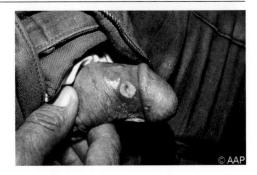

22

Chlamydia trachomatis

Clinical Manifestations

Chlamydia trachomatis causes neonatal conjunctivitis, trachoma (rare in the United States), pneumonia in young infants, genital tract infection, and lymphogranuloma venereum (LGV). Neonatal chlamydial **conjunctivitis** is characterized by ocular congestion, edema, and discharge developing a few days to weeks after birth and lasting for 1 to 2 weeks. Scars and pannus formation are rare. **Trachoma** is a chronic follicular keratoconjunctivitis with neovascularization of the cornea that results from repeated and chronic infection that can lead to blindness. **Pneumonia** in young infants usually is an afebrile illness of insidious onset occurring between 2 and 19 weeks after birth. A repetitive staccato cough, tachypnea, and rales are characteristic but not always present. Wheezing is uncommon. **Vaginitis** in prepubertal girls; urethritis, cervicitis, endometritis, salpingitis, and perihepatitis in postpubertal females; epididymitis in males; and Reiter syndrome also can occur. In postpubertal females, chlamydial infection can progress to acute or chronic pelvic inflammatory disease and result in ectopic pregnancy or infertility. **LGV** classically is an invasive lymphatic infection with an initial ulcerative lesion on the genitalia accompanied by tender, suppurative, inguinal, and/or femoral lymphadenopathy that typically is unilateral.

Etiology

C trachomatis is an obligate intracellular bacterial agent with at least 18 serologic variants (serovars).

Epidemiology

C trachomatis is the most common reportable STI in the United States; median prevalence among 15- to 24-year-old women screened in prenatal clinics was 7%. Oculogenital serovars of *C trachomatis* can be transmitted from the genital tract of infected mothers to their newborn infants. Acquisition occurs in approximately 50% of infants born vaginally to infected mothers and in some infants delivered by cesarean section with intact membranes. The risk of conjunctivitis is 25% to 50%, and the risk of pneumonia is 5% to 20% in infants who are exposed to *C trachomatis*.

Genital tract infection in adolescents and adults is transmitted sexually.

LGV biovars are worldwide in distribution but particularly are prevalent in tropical and subtropical areas, but rare in the United States.

Incubation Period

At least 1 week.

Diagnostic Tests

Definitive diagnosis can be made by isolating the organism, an obligate intracellular bacterium in tissue culture, or by nucleic acid amplification testing.

Treatment

- Young infants with **chlamydial conjunctivitis** are treated with oral erythromycin base or ethylsuccinate. Topical treatment of conjunctivitis is ineffective and unnecessary.
- **Chlamydial pneumonia** is treated with oral azithromycin or erythromycin base or ethylsuccinate.
- Treatment of **trachoma** is topical with erythromycin, tetracycline, or sulfacetamide ointment; or oral erythromycin or doxycycline (for children 8 years of age and older) if the infection is severe. Azithromycin also is effective.
- For uncomplicated *C trachomatis* **genital tract infection** in adolescents or adults, oral doxycycline for 7 days or azithromycin in a single oral dose is recommended. Alternatives include oral erythromycin, ofloxacin, or levofloxacin.
- For **LGV,** doxycycline is the preferred treatment for children 8 years of age and older.

Previously infected adolescents are a high priority for repeat testing for *C trachomatis,* usually 3 to 6 months after initial infection.

Image 22.1

Infected HeLa cells (fluorescent antibody stain). *Chlamydia trachomatis* is the most common reportable STI in the United States, with high rates of infection among sexually active adolescents and young adults.

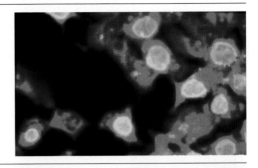

Image 22.2

Conjunctivitis in an infant due to *Chlamydia trachomatis*. The risk of neonatal conjunctivitis is 25% to 50% for infants of untreated, infected mothers.

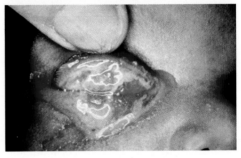

23

Clostridium botulinum
(Botulism and Infant Botulism)

Clinical Manifestations

Three distinct, naturally occurring forms: food-borne, wound, and infant. Cranial nerve palsies always occur in botulism, possibly followed by symmetric, descending, flaccid paralysis of somatic musculature. Infant botulism is preceded by or begins with constipation and manifests as decreased movement, loss of facial expression, poor feeding, weak cry, diminished gag reflex, ocular palsies, truncal weakness, and progressive descending generalized weakness and hypotonia. The spectrum of disease ranges from mild (eg, constipation, slow feeding) to rapidly progressive (eg, apnea, sudden infant death).

Etiology

Botulism results from absorption of botulinum toxins into the circulation from a wound or mucosal surface. *Clostridium botulinum* spores are ubiquitous in soil worldwide.

Epidemiology

Food-borne botulism results when a food contaminated with spores of *C botulinum* is preserved or stored improperly. Outbreaks have occurred after ingestion of restaurant-prepared foods, such as patty melts, potato salad, aluminum foil–wrapped baked potatoes, home-canned foods, bottled garlic, cheese sauce, and tissue from beached whales.

Infant botulism results after ingested spores of *C botulinum* germinate, multiply, and produce botulinum toxin in the intestine. Most cases occur in breastfed infants at the time of first introduction of nonhuman milk sub-

stances, and the source of spores usually is not identified. Honey has been identified as an avoidable source. Rarely, intestinal botulism can occur in older children and adults after intestinal surgery, in the presence of inflammatory bowel disease, and with exposure to antimicrobial agents.

Wound botulism results when *C botulinum* contaminates traumatized tissue, multiplies, and produces toxin. Gross trauma or crush injury can be a predisposing event. During the last decade, injection of contaminated black tar heroin has been associated with virtually all cases.

Incubation Period

Food-borne botulism, 12 to 48 hours; infant botulism, 3 to 30 days; wound botulism, 4 to 14 days.

Diagnostic Tests

A toxin neutralization bioassay identifies botulinum toxin in serum, stool, gastric aspirate, or suspect foods. Enriched and selective media are used to culture *C botulinum* from stool and foods. In infant and wound botulism, the diagnosis is made by demonstrating *C botulinum* toxin or organisms in feces, wound exudate, or tissue specimens.

Treatment

Respiratory and nutritional support, and administration of antitoxin. Because results of laboratory testing can be delayed by several days, treatment with antitoxin should be initiated promptly on the basis of clinical suspicion. Antimicrobial therapy is not indicated. Aminoglycoside agents potentiate the paralytic effects of the toxin and should be avoided.

Image 23.1
An infant with mild botulism depicting the loss of facial expression. This infant also had a weak cry, poor feeding, diminished gag reflex, and hypotonia. Infant botulism most often occurs in infants younger than 6 months.

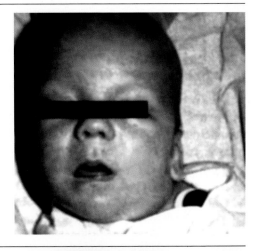

Image 23.2
Botulism with ocular muscle paralysis in an adolescent female. She also had respiratory muscle weakness but did not require ventilatory support.

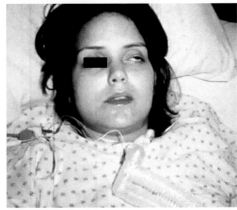

Image 23.3
Wound botulism in the compound fracture of the right arm of a 14-year-old boy. The patient fractured his right ulna and radius and subsequently developed wound botulism.

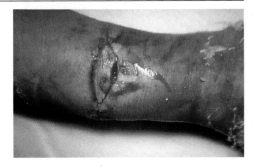

24

Clostridium difficile

Clinical Manifestations

Syndromes associated with infections include pseudomembranous colitis and antimicrobial-associated diarrhea. Pseudomembranous colitis generally is characterized by diarrhea, abdominal cramps, fever, systemic toxicity, abdominal tenderness, and passage of stools containing blood and mucus. Occasionally children can have marked abdominal tenderness and distention with minimal diarrhea. The colonic mucosa often contains small (2- to 5-mm), raised, yellowish plaques. Characteristically, disease begins while the child is in a hospital receiving antimicrobial therapy, but disease can occur days or weeks after hospital discharge or after cessation of therapy. Severe or fatal disease is more likely to occur in severely neutropenic children with leukemia, in infants with Hirschsprung disease, and in patients with inflammatory bowel disease. Infection also can result only in mild diarrhea or asymptomatic carriage. Carriage is common in newborn infants and in children younger than 1 year, and is of no clinical significance.

Etiology

Clostridium difficile is a spore-forming, obligate anaerobic, gram-positive bacillus. Disease is related to the action of toxin(s) produced by these organisms. Although other toxins also exist, toxins A and B have been associated most strongly with human disease.

Epidemiology

C difficile can be isolated from soil and commonly is present in the environment. *C difficile* is acquired from the environment or from the stool of other colonized or infected people by the fecal-oral route. Intestinal colonization rates in healthy neonates and young infants can be as high as 50% but usually are less than 5% in children older than 2 years and in adults. Hospitals, nursing homes, and child care facilities are major reservoirs for *C difficile*. Risk factors for disease are those that increase exposure to organisms and those that diminish the barrier effect of the normal intestinal flora, allowing *C difficile* to proliferate and elaborate toxin(s) in vivo. Risk factors for acquisition include experiencing prolonged hospitalization, having an infected hospital roommate, and having symptomatically infected patients on the same hospital ward. Risk factors for developing disease include antimicrobial therapy, repeated enemas, prolonged nasogastric tube insertion, and gastrointestinal tract surgery and having renal insufficiency. Penicillins, clindamycin, and cephalosporins are the antimicrobial drugs most commonly associated with *C difficile* colitis, but colitis has been associated with almost every antimicrobial agent. A previously uncommon strain of *C difficile* with variations in toxin genes has become more resistant to fluoroquinolones and has emerged as a cause of outbreaks of *C difficile*–associated diarrhea with significantly greater morbidity and mortality in adults.

Incubation Period

Unknown.

Diagnostic Tests

Endoscopic findings of pseudomembranes and hyperemic, friable rectal mucosa suggest pseudomembranous colitis. To diagnose *C difficile* disease, stool should be tested for presence of *C difficile* toxins. Commercially available enzyme immunoassays (EIAs) detect toxins A and B, or an EIA for toxin A may be used in conjunction with cell culture cytotoxicity assay, the "gold standard" for toxin B detection. Latex agglutination tests should not be used. Real-time PCR assays are investigational but allow greater sensitivity for toxin detection than EIA. Symptomatic infants younger than 1 year should be investigated for causes of diarrhea other than *C difficile* because carriage of *C difficile* is common in this age group. The presence of *C difficile* toxin is not responsible for clinical signs or symptoms.

Treatment

- Antimicrobial therapy should be discontinued as soon as possible.
- Antimicrobial therapy for *C difficile* disease is indicated for patients with severe disease or in whom diarrhea persists after antimicrobial therapy is discontinued.
- Strains of *C difficile* are susceptible to metronidazole and vancomycin, and both

are effective. Metronidazole is the drug of choice for the initial treatment of most patients with colitis. Oral vancomycin is an alternative drug, but use of vancomycin should be discouraged because of the potential for promoting vancomycin-resistant organisms. Vancomycin is indicated for patients who do not respond to metronidazole. Metronidazole is effective when given orally or intravenously; vancomycin is effective only when administered orally or rectally.

- Up to 40% of patients experience a relapse after discontinuing therapy, but the infection usually responds to a second course of the same treatment.
- Drugs that decrease intestinal motility should not be administered.

Follow-up testing for toxin is not recommended if symptoms resolve.

Image 24.1
Clostridium difficile is a gram-positive spore-forming bacteria that can be part of the normal intestinal flora in as many as 50% of children younger than 2 years. It is a major cause of pseudomembranous colitis and antibiotic-associated diarrhea in children and adults.

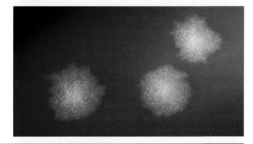

Image 24.2
This photograph depicts *Clostridium difficile* after 24 hours' growth on a blood agar plate (4.8x).

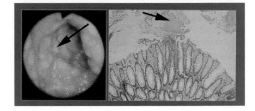

Image 24.3
The right-hand panel shows the typical pseudomembranes of *Clostridium difficile* colitis; the left-hand panel shows the histology, with the pseudomembrane structure at the top middle (arrows).

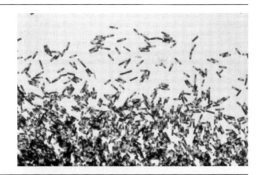

25

Clostridial Myonecrosis
(Gas Gangrene)

Clinical Manifestations

Onset is heralded by acute pain at the site of the wound, followed by edema, tenderness, exudate, and progression of pain. Systemic findings include tachycardia disproportionate to the degree of fever, pallor, diaphoresis, hypotension, renal failure and, later, alterations in mental status. Crepitus is suggestive but not pathognomonic of *Clostridium* infection and is not always present.

Etiology

Clostridial myonecrosis is caused by *Clostridium* species, most often *Clostridium perfringens,* which are large, gram-positive, spore-forming anaerobic bacilli with blunt ends. Mixed infection with other gram-positive and gram-negative bacteria is common.

Epidemiology

Clostridial myonecrosis usually results from contamination of open wounds involving muscle. The sources of *Clostridium* species are soil, contaminated objects, and human and animal feces. Dirty surgical or traumatic wounds with significant devitalized tissue and foreign bodies predispose to disease. Nontraumatic gas gangrene occurs occasionally from *Clostridium* organisms in the gastrointestinal tract and in immunocompromised people.

Incubation Period

Unknown.

Diagnostic Tests

Strict anaerobic cultures of wound exudate, involved soft tissue and muscle, and blood should be performed. Because *Clostridium* species are ubiquitous, their recovery from a wound is not diagnostic unless typical clinical manifestations are present. A Gram-stained smear of wound discharge demonstrating characteristic gram-positive bacilli and absent or sparse polymorphonuclear leukocytes suggests clostridial infection. Tissue specimens and aspirates (not swab specimens) are appropriate for anaerobic culture. A radiograph of the affected site can demonstrate gas in the tissue.

Treatment

- Early and complete surgical excision of necrotic tissue and removal of any foreign material is essential.
- Management of shock, fluid and electrolyte imbalance, hemolytic anemia, and other complications is crucial.
- High-dose penicillin G should be administered intravenously. Clindamycin, metronidazole, imipenem, or meropenem can be considered as alternative drugs for penicillin-allergic patients or for treatment of polymicrobial infections.
- Hyperbaric oxygen may be beneficial, but efficacy data are not available.

Image 25.1
Clostridial omphalitis. Tissue aspirate (Gram stain) showing the characteristic morphology of Clostridial bacilli, erroneously stained gram-negative, and sparse polymorphonuclear leukocytes.

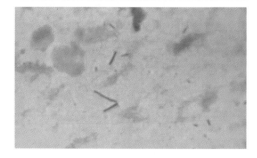

Image 25.2

Clostridial omphalitis in an infant with myonecrosis of the abdominal wall (periumbilical). Early and complete surgical excision of necrotic tissue and careful management of shock, fluid balance, and other complications are crucial for survival.

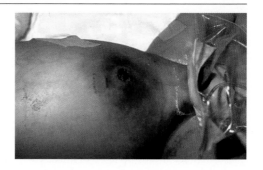

26

Coccidioidomycosis

Clinical Manifestations

Symptomatic disease can resemble influenza, with malaise, fever, cough, myalgia, headache, and chest pain but infection is asymptomatic or self-limited in 60% of children. Diffuse erythematous maculopapular rash, erythema multiforme, erythema nodosum, and arthralgias commonly occur. Up to 5% of infected people develop asymptomatic pulmonary radiographic residua (eg, cysts, coin lesions). Nonpulmonary primary infection is rare, usually follows trauma, and includes cutaneous lesions or soft tissue infections with associated regional lymphadenitis. Infection disseminates hematogenously to skin, bones and joints, CNS, and lungs in less than 1% of infected people: Dissemination is common in infants.

Etiology

Coccidioides immitis is a dimorphic fungus. In soil, it exists in hyphal phase. Infectious arthroconidia (ie, spores) produced in some hyphae become airborne, infecting the host after inhalation or inoculation.

Epidemiology

C immitis is found extensively in soil and is endemic in the southwestern United States, including California, Arizona, New Mexico, West Texas, and Utah; northern Mexico; and certain areas of Central and South America. In areas with endemic infection, clusters of cases of coccidioidomycosis can follow dust storms, seismic events, archaeologic digging, or recreational activities. Infection provides lifelong immunity. Black and Filipino people, pregnant women, neonates, elderly people, and immunocompromised people have an increased risk of dissemination and fatal outcome.

Incubation Period

Typically 10 to 16 days.

Diagnostic Tests

The diagnosis of coccidioidomycosis is best established using serologic, histopathologic, and culture methods. Serologic tests are useful to confirm diagnosis and provide prognostic information. The IgM response can be detected by latex agglutination test, enzyme immunoassay (EIA), or immunodiffusion. An IgM response is detectable 1 to 3 weeks after symptoms appear. IgG response can be detected by immunodiffusion, EIA, or complement fixation test. Complement fixation antibodies in serum usually are of low titer and are transient if the disease is asymptomatic or mild. High (≥1:32) persistent titers occur with severe disease and almost always in disseminated infection. CSF antibodies also are detectable by complement fixation test. Increasing serum and CSF titers indicate progressive disease, and decreasing titers suggest improvement. Low or nondetectable titers in immunocompromised patients should be interpreted with caution. Positive results should be confirmed in a reference laboratory.

Spherules as large as 80 μm in diameter may be visualized in infected body fluid specimens (eg, pleural fluid, bronchoalveolar lavage) and biopsy specimens of skin lesions or organs. The presence of a mature spherule with endospores is pathognomonic of infection.

Treatment

Antifungal therapy is not indicated for uncomplicated primary infection.

Amphotericin B is the recommended initial therapy for severe and progressive (non-CNS) infection. Fluconazole is recommended for CNS infections. Itraconazole and fluconazole also are useful for treatment of less severe infections. For CNS infections unresponsive to fluconazole, intravenous and intrathecal amphotericin B therapy is indicated. Surgical debridement or excision of lesions in bone and lung has been advocated for localized, symptomatic, persistent, resistant, or progressive lesions.

Image 26.1
Histopathologic features of coccidioidomycosis of lung showing spherule and endospore forms of *Coccidioides immitis* (methenamine silver stain).

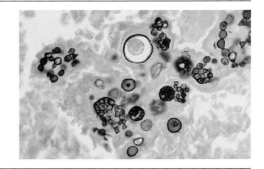

Image 26.2
Coccidioidomycosis of the tongue in an adult male.

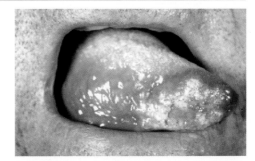

Image 26.3
Erythema nodosum in a preadolescent girl with primary pulmonary coccidioidomycosis.

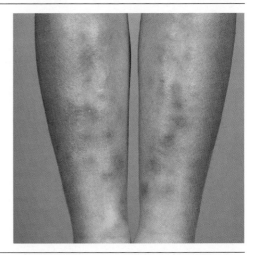

Image 26.4
Coccidioides immitis spherule with endospores from a mass located in the left subcutaneous flank in the patient in Image 26.6 (hematoxylin-eosin stain, 40x).

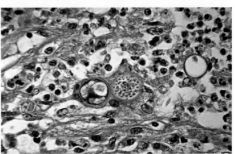

Image 26.5

Primary pulmonary coccidioidomycosis in an 11-year-old boy who recovered spontaneously. The acute disease is usually self-limited in otherwise healthy children. The patient also had erythema nodosum lesions over the tibial area.

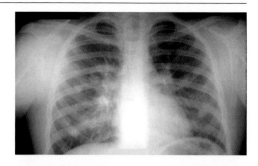

Image 26.6

Spondylitis due to *Coccidioides immitis* in a 2-year-old white male with disseminated disease.

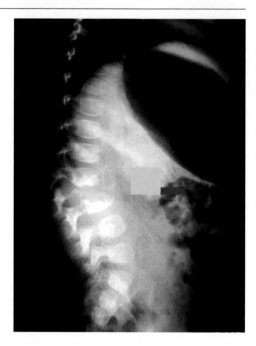

27

Cryptococcus neoformans Infections
(Cryptococcosis)

Clinical Manifestations

Primary infection is acquired by inhalation of aerosolized fungal elements and often is asymptomatic or mild. Pulmonary disease, when symptomatic, is characterized by cough, chest pain, and constitutional symptoms. Chest radiographs may reveal a solitary nodule or mass or focal or diffuse infiltrates. Hematogenous dissemination to the CNS, bones, skin, and other sites can occur, but dissemination is rare in children without defects in cell-mediated immunity (eg, children with leukemia, systemic lupus erythematosus, chronic cutaneous candidiasis, congenital immunodeficiency, or AIDS or people who have undergone solid organ transplantation).

Etiology

Cryptococcus neoformans, an encapsulated yeast, is, with rare exceptions, the only species of the genus *Cryptococcus* considered to be a human pathogen.

Epidemiology

C neoformans variety *neoformans* is isolated primarily from soil contaminated with bird droppings and causes most human infections. Person-to-person transmission does not occur.

Incubation Period

Unknown.

Diagnostic Tests

Encapsulated yeast cells can be visualized using India ink or other stains of CSF. Definitive diagnosis requires isolation of the organism from body fluid or tissue specimens. Blood should be cultured by lysis-centrifugation. The latex agglutination test and enzyme immunoassay for detection of cryptococcal capsular polysaccharide antigen in serum or CSF specimens are excellent rapid diagnostic tests. Antigen is detected in CSF or serum specimens from more than 90% of patients with cryptococcal meningitis.

Treatment

Amphotericin B, in combination with oral flucytosine or fluconazole, is indicated as initial therapy for patients with meningeal and other serious cryptococcal infections. Combination therapy for at least 2 weeks, and then fluconazole, is recommended. Lipid formulations of amphotericin B can be substituted for conventional amphotericin B in children with renal impairment. A lumbar puncture should be performed after 2 weeks of therapy. The 20% to 40% of patients in whom culture is positive at 2 weeks will require a more prolonged treatment course. Patients with less severe disease may be treated with fluconazole or itraconazole, but data on use of these drugs for children with *C neoformans* infection are limited. Children with HIV infection who have completed initial therapy for cryptococcosis should receive lifelong suppressive therapy with fluconazole daily.

Image 27.1

Cryptococcus neoformans. Thin-walled encap-sulated yeast in CSF (India ink preparation, 450x).

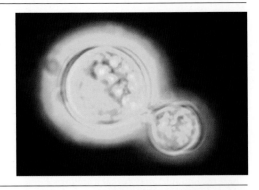

Image 27.2

Cryptococcosis of lung in patient with AIDS (mucicarmine stain). Histopathology of lung shows widened alveolar septum containing a few inflammatory cells and numerous yeasts of *Cryptococcus neoformans.* The inner layer of the yeast capsule stains red.

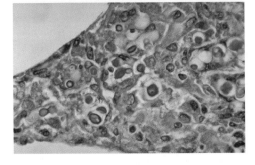

28

Cutaneous Larva Migrans

Clinical Manifestations

Nematode larvae produce pruritic, reddish papules at the site of skin entry, a condition referred to as creeping eruption. An advancing serpiginous tunnel in the skin with an associated intense pruritus is virtually pathognomonic. Rarely, in infections with a large burden of parasites, pneumonitis (Löffler syndrome), and myositis may follow skin lesions. Occasionally, the larvae reach the intestine and may cause eosinophilic enteritis.

Etiology

Infective larvae of cat and dog hookworms (ie, *Ancylostoma braziliense* and *Ancylostoma caninum*) are the usual causes.

Epidemiology

Cutaneous larva migrans is a disease of children, utility workers, gardeners, sunbathers, and others who come in contact with soil contaminated with cat and dog feces. In the United States, the disease is most prevalent in the Southeast.

Diagnostic Tests

Because the diagnosis usually is made clinically, biopsies are not indicated.

Treatment

The disease usually is self-limited, with spontaneous cure after several weeks or months. Orally administered albendazole or ivermectin or topically administered thiabendazole is the recommended therapy.

Image 28.1
Cutaneous larva migrans lesions on lower leg (caused by hookworm larvae of *Ancylostoma braziliense* and *Ancylostoma caninum*).

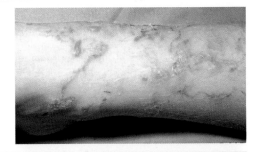

Image 28.2
Cutaneous larva migrans infection of the foot in an adolescent male.

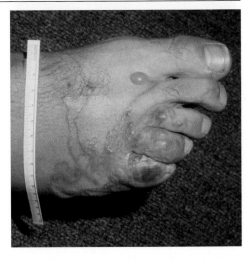

29

Cytomegalovirus Infection

Clinical Manifestations

Manifestations of acquired human CMV infection vary with age and host immunocompetence. Asymptomatic infections are the most common, particularly in children. An infectious mononucleosis-like syndrome with prolonged fever and mild hepatitis can occur in adolescents and adults. Pneumonia, colitis, and retinitis occur in immunocompromised hosts.

Congenital infection has a spectrum of manifestations but usually is silent clinically. Some congenitally infected infants who appear healthy at birth are later found to have hearing loss or learning disability. Approximately 10% of infants with congenital CMV infection have profound involvement evident at birth, with manifestations including intrauterine growth retardation, jaundice, purpura, hepatosplenomegaly, microcephaly, intracerebral calcifications, and retinitis.

Infection acquired intrapartum from maternal cervical secretions or postpartum from human milk usually is not associated with clinical illness.

Etiology

Human CMV, a DNA virus, is a member of the herpesvirus group.

Epidemiology

CMV is ubiquitous and is transmitted horizontally (by direct person-to-person contact with virus-containing secretions); vertically (from mother to infant before, during, or after birth); and via transfusions of blood, platelets, and white blood cells from previously infected people. CMV persists in latent form after a primary infection, and reactivation can occur years later, particularly under conditions of immunosuppression.

Horizontal transmission probably is the result of salivary contamination, but contact with infected urine also can have a role. Spread of CMV in households and child care centers is well documented. CMV excretion rates in child care centers can be as high as 70% in children 1 to 3 years of age. In adolescents and adults, sexual transmission also occurs.

Seropositive healthy people have latent CMV in their leukocytes and tissues; hence, blood transfusions and organ transplantation can result in viral transmission. Severe CMV disease is more likely to occur if the recipient is seronegative. Latent CMV commonly will reactivate in immunosuppressed people and can result in disease if immunosuppression is severe. Vertical transmission of CMV to an infant occurs by one of the following routes: (1) in utero by transplacental passage of maternal blood-borne virus, (2) at birth by passage through an infected maternal genital tract, or (3) postnatally by ingestion of CMV-positive human milk. Approximately 1% of all live-born infants are infected in utero and excrete CMV at birth. Risk to the fetus is greatest during the first half of gestation. Sequelae are far more common in infants exposed to maternal primary infection, with 10% to 20% diagnosed with mental retardation or sensorineural deafness in childhood and 10% having manifestations evident at birth.

Maternal cervical infection is common. Cervical CMV excretion rates are highest among young mothers in lower socioeconomic groups. Although interstitial pneumonia caused by CMV can develop during the early months of life, most infected infants remain well. Similarly, although disease can occur in seronegative infants fed CMV-infected milk, most infants infected from ingestion of human milk do not develop clinical illness, most likely because of the presence of passively transferred maternal antibody. Of infants who acquire infection from maternal cervical secretions or human milk, preterm infants are at greater risk of CMV illness and sequelae than are full-term infants.

Incubation Period

Unknown for horizontally transmitted CMV infections. Infection usually manifests 3 to 12 weeks after blood transfusions and between 1 and 4 months after tissue transplantation.

Diagnostic Tests

Diagnosis of CMV disease is confounded by ubiquity of the virus, high rate of asymptomatic excretion, frequency of reactivated infections, development of serum IgM CMV-specific antibody in some episodes of reactivation, and concurrent infection with other pathogens.

Virus can be isolated in cell culture from urine, pharynx, peripheral blood leukocytes, human milk, semen, cervical secretions, and other tissues and body fluids. Recovery of virus from tissue provides strong evidence that the disease is caused by CMV infection. A presumptive diagnosis can be made on the basis of a 4-fold antibody titer increase in paired serum specimens or by demonstration of virus excretion. Techniques for detection of viral DNA in tissues and some fluids, especially CSF, by PCR assay is available in reference laboratories.

Various immunofluorescent assays, indirect hemagglutination assays, latex agglutination assays, and enzyme immunoassays are preferred for detecting CMV-specific antibodies.

Amniocentesis has been used to establish the diagnosis of intrauterine infection. Proof of congenital infection requires isolation of CMV from urine, stool, respiratory tract secretions, or CSF obtained within 3 weeks of birth. A strongly positive CMV-specific IgM is suggestive during early infancy, but IgM antibody assays vary in accuracy for identification of primary infection.

Treatment

Ganciclovir is recommended for induction and maintenance treatment of retinitis caused by acquired or recurrent CMV infection in immunocompromised patients, including HIV-infected adults, and for prevention of CMV infection in transplant recipients. Ganciclovir also is used to treat CMV infections of other sites (esophagus, colon, lungs) and for preemptive treatment of immunosuppressed adults with CMV antigenemia or viremia. Limited data in children suggest that safety and efficacy are similar to those in adults. Oral ganciclovir is less effective than intravenous ganciclovir because of lower bioavailability. Although ganciclovir has been used to treat some congenitally infected infants, it is not recommended routinely because of insufficient efficacy data. Cidofovir has not been studied in children and is nephrotoxic.

CMV disease in HIV-infected patients is not cured by currently available antiviral agents. Chronic suppressive therapy should be administered to HIV-infected patients with a history of CMV disease to prevent recurrence. For children with CMV disease, no data are available to guide decisions concerning discontinuing secondary prophylaxis (chronic maintenance therapy) when CD4 T-lymphocyte count has increased in response to highly active antiretroviral therapy.

Image 29.1
Infant with lethal congenital CMV disease, purpuric skin lesions, and striking hepatosplenomegaly.

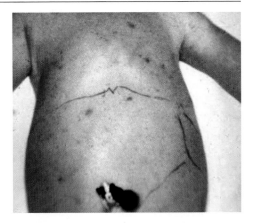

Image 29.2
Characteristic white perivascular infiltrates
in the retina of an infant with congenital
CMV infection.

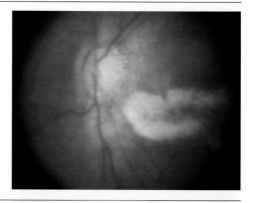

Image 29.3
Axial T2 weighted MR image demonstrates
periventricular germinolytic cysts (arrows).
Also note the periventricular white matter
hyperintensities that are representative of
demyelination and gliosis.

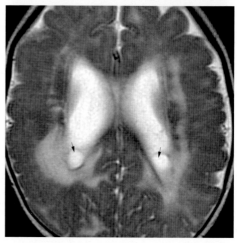

Image 29.4
Active CMV infection of lung in a patient with
AIDS. Histopathology of lung shows cytomegalic
pneumocyte containing characteristic intranu-
clear inclusion.

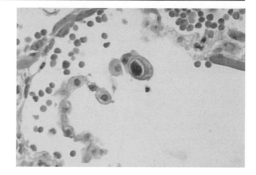

30
Diphtheria

Clinical Manifestations

Respiratory diphtheria usually occurs as membranous nasopharyngitis or obstructive laryngotracheitis. Local infections are associated with a low-grade fever and gradual onset of manifestations over 1 to 2 days. Less commonly, diphtheria presents as cutaneous, vaginal, conjunctival, or otic infection. Cutaneous diphtheria is more common in tropical areas and among the urban homeless. Serious complications of diphtheria include severe neck swelling (bull neck) accompanying upper airway obstruction caused by extensive membrane formation, myocarditis, and peripheral neuropathies.

Etiology

Diphtheria is caused by toxigenic strains of *Corynebacterium diphtheriae* and, rarely, *Corynebacterium ulcerans.* The exotoxin inhibits protein synthesis in all cells, including myocardial, renal, and peripheral nerve cells, resulting in myocarditis, acute tubular necrosis, and delayed peripheral nerve conduction.

Epidemiology

Humans are the sole reservoir of *C diphtheriae.* The organisms are spread by respiratory droplets and by contact with discharges from skin lesions. In untreated people, organisms can be present in discharges from the nose and throat and from eye and skin lesions for 2 to 6 weeks after infection. Rarely, fomites and raw milk or milk products can serve as vehicles of transmission.

Incubation Period

Usually 2 to 7 days.

Diagnostic Tests

Specimens for culture should be obtained from the nose or throat or any mucosal or cutaneous lesion. Material should be obtained from beneath the membrane, or a portion of the membrane itself should be submitted for culture. Tellurite medium is required.

Treatment

Antitoxin. A single intravenous dose of equine antitoxin should be administered on the basis of clinical diagnosis, even before culture results are available. Testing for sensitivity to horse serum before administering antitoxin should be performed. The site and size of the diphtheria membrane, the degree of toxic effects, and the duration of illness are guides for estimating the dose of antitoxin; the presence of soft, diffuse cervical lymphadenitis suggests moderate to severe toxin absorption.

Antimicrobial Therapy. Erythromycin given orally or parenterally, penicillin G given intramuscularly or intravenously for 14 days, or penicillin G procaine given intramuscularly constitutes acceptable therapy. Antimicrobial therapy is required to stop toxin production, eradicate *C diphtheriae,* and prevent transmission but it is not a substitute for antitoxin, which is the primary therapy.

Immunization. Active immunization against diphtheria should be undertaken during convalescence from diphtheria; disease does not necessarily confer immunity.

Cutaneous Diphtheria. Thorough cleansing of the lesion with soap and water with administration of an appropriate antimicrobial agent is recommended.

Carriers. If not immunized, carriers should receive active immunization promptly. Carriers should be given oral erythromycin or penicillin or a single intramuscular dose of benzathine penicillin G. Two follow-up cultures should be obtained after completing antibiotic treatment to ensure detection of relapse, which occurs in as many as 20% of patients treated with erythromycin.

Image 30.1
Pharyngeal diphtheria with membranes covering the tonsils and uvula in a 15-year-old girl.

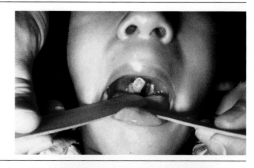

Image 30.2
Bull neck appearance of diphtheritic cervical lymphadenopathy in a 13-year-old boy.

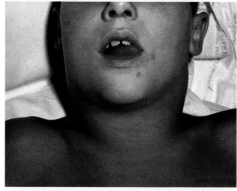

Image 30.3
Nasal membrane of diphtheria in a preschool-aged white male.

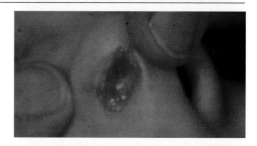

Image 30.4
Diphtheria pneumonia (hemorrhagic) with bronchiolar membranes (hematoxylin-eosin stain).

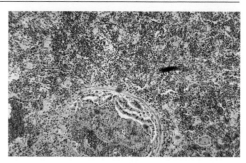

31

Ehrlichia and *Anaplasma* Infections
(Human Ehrlichioses)

Clinical Manifestations

Human monocytotrophic ehrlichiosis (HME) and human granulocytotrophic anaplasmosis (HGA) are acute, systemic, febrile illnesses that are similar clinically to Rocky Mountain spotted fever but differ in that infections often demonstrate (1) leukopenia, absolute lymphopenia, and neutropenia (HME); (2) neutropenia (HGA); (3) anemia; (4) hepatitis; (5) lack of vasculitis; and (6) rash less commonly. Headache, chills or rigors, malaise, myalgia, arthralgia, nausea, vomiting, anorexia, and acute weight loss can accompany the febrile illness. Rash, when present, is variable in appearance and location, typically develops approximately 1 week after onset of illness, and occurs only in approximately 60% of children and 25% of adults with HME and less than 10% of people with HGA. Diarrhea, abdominal pain, cough, or change in mental status occurs less frequently. More severe manifestations include pulmonary infiltrates, bone marrow hypoplasia, respiratory failure, encephalopathy, meningitis, disseminated intravascular coagulation, spontaneous hemorrhage, and renal failure. Anemia, hyponatremia, thrombocytopenia, increased serum hepatic transaminase concentrations, and CSF abnormalities are common. Symptoms typically last 1 to 2 weeks, and recovery generally occurs without sequelae.

Etiology

Ehrlichia and *Anaplasma* species are gram-negative cocci. In the United States, human ehrlichioses are caused by at least 3 distinct species of obligate intracellular bacteria. HME results from infection with *Ehrlichia chaffeensis*. HGA is caused by *Anaplasma phagocytophilum*. *Ehrlichia ewingii* also causes ehrlichiosis.

Epidemiology

Ehrlichial infections are tick-borne. Various mammalian reservoirs for the agents of human ehrlichioses have been identified, including white-tailed deer, white-footed mice, and *Neotoma* woodrats. Compared with patients with Rocky Mountain spotted fever, reported cases of symptomatic ehrlichioses characteristically are in individuals older than 40 years. Most human infections occur between April and September, with peak occurrence from May through July. Coinfections of anaplasmosis with other tick-borne diseases, including babesiosis and Lyme disease, can occur.

Incubation Period

5 to 10 days after a tick bite.

Diagnostic Tests

A confirmed case of human ehrlichioses or anaplasmosis is defined as isolation of *Ehrlichia* or *Anaplasma* organisms from blood or CSF, a 4-fold or greater change in antibody titer by indirect immunofluorescent antibody (IFA) assay between acute and convalescent serum specimens (ideally collected 2–3 weeks apart), PCR assay amplification of specific DNA from a clinical specimen, or detection of intraleukocytoplasmic microcolonies of bacteria (morulae) in conjunction with a single IFA titer of 64 or higher. A probable case is defined as a single IFA titer of 64 or higher or the presence of morulae within infected leukocytes. These tests are available in reference laboratories, in some commercial laboratories and state health departments, and at the CDC.

Treatment

Doxycycline is the drug of choice for treatment of human ehrlichioses and anaplasmosis and should be initiated on presumptive diagnosis. Failure to respond to doxycycline within the first 3 days suggests infection with an agent other than *Ehrlichia* or *Anaplasma* species. Unequivocal evidence of clinical improvement generally is evident after 1 week of therapy.

Table 31.1
Human Ehrlichioses and Anaplasmosis in the United States

Disease	Causal Agent	Major Target Cell	Tick Vector	Geographic Distribution
Human monocytotrophic ehrlichiosis	*Ehrlichia chaffeensis*	Macrophages	Lone star tick *(Amblyomma americanum)*, American dog tick *(Dermacentor variabilis)*, Western black-legged tick *(Ixodes pacificus)*	Predominately southeastern, south central, and midwestern states
Human granulocytotrophic anaplasmosis	*Anaplasma phagocytophilum*	Granulocytes	Black-legged or deer tick *(Ixodes scapularis)* or western black-legged tick *(I pacificus)*	Northeastern and north central states and northern California
Ehrlichia ewingii ehrlichiosis	*E ewingii*	Granulocytes	Lone star tick *(A americanum)*, American dog tick *(D variabilis)*	Southeastern, south central, and midwestern states

Figure 31.1
Reported Human Granulocytic Ehrlichiosis Cases by State, 2003

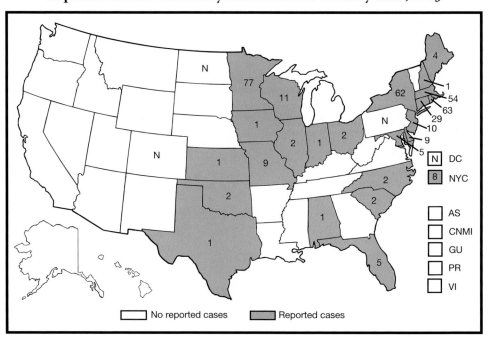

Human ehrlichiosis is an emerging tick-borne disease that became nationally notifiable in 1999 (in certain states, ehrlichiosis is not a notifiable disease). Identification and reporting of human ehrlichioses are incomplete, and numbers of cases reported here are not indicative of the overall distribution or regional prevalence of disease.

Courtesy of the Centers for Disease Control and Prevention.

Figure 31.2
Reported Human Monocytic Ehrlichiosis Cases by State, 2003

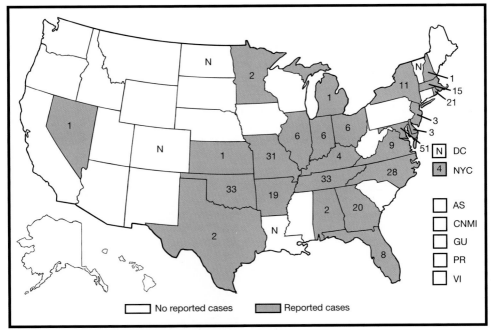

No reported cases   Reported cases

Human ehrlichiosis is an emerging tick-borne disease that became nationally notifiable in 1999 (in certain states, ehrlichiosis is not a notifiable disease). Identification and reporting of human ehrlichioses are incomplete, and numbers of cases reported here are not indicative of the overall distribution or regional prevalence of disease.

Courtesy of the Centers for Disease Control and Prevention.

Image 31.1
Etiologic agents of ehrlichioses. Photomicro-graphs of (1) human white blood cells infected with the agent of human granulocytic ehrlichiosis (sometimes referred to as *Ehrlichia phagocytophila*) and (2) the agent of human monocytic ehrlichiosis *(Ehrlichia chaffeensis)*.

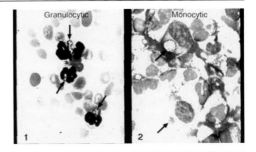

Image 31.2
The intracytoplasmic inclusion, or morula, of human monocytic ehrlichiosis in a cyto-centrifuge preparation of CSF from a patient with CNS involvement.

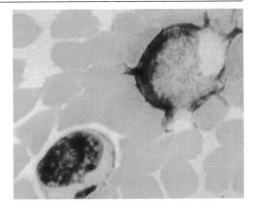

Image 31.3

The characteristic rash of human monocytic ehrlichiosis. The differential diagnosis of this rash includes Rocky Mountain spotted fever, meningococcemia, and Stevens-Johnson syndrome. Other tick-borne diseases such as Lyme disease, babesiosis, Colorado tick fever, relapsing fever, and tularemia may need to be considered.

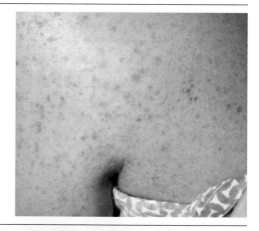

Image 31.4

Human monocytic ehrlichiosis (HME) in a semi-comatose 16-year-old girl with leukopenia, lymphopenia, thrombocytopenia, and elevated transaminase levels. The PCR and serologic test results were positive for HME.

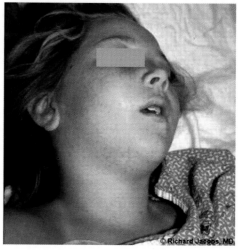

32

Enterovirus (Nonpolio-virus) Infections

(Group A and B Coxsackieviruses, Echoviruses, and Numbered Enteroviruses)

Clinical Manifestations

The most common manifestation of nonpolio enterovirus infection is nonspecific febrile illness, which, in young infants, can lead to evaluation for bacterial sepsis. Neonates without maternal antibodies who acquire infection are at risk of disseminated disease with a high mortality rate. Manifestations in children include the following: (1) respiratory: common cold, pharyngitis, herpangina, stomatitis, pneumonia, and pleurodynia; (2) skin: exanthem; (3) neurologic: aseptic meningitis, encephalitis, and paralysis; (4) gastrointestinal: vomiting, diarrhea, abdominal pain, and hepatitis; (5) eye: acute hemorrhagic conjunctivitis; and (6) heart: myopericarditis.

Patients with humoral immune deficiencies can have persistent CNS infections or a dermatomyositis-like syndrome lasting for several months or more.

Etiology

The nonpolio enteroviruses are RNA viruses, which include 24 group A coxsackieviruses, 6 group B coxsackieviruses, 34 echoviruses, and 5 enteroviruses.

Epidemiology

Enterovirus infections are common and are spread by fecal-oral and respiratory routes, fomites, and from mother to infant in the peripartum period. In temperate climates, enteroviral infections are most common during summer and early fall, but seasonal patterns are less evident in the tropics. Fecal viral shedding can continue for several weeks after onset of infection, but respiratory tract shedding usually is limited to a week or less. Viral shedding can occur without signs of clinical illness.

Incubation Period

3 to 6 days, except for acute hemorrhagic conjunctivitis, in which the incubation period is 24 to 72 hours.

Diagnostic Tests

Isolation of enteroviruses in cell culture is the standard diagnostic method. In general, stool, rectal swab, and throat specimens produce the highest yield, but enteroviruses also may be recovered from urine and blood during the acute illness and from CSF when meningitis is present. Note that many group A coxsackieviruses grow poorly or not at all in vitro. PCR assay for detection of enterovirus RNA is available at many reference and commercial laboratories for CSF specimens. PCR assay is more rapid and more sensitive than cell culture and can detect all enteroviruses, including enteroviruses that are difficult to culture. Commercially available serologic assays are standardized poorly and lack specificity.

Treatment

No specific therapy is available. IGIV may be beneficial for chronic enteroviral meningoencephalitis in immunodeficient patients. IGIV also has been used in life-threatening neonatal infections and cases of suspected viral myocarditis, although there is little evidence of efficacy for these uses.

Image 32.1
Enterovirus infection (hand-foot-and-mouth disease caused by coxsackievirus A16) affecting the hands.

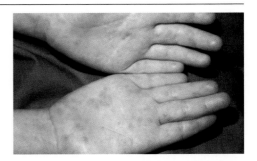

Image 32.2
Enterovirus infection (hand-foot-and-mouth disease) affecting the feet.

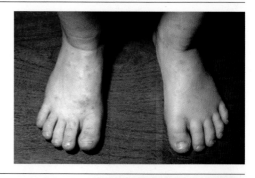

Image 32.3
Enterovirus infection (hand-foot-and-mouth disease) affecting the anterior bucosal mucosa. These lesions generally are less painful than herpes simplex lesions.

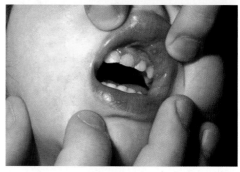

Image 32.4
Newborn with generalized enteroviral exanthem.

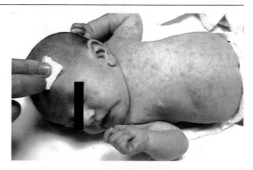

Image 32.5
Herpangina (coxsackievirus) lesions on the posterior palate of a young adult male. Coxsackievirus lesions usually are found in the posterior aspect of the oropharynx and may progress rapidly to painful ulceration.

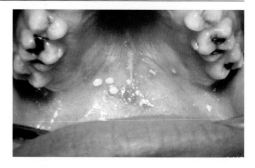

33

Epstein-Barr Virus Infections

(Infectious Mononucleosis)

Clinical Manifestations

Infectious mononucleosis manifests typically as fever, exudative pharyngitis, lymphadenopathy, hepatosplenomegaly, and atypical lymphocytosis. The spectrum of infection is wide, ranging from asymptomatic to fatal disease. Infections commonly are unrecognized in infants and young children. Rash can occur and is more common in patients treated with penicillins. CNS complications include aseptic meningitis, encephalitis, myelitis, optic neuritis, cranial nerve palsies, transverse myelitis, and Guillain-Barré syndrome. Hematologic complications include splenic rupture, thrombocytopenia, agranulocytosis, hemolytic anemia, and hemophagocytic syndrome. Pneumonia, orchitis, and myocarditis are observed infrequently. Fatal disseminated infection or B- or T-lymphocyte lymphomas can occur in children with no detectable immunologic abnormality as well as in children with congenital or acquired cellular immune deficiencies.

Epstein-Barr virus (EBV) is associated with several other distinct disorders, including X-linked lymphoproliferative syndrome, posttransplantation lymphoproliferative disorders, Burkitt lymphoma, nasopharyngeal carcinoma, and undifferentiated B- or T-lymphocyte lymphomas of the CNS.

Chronic fatigue syndrome is not related specifically to EBV infection; however, a postinfectious fatigue state follows approximately 10% of cases of classic infectious mononucleosis and other infectious diseases.

Etiology

EBV is a gammaherpesvirus of the *Lymphocryptovirus* genus and is the most common cause of infectious mononucleosis.

Epidemiology

Humans are the only source of EBV. Close personal contact usually is required for transmission. The virus is viable in saliva for several hours outside the body, but the role of fomites in transmission is unknown. EBV also is transmitted occasionally by blood transfusion. Infection commonly is contracted early in life, particularly among members of lower socioeconomic groups, in which intrafamilial spread is common. Endemic infectious mononucleosis is common in group settings of adolescents, such as in educational institutions. No seasonal pattern has been documented. Respiratory tract viral excretion can occur for many months after infection, and asymptomatic carriage is common. Intermittent excretion is lifelong. The period of communicability is indeterminate.

Incubation Period

An estimated 30 to 50 days.

Diagnostic Tests

Routine diagnosis depends on serologic testing. Nonspecific tests for heterophil antibody are available most commonly. The heterophil antibody response primarily is IgM, which appears during the first 2 weeks of illness and gradually disappears over a 6-month period. Heterophil antibody tests often are negative in children younger than 4 years with EBV infection; they identify approximately 85% of cases of classic infectious mononucleosis in older children and adults during the second week of illness. An absolute increase in atypical lymphocytes is a characteristic but nonspecific finding. However, the finding of more than 10% atypical lymphocytes together with a positive heterophil antibody test result is considered diagnostic of acute infection.

Multiple specific serologic antibody tests for EBV infection are available. (See Table 33.1.)

Serologic tests for EBV are useful particularly for evaluating patients who have heterophil-negative infectious mononucleosis. Testing for other viral agents, especially CMV and HIV, also may be indicated for some of these patients. Diagnosis of the entire range of EBV-associated illness requires use of molecular and antibody techniques, particularly for patients with immune deficiencies.

Treatment

Contact sports should be avoided until the patient is recovered fully from infectious mononucleosis and the spleen no longer is palpable. Patients suspected to have infectious mononucleosis should not be given ampicillin or amoxicillin, which cause nonallergic morbilliform rashes in a high proportion of patients with mononucleosis. A short course of corticosteroids should be considered only for patients with marked tonsillar inflammation with impending airway obstruction, massive splenomegaly, myocarditis, hemolytic anemia, or hemophagocytic syndrome. Life-threatening hemophagocytic syndrome has been treated with cytotoxic agents and immunomodulators, including cyclosporin and corticosteroids. Decreasing immunosuppressive therapy is beneficial for patients with EBV-induced post-transplant lymphoproliferative disorders, whereas an antiviral drug, such as acyclovir or valacyclovir, sometimes is used in patients with active replicating EBV infection with or without passive antibody therapy provided by IGIV.

Table 33.1
Serum Epstein-Barr Virus (EBV) Antibodies in EBV Infection

Infection	VCA IgG	VCA IgM	EA (D)	EBNA
No previous infection	-	-	-	-
Acute infection	+	+	+/-	-
Recent infection	+	+/-	+/-	+/-
Past infection	+	-	+/-	+

VCA IgG indicates immunoglobulin (Ig) G class antibody to viral capsid antigen; VCA IgM, IgM class antibody to VCA; EA (D), early antigen diffuse staining; and EBNA, EBV nuclear antigen.

Image 33.1
Atypical lymphocyte in a peripheral blood smear of a patient with infectious mononucleosis. This lymphocyte is larger than normal lymphocytes, with a higher ratio of cytoplasm to nucleus. The cytoplasm is vacuolated and basophilic. This can also be present in CMV infections.

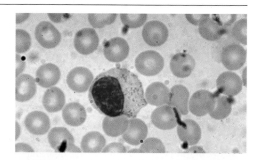

Image 33.2
Epstein-Barr virus disease. Bilateral cervical lymphadenopathy.

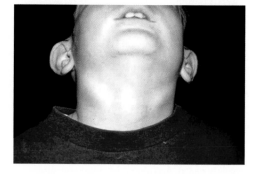

35

Escherichia coli Diarrhea

(Including Hemolytic-Uremic Syndrome)

Clinical Manifestations

At least 5 pathotypes of diarrhea-producing *Escherichia coli* strains have been identified. Clinical features of disease caused by each pathotype are summarized below. (See Table 35.1.)

- Shiga toxin-producing *E coli* (**STEC**) organisms are associated with diarrhea, hemorrhagic colitis, hemolytic-uremic syndrome (HUS), and postdiarrheal thrombotic thrombocytopenic purpura (TTP). STEC O157:H7 is the prototype and the most virulent member of this *E coli* pathotype. Illness caused by STEC often begins as non-bloody diarrhea, but usually progresses to diarrhea with visible or occult blood. Severe abdominal pain is typical; fever occurs in less than one third of cases. Severe infection can result in hemorrhagic colitis.
- Diarrhea caused by enteropathogenic *E coli* (**EPEC**) is watery and often is severe enough to result in dehydration and even death. Chronic EPEC diarrhea characteristically is persistent and leads to growth retardation. Illness occurs almost exclusively in children younger than 2 years and predominantly (but not exclusively) in resource-limited countries, either sporadically or in epidemics.
- Diarrhea caused by enterotoxigenic *E coli* (**ETEC**) is a brief (1–5 days), self-limited illness of moderate severity, typically with watery stools and abdominal cramps.
- Diarrhea caused by enteroinvasive *E coli* (**EIEC**) is similar clinically to infection caused by *Shigella* species. Although dysentery can occur, diarrhea usually is watery without blood or mucus. Patients often are febrile, and stools may contain leukocytes.
- Enteroaggregative *E coli* (**EAEC**) organisms cause watery diarrhea, predominantly in infants and young children in resource-limited countries, but all ages can be affected. EAEC organisms have been associated with prolonged diarrhea (>14 days). Asymptomatic infection can be accompanied by a subclinical inflammatory enteritis, which can cause growth disturbances.

Late Sequelae of STEC Infection. HUS is a serious sequela of STEC enteric infection and seems to occur more frequently in the United States with *E coli* O157:H7 than with other STEC serotypes. HUS is defined by the triad of microangiopathic hemolytic anemia, thrombocytopenia, and acute renal dysfunction. HUS occurs in 8% of children with *E coli* O157:H7 diarrhea and in very few adults. The illness develops during the 2 weeks after onset of diarrhea. Fifty percent of patients require dialysis, and 3% to 5% die. TTP occurs in adults and, in addition to the manifestations of HUS, includes neurologic abnormalities and fever and is part of a disease spectrum often designated as TTP-HUS. STEC disease in children can result in HUS and in adults can manifest as TTP. Children with diarrhea-associated HUS should be observed for diabetes mellitus during their acute illness.

Etiology

Each *E coli* pathotype has specific virulence characteristics, some of which are encoded on pathotype-specific plasmids. Each pathotype has a distinct set of somatic (O) and flagellar (H) antigens. Pathogenic characteristics are as follows:

- Illness caused by *E coli* O157:H7 occurs in a 2-step process. The intestinal phase is characterized by formation of the so-called attaching and effacing (AE) lesion, resulting in secretory diarrhea. This phase is followed by elaboration of Shiga toxin, a potent cytotoxin, one form of which also is elaborated by *Shigella dysenteriae* type 1. The action of Shiga toxin on intestinal cells can result in hemorrhagic colitis, and absorption of the toxin in the circulation can result in systemic complications including HUS and neurologic sequelae.
- Strains of **EPEC** adhere to the small bowel mucosa and, like *E coli* O157:H7, produce AE lesions.
- Strains of **ETEC** colonize the small intestine without invading and produce heat-labile enterotoxin, heat-stable enterotoxin, or both.
- **EIEC** organisms invade the colonic mucosa, where they spread laterally and induce a local inflammatory response.

- **EAEC** organisms are defined by their characteristic "stacked brick" adherence pattern in cell culture–based assays. These organisms elaborate one or more enterotoxins and elicit damage to the intestinal mucosa.

Epidemiology

Transmission of most diarrhea-associated *E coli* strains is from food or water contaminated with human or animal feces or from infected symptomatic people or carriers. The only *E coli* pathotype that commonly causes diarrhea in children living in the United States is STEC, especially *E coli* O157:H7, which is shed in feces of cattle and, to a lesser extent, of sheep, deer, and other ruminants. STEC can be transmitted by undercooked ground beef, contaminated water or produce, unpasteurized milk, and a wide variety of vehicles contaminated with bovine feces. Contact with animals and their environment and person-to-person or fomite spread are other modes of transmission. Infections caused by E *coli* O157:H7 are detected sporadically or during outbreaks. Outbreaks have been linked to ground beef, petting zoos, contaminated apple cider, raw fruits and vegetables, salami, yogurt, drinking water, and ingestion of water in recreational areas. The infectious dose is low (approximately 100 organisms), and person-to-person transmission is common during outbreaks. Less is known about the epidemiology of STEC strains other than O157:H7.

Non-STEC pathotypes are associated with disease predominantly in resource-limited countries.

Incubation Period

Most *E coli* strains, 10 hours to 6 days; *E coli* O157:H7, usually 3 to 4 days (range, 1 to 8 days).

Diagnostic Tests

Diagnosis of infection caused by diarrhea-associated *E coli* usually is difficult because most clinical laboratories cannot differentiate diarrhea-associated *E coli* strains from stool flora *E coli* strains. The exception is *E coli* O157:H7, which can be identified specifically. Clinical laboratories can screen for *E coli* O157:H7 by using MacConkey agar base with sorbitol substituted for lactose. Approximately 90% of human intestinal *E coli* strains rapidly ferment sorbitol, whereas *E coli* O157:H7 strains do not. Sorbitol-negative *E coli* then can be serotyped, using commercially available antisera, to determine whether they are O157:H7. If a case or outbreak attributable to diarrhea-associated *E coli* other than O157:H7 is suspected, *E coli* isolates should be sent to the state health laboratory or another reference laboratory for serotyping and identification of pathotypes.

Strains of STEC should be sought for patients with bloody diarrhea (indicated by history, inspection of stool, or guaiac), HUS, and post-diarrheal TTP as well as for contacts of patients with HUS who have any type of diarrhea. People with presumptive diagnoses of intussusception, inflammatory bowel disease, or ischemic colitis sometimes have disease caused by *E coli* O157:H7. Methods of definitive identification of STEC that are used in reference or research laboratories include DNA probes, PCR assay, enzyme immunoassay, and phenotypic testing of strains or stool specimens for Shiga toxin.

Hemolytic-Uremic Syndrome. For all patients with HUS, stool specimens should be cultured for *E coli* O157:H7 and, if results are negative, for other STEC serotypes. However, the absence of STEC in feces does not preclude the diagnosis of STEC-associated HUS because HUS typically is diagnosed a week or more after onset of diarrhea, when the organism no longer may be detectable. When STEC infection is considered, a stool culture should be obtained as early in the illness as possible.

Treatment

Dehydration and electrolyte abnormalities should be prevented if possible or corrected quickly. Orally administered solutions usually are adequate. Antimotility agents should not be administered to children with inflammatory or bloody diarrhea. Careful follow-up of patients with hemorrhagic colitis (including complete blood cell count with smear, blood urea nitrogen, and creatinine concentrations) is recommended to detect changes suggestive of HUS. If patients have no laboratory evidence of hemolysis, thrombocytopenia, or nephropathy 3 days after resolution of diarrhea, their risk of developing HUS is low.

Antimicrobial Therapy. Although some studies have suggested that children with hemorrhagic colitis caused by STEC have a greater risk of developing HUS if treated with antimicrobial agents when compared with children not treated with antimicrobial agents, a meta-analysis failed to confirm this increased risk or to show a benefit of antimicrobial therapy. However, most experts would not treat children with *E coli* O157:H7 enteritis with an antimicrobial agent because no benefit has been proven. If severe watery ETEC diarrhea is suspected in a traveler to a resource-limited country, therapy can be provided. The optimal therapies for ETEC and EAEC are not established. Trimethoprim-sulfamethoxazole, azithromycin, or ciprofloxacin should be considered if diarrhea is severe. For dysentery caused by EIEC strains, antimicrobial agents, such as trimethoprim-sulfamethoxazole, azithromycin, or ciprofloxacin, can be given orally.

Table 35.1
Classification of *Escherichia coli* Associated With Diarrhea

E coli Pathotype	Epidemiology	Type of Diarrhea	Mechanism of Pathogenesis
Shiga toxin–producing	Hemorrhagic colitis and hemolytic-uremic syndrome in all ages and postdiarrheal thrombotic thrombocytopenic purpura in adults	Bloody or non-bloody	Large bowel adherence and effacement (AE)
Enteropathogenic	Acute and chronic endemic and epidemic diarrhea in infants	Watery	Small bowel AE
Enterotoxigenic	Infantile diarrhea in resource-limited countries and traveler's diarrhea in all ages	Watery	Small bowel AE, heat stable/heat labile enterotoxin production
Enteroinvasive	Diarrhea with fever in all ages	Bloody or non-bloody; dysentery	Adherence, mucosal invasion and inflammation of large bowel
Enteroaggregative	Acute and chronic diarrhea in infants	Watery, occasionally bloody	Small and large bowel adherence, enterotoxin and cytotoxin production

Figure 35.1

Number of Reported Cases of Enterohemorrhagic *Escherichia coli* in the United States and US Territories, 2003

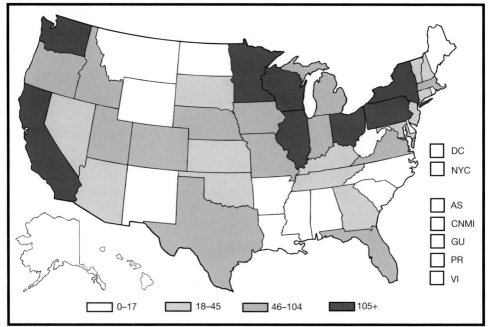

Escherichia coli O157:H7 constitutes the major serotype of enterohemorrhagic *E coli*, although many other *E coli* serotypes can produce Shiga toxin and cause hemorrhagic colitis. *E coli* O157:H 7 has been a nationally notifiable disease since 1994. In 2001 surveillance was expanded to include all serotypes of enterohemorrhagic *E coli*; however, certain laboratories still lack the capacity to isolate and identify *E coli* serotypes other than O157:H7.

Courtesy of the Centers for Disease Control and Prevention.

Figure 35.2

Number of Reported Cases of Postdiarrheal Hemolytic-Uremic Syndrome in the United States and US Territories, 2003

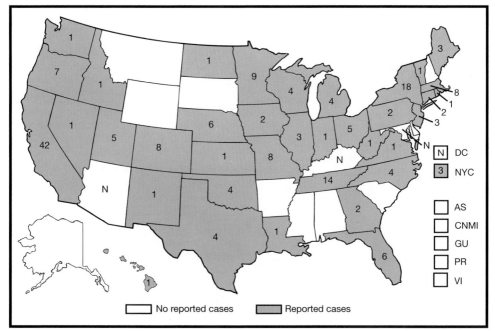

In the United States, most cases of postdiarrheal hemolytic-uremic syndrome are caused by infection with *Escherichia coli* O157:H7. Approximately 50% of cases occur among children younger than 5 years.

Courtesy of the Centers for Disease Control and Prevention.

Image 35.1

Ultrasound of a 6-year-old boy with hemorrhagic colitis from *Escherichia coli* O157:H7 developed hemolytic-uremic syndrome. Note the bowel wall edema indicated by the arrows.

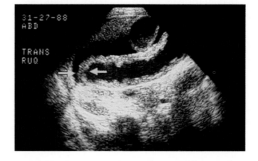

36

Giardia intestinalis Infections

(Giardiasis)

Clinical Manifestations

Symptomatic infection causes a broad spectrum of clinical manifestations. Children can have occasional days of acute watery diarrhea with abdominal pain, or they may experience a protracted, intermittent, often debilitating disease, which is characterized by passage of foul-smelling stools associated with flatulence, abdominal distention, and anorexia. Anorexia combined with malabsorption can lead to significant weight loss, failure to thrive, and anemia. Asymptomatic infection is common.

Etiology

Giardia intestinalis is a flagellate protozoan that exists in trophozoite and cyst forms; the infective form is the cyst. Infection is limited to the small intestine and biliary tract.

Epidemiology

Giardiasis has a worldwide distribution. Humans are the principal reservoir of infection, but *Giardia* organisms can infect dogs, cats, beavers, and other animals. These animals can contaminate water with feces containing cysts that are infectious for humans. People become infected directly (by hand-to-mouth transfer of cysts from feces of an infected person) or indirectly (by ingestion of fecally contaminated water or food). Most community-wide epidemics have resulted from a contaminated water supply. Epidemics resulting from person-to-person transmission occur in child care centers and in institutions for people with developmental disabilities. Humoral immunodeficiencies predispose to chronic symptomatic *G intestinalis* infections. Surveys conducted in the United States have demonstrated prevalence rates of *Giardia* organisms in stool specimens that range from 1% to 20%, depending on geographic location and age. Duration of cyst excretion is variable but can be months.

Incubation Period

1 to 4 weeks.

Diagnostic Tests

Identification of trophozoites or cysts in direct smear examination or immunofluorescent antibody testing of stool specimens or duodenal fluid is diagnostic. Single direct smear examination of stool has a sensitivity of 75% to 95%. Sensitivity is higher for diarrheal stool specimens. Sensitivity is increased by examining 3 or more specimens collected every other day. To enhance detection, microscopic examination of stool specimens or duodenal fluid should be performed soon after collection, or stool should be placed in fixative, concentrated, and examined by wet mount using a permanent stain such as trichrome. Commercially available stool collection kits are convenient for preserving stool specimens collected at home. Sensitive and specific enzyme immunoassay kits are available commercially. When giardiasis is suspected clinically but the organism is not found on repeated stool examination, examination of duodenal contents obtained by direct aspiration or by using a commercially available string test (Enterotest) may be diagnostic.

Treatment

Dehydration and electrolyte abnormalities should be corrected. Metronidazole, tinidazole, or nitazoxanide is the drug of choice. Tinidazole, a nitroimidazole, has a similar cure rate. Nitazoxanide oral suspension is as effective as metronidazole and has the advantage of treating multiple other intestinal parasites. Furazolidone and quinacrine are alternatives. Albendazole and mebendazole have been shown to be as effective as metronidazole for treating giardiasis in children and have fewer adverse effects.

If therapy fails, a course can be repeated with the same drug. Relapse is common in immunocompromised patients who may require prolonged treatment.

Treatment of asymptomatic carriers generally is not recommended. Possible exceptions to prevent transmission are carriers in households of patients with hypogammaglobulinemia or cystic fibrosis and pregnant women with toddlers.

Figure 36.1
Reported Giardiasis Cases by State, 2003[1]

DC	
NYC	
AS	
CNMI	
GU	
PR	
VI	

0–3.71   3.72–8.11   8.12–11.31   11.32+

[1] Per 100,000 population.

Surveillance data from 2003 indicate that infection with *Giardia intestinalis* is geographically widespread in the United States. The diagnosis or transmission of giardiasis might be higher in the northern states; however, state-by-state differences should be interpreted with caution because different state surveillance systems have varying capabilities to detect cases. Reported illness onset dates exhibited a seasonal increase from early summer through early fall.

Courtesy of the Centers for Disease Control and Prevention.

Image 36.1

Photomicrograph of a *Giardia lamblia* cyst using a trichrome stain.

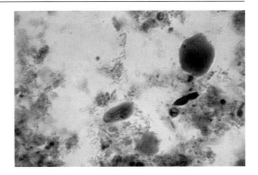

37

Gonococcal Infections

Clinical Manifestations

Gonococcal infections in children occur in 3 distinct age groups. Infection in the **newborn** usually involves the eyes. Other types of infections include scalp abscess (associated with fetal monitoring), vaginitis, and disseminated disease with bacteremia, arthritis, or meningitis. In children beyond the newborn period, including **prepubertal children,** gonococcal infection may occur in the genital tract and almost always is sexually transmitted. Vaginitis is the most common manifestation. Gonococcal urethritis in prepubertal males is uncommon. Anorectal and tonsillopharyngeal infection also can occur in prepubertal children.

In **sexually active adolescents,** gonococcal infection of the genital tract in females often is asymptomatic; common clinical syndromes are vaginitis, urethritis, endocervicitis, and salpingitis. In males, infection often is symptomatic, and the primary site is the urethra. Infection of the rectum and pharynx can occur alone or with genitourinary tract infection in either gender. Rectal and pharyngeal infections often are asymptomatic. Extension from primary genital mucosal sites can lead to epididymitis in males and bartholinitis, pelvic inflammatory disease (PID), and perihepatitis (Fitz-Hugh-Curtis syndrome) in females. Even asymptomatic infection in females can progress to PID, with tubal scarring that can result in ectopic pregnancy or infertility. Infection involving other mucous membranes can produce conjunctivitis, pharyngitis, or proctitis. Hematogenous spread can involve skin and joints (arthritis-dermatitis syndrome) and occurs in up to 3% of untreated people with mucosal gonorrhea. Bacteremia causes a maculopapular rash with necrosis, tenosynovitis, and migratory arthritis. Arthritis may be reactive (sterile) or septic in nature. Meningitis and endocarditis occur rarely.

Etiology

Neisseria gonorrhoeae is a gram-negative oxidase-positive diplococcus.

Epidemiology

Transmission of *N gonorrhoeae* results from intimate contact, such as sexual acts, parturition and, rarely, household exposure in prepubertal children. Sexual abuse should be considered strongly when genital, rectal, or pharyngeal colonization or infection are diagnosed in prepubertal children beyond the newborn period. Reported incidence of infection is highest in females 15 to 19 years of age and in males 20 to 24 years of age. Concurrent infection with *Chlamydia trachomatis* is common.

Incubation Period

Usually 2 to 7 days.

Diagnostic Tests

Microscopic examination of Gram-stained smears of exudate from the eyes; vagina of prepubertal girls; male urethra; skin lesions; synovial fluid; and, when clinically warranted, CSF may be useful in the initial evaluation. Identification of gram-negative intracellular diplococci in these smears can be helpful, particularly if the organism is not recovered in culture.

N gonorrhoeae can be cultured from normally sterile sites, such as blood, CSF, or synovial fluid, using nonselective chocolate agar with incubation in 5% to 10% CO_2. Selective media that inhibit normal flora and nonpathogenic *Neisseria* organisms are used for culture from nonsterile sites, such as the cervix, vagina, rectum, urethra, and pharynx. Specimens for *N gonorrhoeae* culture from mucosal sites should be inoculated immediately onto the appropriate agar because *N gonorrhoeae* is extremely sensitive to drying and temperature changes.

N gonorrhoeae can be confused with other *Neisseria* species that colonize the genitourinary tract or pharynx. At least 2 confirmatory bacteriologic tests involving different principles (eg, biochemical, enzyme substrate, or serologic) should be performed.

Nucleic acid amplification (NAA) tests are highly sensitive and specific when used on urethral (males), endocervical swab, and urine specimens. These tests include PCR, transcription-mediated amplification (TMA), and strand-displacement assays. Only the TMA assay is approved by the FDA for testing vaginal swabs from postmenarcheal females. Other *Neisseria* species and gram-negative cocci can be present in the female genital tract and result in a false-positive NAA test result. Use of urine specimens increases feasibility of initial testing and follow-up of hard-to-access populations, such as adolescents. These techniques also permit dual testing of urine for *C trachomatis* and *N gonorrhoeae.* These NAA tests are not recommended for rectal or pharyngeal swabs. A limited number of nonculture tests are approved by the FDA for conjunctival specimens.

Sexual Abuse. In all prepubertal children beyond the newborn period and in non–sexually active adolescents who have gonococcal infection, sexual abuse must be considered to have occurred unless proven otherwise. Genital, rectal, and pharyngeal secretion cultures should be performed for all patients before antimicrobial treatment is given.

Treatment

Because of the prevalence of penicillin- and tetracycline-resistant *N gonorrhoeae,* an extended-spectrum cephalosporin (eg, ceftriaxone, cefixime, or cefpodoxime) is recommended as initial therapy for children, and either an extended-spectrum cephalosporin or fluoroquinolone (ciprofloxacin, levofloxacin, ofloxacin) is recommended for adults.

All patients with presumed or proven gonorrhea should be evaluated for concurrent syphilis, hepatitis B virus, HIV, and *C trachomatis* infections. All patients beyond the neonatal period with gonorrhea should be treated presumptively for *C trachomatis* infection.

Specific recommendations for management and antimicrobial therapy are as follows:

Neonatal Disease. Infants with clinical evidence of ophthalmia neonatorum, scalp abscess, or disseminated infections should be hospitalized. Cultures of blood, eye discharge, or other sites of infection, such as CSF, should be performed for infants to confirm the diagnosis and determine antimicrobial susceptibility. Tests for concomitant infection with *C trachomatis,* syphilis, and HIV should be performed. Results of the maternal test for hepatitis B surface antigen should be confirmed. The mother and her partner(s) also need appropriate examination and management for *N gonorrhoeae.*

Nondisseminated Infections. Recommended antimicrobial therapy, including that for ophthalmia neonatorum, is ceftriaxone given once. Infants with gonococcal ophthalmia should receive eye irrigations with saline solution immediately and at frequent intervals until the discharge is eliminated. Topical antimicrobial treatment is unnecessary. Infants with gonococcal ophthalmia should be hospitalized and evaluated for disseminated infection (sepsis, arthritis, meningitis).

Disseminated Infections. Recommended therapy for arthritis and septicemia is ceftriaxone or cefotaxime. Cefotaxime is recommended for infants with hyperbilirubinemia.

Special Problems in Treatment of Children (Beyond the Neonatal Period) and Adolescents. Patients with uncomplicated endocervical infection, urethritis, or proctitis who are allergic to cephalosporins should be treated with spectinomycin if they are not old enough to receive a fluoroquinolone (≥18 years of age) or if infection was acquired in an area with high prevalence of quinolone-resistant *N gonorrhoeae.* Doxycycline or azithromycin should be used for the concurrent treatment of presumptive *C trachomatis* infection depending on the age of the patient.

Patients with uncomplicated pharyngeal gonococcal infection should be treated with ceftriaxone in a single intramuscular dose. People older than 17 years who are not pregnant and who cannot tolerate ceftriaxone should be treated with ciprofloxacin if infection was not acquired in an area with high prevalence of quinolone-resistant *N gonorrhoeae.* Spectinomycin is approximately 50% effective for treatment of pharyngeal gonorrhea, so it should be used only in people who are unable to take ceftriaxone or ciprofloxacin, and a pharyngeal culture should be obtained 3 to 5 days after treatment to verify eradication.

A single dose of ceftriaxone or azithromycin is not effective treatment for concurrent infection with syphilis.

Acute PID. *N gonorrhoeae* and *C trachomatis* are implicated in many cases of PID; all cases have a polymicrobial etiology. No reliable clinical criteria distinguish gonococcal from nongonococcal-associated PID. Hence, broad-spectrum treatment regimens are recommended.

Acute Epididymitis. Sexually transmitted organisms, such as *N gonorrhoeae* or *C trachomatis,* can cause acute epididymitis in sexually active adolescents and young adults but rarely cause acute epididymitis in prepubertal children. The recommended regimen for sexually transmitted epididymitis is ceftriaxone plus erythromycin, or doxycycline, depending on the patient's age.

Image 37.1
A Gram-stain of a urethral exudate showing typical intracellular gram-negative diplococci and pleomorphic extracellular gram-negative *Neisseria gonorrhoeae* organisms. Of the *Neisseria* and related species, only *N gonor-rhoeae* is considered always to be pathogenic. *N gonorrhoeae* is not considered to be normal flora under any circumstances, and some strains can infect the mucosal surfaces of urogenital sites (ie, cervix, urethra, rectum) and the oro-pharynx and nasopharynx (ie, throat) causing symptomatic or asymptomatic infections.

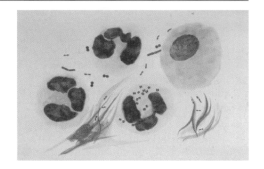

Image 37.2
A newborn with gonococcal ophthalmia neo-natorum caused by a maternally transmitted gonococcal infection. Unless preventive mea-sures are taken, it is estimated that gonococcal ophthalmia neonatorum will develop in 28% of infants born to women with gonorrhea. It affects the corneal epithelium, causing microbial kerati-tis, ulceration, and perforation.

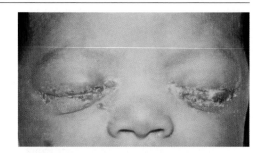

Image 37.3
This patient presented with a cutaneous gono-coccal lesion due to a disseminated *Neisseria gonorrhoeae* bacteremia. Though an STI, if a gonorrhea infection is allowed to go untreated, *N gonorrhoeae* can become disseminated throughout the body, forming lesions in extra-genital locations.

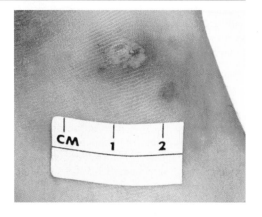

Image 37.4

Intracellular gram-negative diplococci *(Neisseria gonorrhoeae)* isolated on culture of a skin lesion that resembles a fire ant bite.

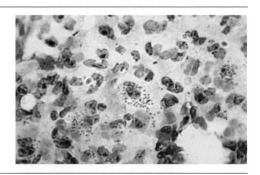

Image 37.5

This male presented with purulent penile discharge due to gonorrhea with an overlying penile pyodermal lesion.

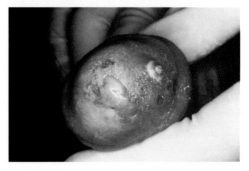

38

Granuloma Inguinale
(Donovanosis)

Clinical Manifestations

Initial lesions are single or multiple subcutaneous nodules that progress to form painless, highly vascular, friable, granulomatous ulcers without regional adenopathy. Lesions usually involve the genitalia, but anal infections occur in 5% to 10% of patients; lesions at distant sites (eg, face, mouth, or liver) are rare. Subcutaneous extension into the inguinal area results in induration that can mimic inguinal adenopathy (ie, "pseudobubo"). Fibrosis manifests as sinus tracts, adhesions, and lymphedema, resulting in extreme genital deformity. Urethral obstruction can occur.

Etiology

The disease is caused by *Calymmatobacterium granulomatis,* an intracellular gram-negative bacillus.

Epidemiology

Indigenous granuloma inguinale occurs only rarely in the United States and most developed countries. Donovanosis is endemic in Papua, New Guinea, and parts of India, southern Africa, central Australia and, to a much lesser extent, the Caribbean and parts of South America, most notably Brazil. The highest incidence of disease occurs in tropical and subtropical environments. The incidence of infection seems to correlate strongly with sustained high temperatures and high relative humidity. Infection usually is acquired by sexual intercourse, most commonly with a person with active infection, but possibly also from a person with asymptomatic rectal infec-

tion. Young children can acquire infection by contact with infected secretions. The period of communicability extends throughout the duration of active lesions or rectal colonization.

Incubation Period

8 to 80 days.

Diagnostic Tests

The causative organism is difficult to culture, and diagnosis requires microscopic demonstration of dark staining intracytoplasmic Donovan bodies on Wright or Giemsa staining of a crush preparation from subsurface scrapings of a lesion or tissue. The microorganism also can be detected by histologic examination of biopsy specimens. Lesions should be cultured for *Haemophilus ducreyi* to exclude chancroid (pseudogranuloma inguinale). Granuloma inguinale often is misdiagnosed as carcinoma, which can be excluded by histologic examination of tissue or by response of the lesion to antimicrobial agents.

Treatment

Ciprofloxacin, which generally is not recommended for use in pregnant or lactating women or children younger than 18 years, is the recommended treatment. Gentamicin may be added if no improvement is evident in several days. Doxycycline (which ordinarily should not be given to children younger than 8 years) and trimethoprim-sulfamethoxazole have been reported to be effective. Erythromycin base or azithromycin also are alternative therapies and are appropriate for pregnant patients. Antimicrobial therapy is continued until the lesions have resolved. Complicated or long-standing infection may require surgical intervention.

Image 38.1
Giemsa-stained Donovan bodies of granuloma inguinale.

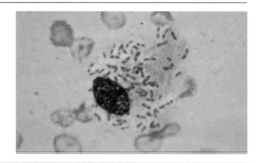

Image 38.2
Penile lesions due to gram-negative *Calymmato-bacterium granulomatis* bacteria. *C granulomatis* bacteria cause what is known as donovanosis, or granuloma inguinale, an STI that is a slowly progressive, ulcerative condition of the skin and lymphatics of the genital and perianal area. A definitive diagnosis is achieved when a tissue smear tests positive for the presence of Donovan bodies.

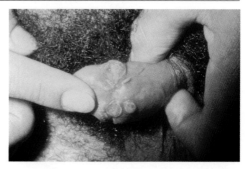

Image 38.3
This 19-year-old white female presented with a perianal granuloma inguinale lesion of about 8 months' duration. A genital ulcerative disease caused by the intracellular gram-negative bacterium *Calymmatobacterium granulomatis,* granulomatis inguinale, also known as donovanosis, only occurs rarely in the United States.

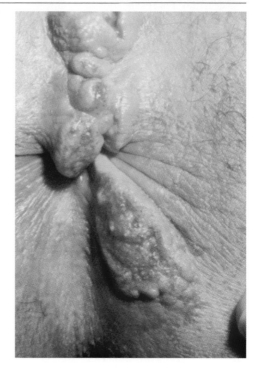

39

Haemophilus influenzae Infections

Clinical Manifestations

Haemophilus influenzae type b (Hib) causes pneumonia, occult febrile bacteremia, meningitis, epiglottitis, septic arthritis, cellulitis, otitis media, purulent pericarditis, and other less common infections, such as endocarditis, endophthalmitis, osteomyelitis, and peritonitis. Non–type b encapsulated strains occasionally cause invasive disease similar to type b infections. Nontypeable strains more commonly cause infections of the respiratory tract (eg, conjunctivitis, otitis media, sinusitis, pneumonia) and, less often, bacteremia, meningitis, chorioamnionitis, and neonatal septicemia.

Etiology

H influenzae is a pleomorphic, gram-negative coccobacillus. Encapsulated strains express 1 of 6 antigenically distinct capsular polysaccharides (a–f); nonencapsulated strains fail to react with typing antisera against capsular serotypes a through f and are designated nontypeable.

Epidemiology

The natural habitat of the organism is the upper respiratory tract of humans. The mode of transmission is person to person by inhalation of respiratory droplets or by direct contact with respiratory tract secretions. In neonates, infection with nonencapsulated strains is acquired intrapartum by aspiration of amniotic fluid or by contact with genital tract secretions containing the organism. Asymptomatic colonization by non-encapsulated *H influenzae* is common, which are recovered from the nasopharynx of 40% to 80% of children. Nasopharyngeal colonization by type b organisms is rare, occurring in 2% to 5% of children in the prevaccine era and even fewer children after widespread immunization. Colonization by strains expressing non–type b capsules also is uncommon.

Before introduction of effective Hib conjugate vaccines, Hib was the most common cause of bacterial meningitis in children in the United States. The peak incidence of meningitis and most other invasive Hib infections occurred between 6 and 18 months of age. In contrast, the peak age for epiglottitis was 2 to 4 years of age.

Since 1988, when Hib conjugate vaccines were introduced, the incidence of invasive Hib disease in infants and young children has decreased by 99% to fewer than 1 case per 100 000 children younger than 5 years. The incidence of invasive infections caused by all other encapsulated and nontypeable strains combined also is low. In the United States, invasive Hib disease occurs primarily in underimmunized children and among infants too young to have completed the primary immunization series. Hib remains an important pathogen in economically developing countries where routine vaccines are not available to most of the population.

Incubation Period

Unknown.

Diagnostic Tests

CSF, blood, synovial fluid, pleural fluid, and middle ear aspirates should be cultured on a medium such as chocolate agar, a medium enriched with factors X and V. Gram stain of an infected body fluid specimen can facilitate presumptive diagnosis. Latex particle agglutination for detection of type b capsular antigen in CSF can be helpful, but a negative test result does not exclude the diagnosis, and false-positive results have been recorded.

Treatment

Initial therapy for children with meningitis possibly caused by Hib is cefotaxime or ceftriaxone. Meropenem or the combination of ampicillin and chloramphenicol is an alternative empiric regimen. For antimicrobial treatment of epiglottitis, arthritis, and other invasive *H influenzae* infections, recommendations are similar. Epiglottitis is a medical emergency. An airway must be established promptly with an endotracheal tube or by tracheostomy. Infected synovial, pleural, or pericardial fluid should be removed.

Dexamethasone may be beneficial for treatment of infants and children with Hib meningitis to diminish the risk of neurologic sequelae, including hearing loss, if given before or concurrently with the first dose of an antimicrobial agent(s). There probably is no benefit if dexamethasone is given more than 1 hour after an antimicrobial agent(s).

Oral amoxicillin is given for empiric treatment of acute otitis media in children younger than 2 years or in children 2 years or older with severe disease. Alternative treatments for refractory or recurrent infections include amoxicillin-clavulanate; an oral cephalosporin, such as cefuroxime or cefpodoxime; or a newer macrolide.

Image 39.1
An infant girl with periorbital cellulitis and meningitis caused by *Haemophilus influenzae* type b.

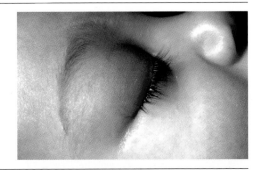

Image 39.2
A classic presentation of *Haemophilus influenzae* type b (Hib) facial cellulitis in a 10-month-old white female. This once common infection has been nearly eliminated among children who have been immunized with the Hib vaccine.

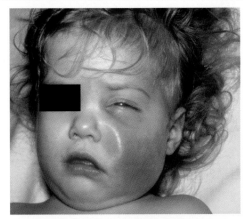

Image 39.3
Acute *Haemophilus influenzae* type b epiglottitis with striking erythema and swelling of the epiglottis.

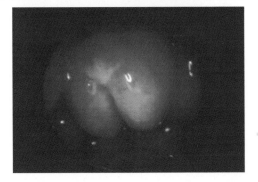

Image 39.4
Haemophilus influenzae type b pneumonia
(proven by blood culture).

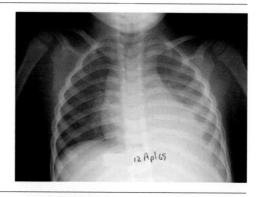

Image 39.5
Haemophilus influenzae type b pneumonia, bilateral, in a patient with acute epiglottitis (proven by blood culture).

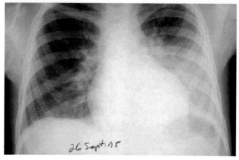

Image 39.6
A 12-year-old male with periorbital cellulitis and ethmoid sinusitis caused by *Haemophilus influenzae*.

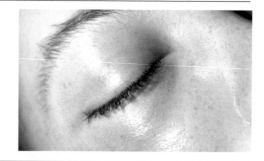

Image 39.7
MRI showing localized cerebritis and vasculitis in a patient with *Haemophilus influenzae* type b meningitis.

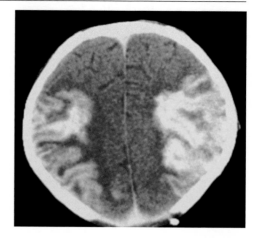

40

Hantavirus Pulmonary Syndrome

Clinical Manifestations

Hantaviruses in humans cause 2 syndromes: hantavirus pulmonary syndrome (HPS), a noncardiogenic pulmonary edema, and hemorrhagic fever with renal syndrome. The prodromal illness of HPS is 3 to 7 days and is characterized by fever; chills; headache; myalgias of the shoulders, lower back, and thighs; nausea; vomiting; diarrhea; dizziness; and sometimes cough. Respiratory tract symptoms or signs usually do not occur for the first 3 to 7 days until pulmonary edema and severe hypoxemia appear abruptly after the onset of cough and dyspnea, and the disease progresses over a few hours. In severe cases, persistent hypotension caused by myocardial dysfunction is present.

The extensive bilateral interstitial and alveolar pulmonary edema and pleural effusions are the result of a diffuse pulmonary capillary leak and seem to be caused by immune responses to hantavirus in endothelial cells of the microvasculature. Intubation and assisted ventilation usually are required for 2 to 4 days, with resolution heralded by the onset of diuresis and rapid clinical improvement. The severe myocardial depression is different from that of septic shock; the cardiac indices and the stroke volume index are low, the pulmonary wedge pressure is normal, and systemic vascular resistance is increased.

The mortality rate for patients with HPS in recent years has been 30% to 40%. Asymptomatic and mild forms of disease are rare in adults, but limited information suggests they may be more common in children. Serious sequelae are uncommon.

Etiology

Hantaviruses are RNA viruses of the Bunyaviridae family. Within the Hantavirus genus, Sin Nombre virus (SNV) is the major cause of HPS in the 4-corners region of the United States. Bayou virus, Black Creek Canal virus, Monongahela virus, and New York virus are responsible for sporadic cases in Louisiana, Texas, Florida, New York, and other areas of the eastern United States. In recent years, new hantavirus serotypes associated with an HPS syndrome, including Andes virus, Oran virus, Laguna Negra virus, and Choclo virus, have been reported in South America and Panama.

Epidemiology

Rodents, the natural hosts for hantaviruses, acquire a lifelong, asymptomatic, chronic infection with prolonged viruria and virus in saliva, urine, and feces. Humans acquire infection through direct contact with infected rodents, rodent droppings, or nests or inhalation of aerosolized virus particles from rodent urine, droppings, or saliva. Rarely, infection may be acquired from rodent bites or contamination of broken skin with excreta. Person-to-person transmission of hantaviruses has not been demonstrated. Risk activities include handling or trapping rodents; cleaning or entering closed, rodent-infested structures; cleaning feed storage or animal shelter areas; hand plowing; and living in a home with an increased density of mice in or around the home. Exceptionally heavy rainfall and improved rodent food supplies can result in a large increase in the rodent population, thus more frequent contact between humans and infected mice. Most cases occur during spring and summer, and the geographic location is determined by the habitat of the rodent carrier.

Incubation Period

1 to 6 weeks after exposure.

Diagnostic Tests

Characteristic laboratory findings include neutrophilic leukocytosis with immature granulocytes, more than 10% immunoblasts (basophilic cytoplasm, prominent nucleoli, and an increased nuclear-cytoplasmic ratio), thrombocytopenia, and increased hematocrit. In fatal cases, SNV can be identified by immunohistochemical staining of capillary endothelial cells in almost every organ in the body. SNV RNA has been detected uniformly by the reverse transcriptase-PCR assay of peripheral blood mononuclear cells and other clinical specimens up to 10 to 21 days after symptom onset, but the duration of viremia is unknown. Viral RNA is not detected readily in broncho-alveolar lavage fluids.

Hantavirus-specific IgG and IgM antibodies are present at the onset of clinical disease. A rapid diagnostic test can facilitate immediate appropriate supportive therapy and early transfer to a tertiary care facility. Enzyme immunoassay and Western blot are assays that use recombinant antigens and have a high degree of specificity for detection of IgG and IgM antibody. Viral culture is not useful for diagnosis.

Treatment

Patients with suspected HPS should be transferred immediately to a tertiary care facility. Supportive management of pulmonary edema, severe hypoxemia, and hypotension during the first 24 to 48 hours is critical for recovery.

A flow-directed pulmonary catheter for monitoring fluid administration and use of inotropic support, vasopressors, and careful ventilatory control are important. ECMO can provide particularly important short-term support for severe capillary leak syndrome in the lungs. Venoarterial ECMO, which also can provide circulatory support, has shown encouraging early results with rapid and dramatic hemodynamic improvement in patients after only 12 hours and a total duration of only 4 to 5 days.

Ribavirin is active against hantaviruses, including SNV, but is ineffective in treatment of HPS in the cardiopulmonary stage. The small number of patients studied and the rapid progression of disease contribute to an inability to assess the efficacy and safety of ribavirin in HPS.

Image 40.1
The deer mouse *(Peromyscus maniculatus)* is a carrier of Sin Nombre virus, a causative agent of hantavirus pulmonary syndrome.

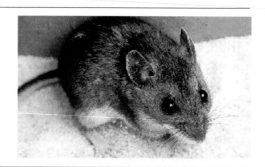

Image 40.2
This photograph depicts the cotton rat, *Sigmodon hispidus,* whose habitat includes the southeastern United States, and Central and South America. Its body is larger than the deer mouse, *Peromyscus maniculatus,* and measures about 5 to 7 inches, which includes the head and body. Its hair is longer and coarser than *P maniculatus,* and is grayish-brown, sometimes grayish-black. The cotton rat prefers overgrown areas with shrubs and tall grasses.

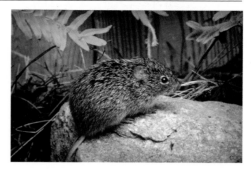

Image 40.3

This micrograph depicts an atypical enlarged lymphocyte found in the blood smear from a patient with hantavirus pulmonary syndrome (HPS). Hematologic findings are important in HPS. The large atypical lymphocyte shown here is an example of one of the laboratory findings, which when combined with a bandemia and dropping platelet count is characteristic of HPS.

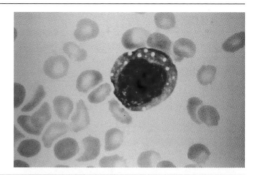

Image 40.4

Hantavirus pulmonary syndrome in a 16-year-old boy with a 36-hour history of fever, myalgia, and shortness of breath. Diffuse interstitial infiltrates with Kerley B lines are shown in addition to diffuse nodular confluent alveolar opacities with some consolidation consistent with adult respiratory distress syndrome. Hantavirus serology confirmed the diagnosis. He recovered with supportive care, including inhaled nitric oxide.

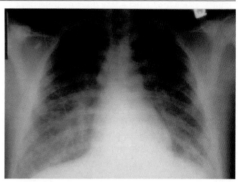

Image 40.5

Histopathologic features of lung in hantavirus pulmonary syndrome include interstitial pneumonitis and intra-alveolar edema.

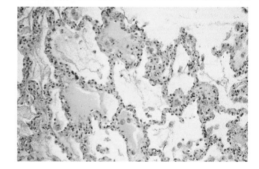

41

Helicobacter pylori Infections

Clinical Manifestations

Helicobacter pylori causes chronic active gastritis and increases the risk of duodenal and gastric ulcers; persistence increases the risk of gastric cancer. Acute infection can manifest as epigastric pain, nausea, vomiting, hematemesis, and guaiac-positive stools. Symptoms usually resolve within a few days despite persistence of the organism for years or for life. H pylori infection is not associated with autoimmune or chemical gastritis.

Etiology

H pylori is a gram-negative and spiral, curved, or U-shaped microaerophilic bacillus.

Epidemiology

H pylori has been isolated only from humans and other primates. Organisms are transmitted from infected humans by the fecal-oral and oral-oral routes. Infection rates are low in children in resource-rich countries, except in children from lower socioeconomic groups; prevalence increases until 60 years of age. Most carriage is asymptomatic, but some colonized people have histologic findings of chronic gastritis. H pylori chiefly is acquired from 1 to 7 years of age in resource-limited countries.

Incubation Period

Unknown.

Diagnostic Tests

H pylori infection can be diagnosed by culture of gastric biopsy tissue on nonselective media or selective media under microaerobic conditions for 2 to 5 days. Organisms usually can be visualized on histologic sections with Warthin-Starry silver, Steiner, Giemsa, or Genta staining. Because of production of urease by organisms, urease testing of a gastric specimen can give a rapid and specific microbiologic diagnosis. Each of these tests requires endoscopy and biopsy. Noninvasive, commercially available tests include breath tests, which detect labeled CO_2 in expired air after oral administration of isotopically labeled urea, and serologic tests for the presence of IgG specific for H pylori. Each of these commercially available tests has a sensitivity and specificity of 95% or more. A stool antigen test also is available commercially.

Treatment

Treatment is recommended only for infected patients who have peptic ulcer disease (currently or in the past), gastric mucosa–associated lymphoid tissue–type lymphoma, or early gastric cancer. Effective regimens include 2 antimicrobial agents (eg, clarithromycin plus either amoxicillin or metronidazole) plus a proton pump inhibitor (lansoprazole, omeprazole, esomeprazole, rabeprazole, or pantoprazole). These regimens are effective in eliminating the organism, healing the ulcer, and preventing recurrence.

Image 41.1
A biopsy of gastric mucosa stained with Warthin-Starry silver stain showing Helicobacter pylori organisms.

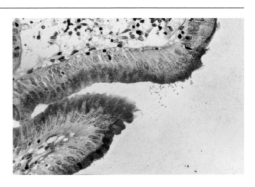

42

Hepatitis A

Clinical Manifestations

Hepatitis A characteristically is an acute, self-limited illness associated with fever, malaise, jaundice, anorexia, and nausea. Symptomatic hepatitis A virus (HAV) infection occurs in approximately 30% of infected children younger than 6 years; few of these children will have jaundice. Among older children and adults, infection usually is symptomatic and typically lasts several weeks, with jaundice occurring in 70% or more. Prolonged or relapsing disease lasting as long as 6 months can occur. Fulminant hepatitis is rare but is more common in people with underlying liver disease. Chronic infection does not occur.

Etiology

HAV is an RNA virus classified as a member of the picornavirus group.

Epidemiology

The most common mode of transmission is person-to-person by the fecal-oral route. Age at infection varies with socioeconomic status and associated living conditions. In developing countries, where infection is endemic, most people are infected during the first decade of life. In the prevaccine era in the United States, hepatitis A was one of the most commonly reported vaccine-preventable diseases, but its incidence has declined in recent years. In 2004, 5683 cases were reported to the CDC, compared with an average of approximately 26 000 cases per year during the prevaccine era. These declining rates have been accompanied by a shift in age-specific rates. Historically, the highest rates occurred among children 5 to 14 years of age, and the lowest rates occurred among adults older than 40 years. However, in recent years the highest rates have occurred among young adults, and rates among children 5 to 14 years of age have been among the lowest.

In addition, the previously observed unequal geographic distribution of hepatitis A incidence, with the highest rates of disease occurring in a limited number of states and communities, has disappeared after introduction of routine immunization.

Among cases of hepatitis A, identified risk factors include close personal contact with a person infected with HAV, household or personal contact with a child care center, international travel, a recognized food-borne or waterborne outbreak, male homosexual activity, and use of injection drugs. Transmission by blood transfusion or from mother to newborn infant (ie, vertical transmission) is rare.

In most infected people, the highest titers of HAV in stool, when patients are most likely to transmit HAV, occur during the 1 to 2 weeks before onset of illness. The risk of transmission subsequently diminishes and is minimal by 1 week after onset of jaundice. However, HAV can be detected in stool for longer periods, especially in neonates and young children.

Incubation Period

15 to 50 days (average of 30 days).

Diagnostic Tests

Serologic tests for HAV-specific total and IgM antibody are available commercially. Serum IgM is present at the onset of illness and usually disappears within 4 months but may persist for 6 months or longer. Presence of serum IgM indicates current or recent infection, although false-positive results can occur. IgG anti-HAV is detectable shortly after the appearance of IgM. The presence of total anti-HAV without IgM anti-HAV indicates past infection and immunity.

Treatment

Supportive.

Figure 42.1
Viral Hepatitis Incidence by Year in the United States, 1973–2003[1]

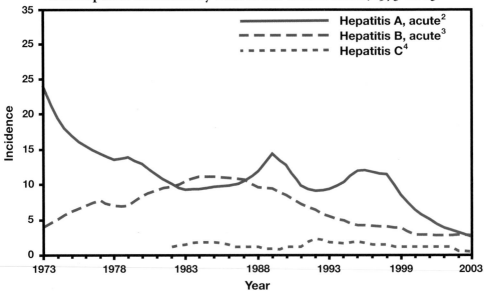

[1]Per 100 000 population.
[2]Hepatitis A vaccine was first licensed in 1995.
[3]Hepatitis B vaccine was first licensed in June 1982.
[4]An anti–hepatitis C antibody test first became available in May 1990.

Hepatitis A incidence continues to decline and in 2003 was the lowest ever recorded. However, cyclic increases in hepatitis A have been observed approximately every 10 years, and incidence could increase again. Hepatitis B incidence, which declined more than 65% during 1990 to 2000, has remained unchanged for the past 4 years, reflecting ongoing transmission in adult populations at high risk. The trend in reported hepatitis C/non-A, non-B (renamed hepatitis C, acute, in 2003) cases after 1990 is misleading because reported cases have included those based only on a positive laboratory test for anti–hepatitis C, and most of these cases represent chronic hepatitis C virus infection.

Courtesy of the Centers for Disease Control and Prevention.

Image 42.1
Acute hepatitis A infection with scleral icterus in a 10-year-old male.

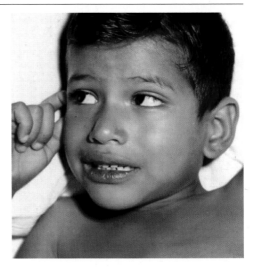

43

Hepatitis B

Clinical Manifestations

People with hepatitis B virus (HBV) infection present with a variety of signs and symptoms, including subacute illness with nonspecific symptoms (eg, anorexia, nausea, or malaise), clinical hepatitis with jaundice, or fulminant fatal hepatitis. Asymptomatic seroconversion is common, and the likelihood of developing symptoms of hepatitis is age dependent. Anicteric or asymptomatic infection is most common in young children. Extrahepatic manifestations, such as arthralgias, arthritis, macular rashes, thrombocytopenia, or papular acrodermatitis (Gianotti-Crosti syndrome), can occur early in the course of the illness and can precede jaundice. Acute HBV infection cannot be distinguished from other forms of acute viral hepatitis on the basis of clinical signs and symptoms or nonspecific laboratory findings. Chronic HBV infection is defined as presence of hepatitis B surface antigen (HBsAg) in serum for at least 6 months or by the presence of HBsAg in a person who tests negative for antibody of the IgM class to hepatitis B core antigen (anti-HBc).

Age at the time of acute infection is the primary determinant of the risk of progressing to chronic infection. More than 90% of infants infected perinatally will develop chronic HBV infection. Between 25% and 50% of children infected between 1 and 5 years of age become chronically infected, whereas only 2% to 6% of acutely infected older children and adults develop chronic HBV infections. Patients who develop acute HBV infection while immuno-suppressed or with an underlying chronic illness have an increased risk of developing chronic infection. Up to 25% of infants and older children who acquire chronic HBV infection eventually develop HBV-related hepatocellular carcinoma or cirrhosis.

Resolved hepatitis B is defined as clearance of HBsAg and normalization of serum transaminase concentrations; development of antibody to HBsAg (anti-HBs) also may be noted. Chronically infected adults clear HBsAg and develop anti-HBs at the rate of 1% to 2% annu-ally; during childhood, the annual clearance rate is less than 1%. Reactivation of resolved chronic infection is possible with immuno-suppression.

Etiology

HBV is a DNA-containing hepadnavirus. Important components of the viral particle include an outer lipoprotein envelope containing HBsAg and an inner nucleocapsid consisting of hepatitis B core antigen. Only IgG anti-HBs provides protection from HBV infection.

Epidemiology

HBV is transmitted through blood or body fluids, including wound exudates, semen, cervical secretions, and saliva. Blood and serum contain the highest concentrations of virus; saliva contains the lowest. People with chronic HBV infection are the primary reservoirs for infection. Common modes of transmission include percutaneous and permucosal exposure to infectious body fluids, sharing or using nonsterilized needles or syringes, sexual contact with an infected person, and perinatal exposure to an infected mother. Transmission by transfusion of contaminated blood or blood products is rare in the United States because of routine screening of blood donors and viral inactivation of certain blood products.

Perinatal transmission of HBV is highly efficient and usually occurs from blood exposures during labor and delivery. In utero transmission of HBV is rare, accounting for less than 2% of perinatal infections. The risk of an infant acquiring HBV from an infected mother as a result of perinatal exposure is 70% to 90% for infants born to mothers who are HBsAg and hepatitis B e antigen (HBeAg) positive; the risk is 5% to 20% for infants born to HBeAg-negative mothers.

Person-to-person spread of HBV can occur in settings involving interpersonal contact over extended periods, such as when a person with chronic HBV infection resides in a household. In household settings, nonsexual transmission occurs primarily from child to child, and young children are at highest risk of infection. The precise mechanisms of transmission from child to child are unknown. Hepatitis B virus can survive in the environment for 1 week or longer but is inactivated by commonly used disinfectants, including household bleach diluted 1:10 with water.

Before implementation of routine childhood hepatitis B immunization, multiple studies documented high rates of early childhood (nonperinatal) HBV transmission within some communities in the United States. The highest risk of early childhood transmission is among children who immigrated to the United States from countries where HBV infection is highly endemic (eg, Southeast Asia, China, Africa). Other children at increased risk of infection include residents of institutions for people with developmental disabilities and patients undergoing hemodialysis.

The frequency of HBV infection and patterns of transmission vary markedly throughout the world. Most areas of the United States, Canada, Western Europe, Australia, and southern South America have a low endemicity of HBV infection. Infection occurs primarily in adolescents and adults; 5% to 8% of the total population has been infected, and 0.2% to 0.9% of the population has chronic infection. However, within these geographic areas are populations with a high endemicity of infection, including Alaska Natives, Asian-Pacific Islanders, and immigrants from other countries with a high endemicity of infection.

Incubation Period

For acute infection: 45 to 160 days (average, 90 days).

Diagnostic Tests

Commercial serologic tests are available to detect HBsAg and HBeAg. Assays also are available for detection of anti-HBs, anti-HBc, IgM anti-HBc, and anti-HBe. In addition, hybridization assays and gene amplification techniques (eg, PCR, branched DNA methods) are available to detect and quantitate HBV DNA. HBsAg is detectable during acute infection. If the infection is self-limited, HBsAg disappears in most patients within a few weeks to several months after infection, followed by appearance of anti-HBs. The brief time between disappearance of HBsAg and appearance of anti-HBs is termed the *window phase* of infection. During the window phase,

the only marker of acute infection is the IgM anti-HBc, which is highly specific for establishing the diagnosis of acute infection. However, IgM anti-HBc usually is not present in infants infected perinatally. People with chronic HBV infection have circulating HBsAg and anti-HBc; on rare occasions, anti-HBs also is present. Both anti-HBs and anti-HBc are detected in people with resolved infection, whereas anti-HBs alone is present in people immunized with hepatitis B vaccine. The presence of HBeAg in serum correlates with higher concentrations of HBV and greater infectivity. Tests for HBeAg and HBV DNA are useful in the selection of candidates to receive antiviral therapy and to monitor the response to therapy.

Treatment

No specific therapy for acute HBV infection is available. Hepatitis B immune globulin (HBIG) and corticosteroids are not effective.

Chronic HBV infection in adults can be treated with interferon-alfa (interferon alfa-2b and peginterferon alfa-2a), lamivudine, adefovir, or entecavir, the latter 3 of which are given orally.

From 25% to 40% of adults with chronic HBV infection and liver disease achieve long-term remission (loss of detectable HBV DNA or loss of HBeAg) after treatment with interferon-alfa. This remission rate is approximately 20% higher than the spontaneous remission rate observed in untreated controls. Adult patients who clear HBeAg have decreases in rates of mortality and clinical complications of cirrhosis. Fewer data are available for treatment of children, but several studies indicate that approximately 30% of children with increased transaminase concentrations who are treated with interferon alfa-2b for 6 months lose HBeAg, compared with approximately 10% of untreated controls. Interferon-alfa is less effective for chronic infections acquired during early childhood, especially if transaminase concentrations are normal. Lamivudine is approved for treatment of chronic HBV infection in people 2 years of age and older. Although resistance to lamivudine develops quickly, therapy is continued. Children coinfected with HIV and HBV should receive lamivudine for treatment of HIV. The FDA has approved adefovir and entecavir for treatment of chronic HBV infection in adults, but safety and effectiveness for children has not been established. Other nucleoside analogues are being developed.

Children and adolescents who have chronic HBV infection are at risk of developing serious liver disease, including primary hepatocellular carcinoma, with advancing age.

Table 43.1
Diagnostic Tests for Hepatitis B Virus (HBV) Antigens and Antibodies[1]

Factor to Be Tested	HBV Antigen or Antibody	Use
HBsAg	Hepatitis B surface antigen	Detection of acutely or chronically infected people; antigen used in hepatitis B vaccine
Anti-HBs	Antibody to HBsAg	Identification of people who have resolved infections with HBV; determination of immunity after immunization
HBeAg	Hepatitis B e antigen	Identification of infected people at increased risk of transmitting HBV
Anti-HBe	Antibody to HBeAg	Identification of infected people with lower risk of transmitting HBV
Anti-HBc	Antibody to hepatitis B core antigen	Identification of people with acute, resolved, or chronic HBV infection (not present after immunization)
IgM anti-HBc	IgM antibody to HBcAg	Identification of people with acute or recent HBV infections (including HBsAg-negative people during the "window" phase of infection)

[1] HBsAg indicates hepatitis B surface antigen; IgM, immunoglobulin M.
[2] No test is available commercially to measure HBcAg.

Image 43.1
This electron micrograph reveals the presence of hepatitis B virus virions, or Dane particles. These particles measure 42 nm in their overall diameter and contain a DNA-based core.

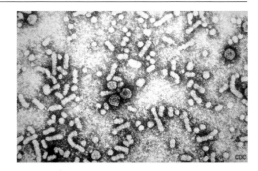

Image 43.2
This female Cambodian patient presented with a
distended abdomen due to a hepatoma resulting
from chronic hepatitis B infection.

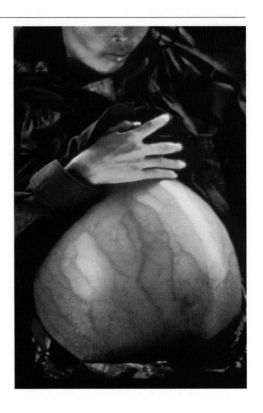

44

Hepatitis C

Clinical Manifestations

Signs and symptoms of hepatitis C virus (HCV) infection are indistinguishable from those of hepatitis A or hepatitis B virus infections. Acute disease tends to be mild and insidious in onset, and most infections are asymptomatic. Jaundice occurs in more than 20% of patients, and abnormalities in liver function tests generally are less pronounced than abnormalities in patients with hepatitis B virus infection. Persistent infection with HCV occurs in 50% to 60% of infected children, even in the absence of biochemical evidence of liver disease. Most children with chronic infection are asymptomatic. Although chronic hepatitis develops in approximately 60% to 70% of infected adults, limited data indicate that chronic hepatitis and cirrhosis are less common in children. Infection with HCV is the leading reason for liver transplantation among adults in the United States.

Etiology

HCV is a small, single-stranded RNA virus and is a member of the Flaviviridae family. Multiple HCV genotypes and subtypes exist.

Epidemiology

The prevalence of HCV infection in the general population of the United States is estimated at 1.8%. The seroprevalence is 0.2% for children younger than 12 years and 0.4% for adolescents 12 to 19 years of age.

Infection is spread primarily by exposure to blood of HCV-infected people. The current risk of HCV infection after blood transfusion in the United States is estimated to be less than 1 in 1 million units transfused because of exclusion of high-risk donors and of HCV-positive units by antibody testing and screening of pools of blood units by some form of nucleic acid amplification (NAA) test.

The highest seroprevalences of HCV infection (60%–90%) are in injection drug users and people with hemophilia who were treated with clotting factor concentrates produced before 1987. Prevalences are moderately high among people with frequent but smaller direct percutaneous exposures, such as patients receiving hemodialysis (10%–20%). Lower prevalences are found among people with inapparent percutaneous or mucosal exposures, such as people with high-risk sexual behaviors (1%–10%), and among people with sporadic percutaneous exposures, such as health care professionals (1%).

Other body fluids contaminated with infected blood can be sources of infection. Sexual transmission among monogamous couples is uncommon. Transmission among family contacts also is uncommon.

Seroprevalence among pregnant women in the United States has been estimated at 1% to 2%. The risk of perinatal transmission averages 5% to 6%, and transmission occurs only from women who are HCV RNA positive at the time of delivery. Maternal coinfection with HIV has been associated with increased risk of perinatal transmission of HCV, which depends in part on the serum titer of maternal HCV RNA. Serum antibody to HCV (anti-HCV) and HCV RNA have been detected in colostrum, but the risk of HCV transmission is similar in breastfed and bottle-fed infants.

All people with HCV RNA in their blood are considered to be infectious.

Incubation Period

Average 6 to 7 weeks (range, 2 weeks–6 months).

Diagnostic Tests

The 2 major types of tests available for the laboratory diagnosis of HCV infections are IgG antibody assays for anti-HCV and NAA tests to detect HCV RNA. The current enzyme immunoassays are at least 97% sensitive and more than 99% specific. False-negative results early in the course of acute infection result from the prolonged interval between exposure and onset of illness and seroconversion. Within 15 weeks after exposure and within 5 to 6 weeks after onset of hepatitis, 80% of patients will have positive test results for serum HCV antibody. Among infants born to anti-HCV–positive mothers, passively acquired maternal antibody may persist for up to 18 months.

FDA-licensed diagnostic NAA tests for qualitative detection of HCV RNA are available. HCV RNA can be detected in serum or plasma within 1 to 2 weeks after exposure to the virus and weeks before onset of liver enzyme abnormalities or appearance of anti-HCV. Assays for detection of HCV RNA are used commonly in clinical practice in the early diagnosis of infection, for identifying infection in infants early in life (ie, perinatal transmission) when maternal serum antibody interferes with the ability to detect antibody produced by the infant, and for monitoring patients receiving antiviral therapy. However, false-positive and false-negative results can occur from improper handling, storage, and contamination of the test specimens.

Treatment

Therapy is aimed at inhibiting HCV replication, eradicating infection, and improving the natural history of disease. Therapies are expensive, can cause significant adverse reactions, and are effective in approximately half of people treated. Interferon-alfa or peginterferon-alfa alone and peginterferon-alfa in combination with ribavirin are recommended for treatment of chronic HCV infection in adults. Given alone, interferon-alfa results in a sustained virologic response (SVR) in 10% to 20% of adult patients treated; peginterferons alfa-2a and alfa-2b, which require only 1 dose weekly, result in average SVR of 39% and 25%, respectively. Lower SVR rates are observed in patients infected with HCV genotype 1, the most common strain in the United States. Combination therapy with interferon alfa-2b and ribavirin results in SVR in 33% of adult patients infected with genotype 1 and approximately 80% in patients with genotypes 2 or 3. Combination therapy with peginterferons results in higher SVR rates, particularly among patients with genotype 1 (40%). Interferon alpha-2b in combination with ribavirin is recommended for treatment of HCV infection in children 3 to 17 years of age. There have been few studies using combination therapy in children, but these studies suggest that children have increased SVR rates and fewer adverse events compared with adults. Major adverse effects of combination therapy include influenza-like symptoms, hematologic abnormalities, and neuropsychiatric symptoms.

Image 44.1
Lichen planus is a skin disorder, the cause of which remains unknown. Suspected causes include stress-related factors, autoimmune origins, or possible viral pathogenic influences such as hepatitis C. It is characterized by scaly, flattened plaques, which appear erythematous, and usually manifests on the wrists and ankles.

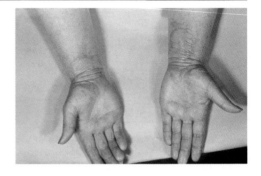

45

Herpes Simplex

Clinical Manifestations

Neonatal. In newborn infants, herpes simplex virus (HSV) infection can manifest as the following: (1) disseminated disease involving multiple organs, most prominently liver and lungs; (2) localized CNS disease; or (3) disease localized to the skin, eyes, and mouth. Approximately one third of cases are disseminated, one third are CNS disease, and one third affect the skin, eyes, or mouth, although there can be clinical overlap among disease types. In many neonates with disseminated or CNS disease, skin lesions do not develop or the lesions appear late in the course of infection. In the absence of skin lesions, the diagnosis of neonatal HSV infection is difficult. Disseminated infection should be considered in neonates with sepsis syndrome with negative bacteriologic culture results and severe liver dysfunction. HSV also should be considered as a causative agent in neonates with fever, irritability, and abnormal CSF findings, especially in the presence of seizures. Although asymptomatic HSV infection is common in older children, it rarely, if ever, occurs in neonates.

Neonatal herpetic infections often are severe, with attendant high mortality and morbidity rates, even when antiviral therapy is administered. Recurrent skin lesions are common in surviving infants and can be associated with CNS sequelae if skin lesions occur frequently during the first 6 months of life.

Initial signs of HSV infection can occur anytime between birth and approximately 4 weeks of age. Disseminated disease has the earliest age of onset, often during the first week of life; CNS disease manifests latest, usually between the second and third weeks of life.

Children Beyond the Neonatal Period and Adolescents. Most primary HSV infections are asymptomatic. Gingivostomatitis, which is the most common clinical manifestation, usually is caused by HSV type 1 (HSV-1). Gingivostomatitis is characterized by fever, irritability, tender submandibular adenopathy, and an ulcerative enanthem involving the gingiva and mucous membranes of the mouth, often with perioral vesicular lesions.

Genital herpes, which is the most common manifestation of HSV infection in adolescents and adults, is characterized by vesicular or ulcerative lesions of the male or female genital organs, perineum, or both. Genital herpes usually is caused by HSV type 2 (HSV-2), but HSV-1 seems to be increasing in frequency.

Eczema herpeticum with vesicular lesions concentrated in the areas of eczematous involvement can develop in patients with dermatitis who are infected with HSV.

In immunocompromised patients, severe local lesions and, less commonly, disseminated HSV infection with generalized vesicular skin lesions and visceral involvement can occur.

After primary infection, HSV persists for life in a latent form. The site of latency for virus causing herpes labialis is the trigeminal ganglion, and the usual site of latency for genital herpes is the sacral ganglia, although any of the sensory ganglia can be involved, depending on the site of primary infection. Reactivation of latent virus most commonly occurs in the absence of symptoms. Symptomatic, recurrent herpes labialis manifests as single or grouped vesicles in the perioral region, usually on the vermilion border of the lips (cold sores). Symptomatic recurrent genital herpes manifests as vesicular lesions on the penis, scrotum, vulva, cervix, buttocks, perianal areas, thighs, or back.

Conjunctivitis and keratitis can result from primary or recurrent HSV infection. Herpetic whitlow consists of single or multiple vesicular lesions on the distal parts of fingers.

HSV encephalitis can result from primary or recurrent infection and usually is associated with fever, alterations in the state of consciousness, personality changes, seizures, and focal neurologic findings. Encephalitis commonly has an acute onset with a fulminant course, leading to coma and death in untreated patients. HSV infection also can cause meningitis with nonspecific clinical manifestations that usually are mild and self-limited. Such episodes of meningitis usually are associated with genital HSV-2 infection. A number of unusual CNS manifestations of HSV have been described, including Bell's palsy, atypical pain syndromes, trigeminal neuralgia, ascending myelitis, and postinfectious encephalomyelitis.

Etiology

HSVs are enveloped, double-stranded DNA viruses. Infections with HSV-1 usually involve the face and skin above the waist; however, an increasing number of genital herpes cases are attributable to HSV-1. Infections with HSV-2 usually involve the genitalia and skin below the waist in sexually active adolescents and adults.

Epidemiology

HSV infections are ubiquitous and are transmitted from people who are symptomatic or asymptomatic with primary or recurrent infections.

Neonatal. The incidence of neonatal HSV infection is estimated to range from 1 in 3000 to 1 in 20 000 live births. Infants in whom HSV infection develops are significantly more likely to have been born preterm. HSV is transmitted to an infant most often during birth through an infected maternal genital tract or by an ascending infection, rarely through apparently intact membranes. Intrauterine infections have been implicated in rare cases. Other less common sources of neonatal infection include postnatal transmission from a parent or other caregiver, most often from a nongenital infection (eg, mouth or hands) or from another infected infant or caregiver in the nursery, probably via the hands of health care professionals attending the infants.

The risk of HSV infection at delivery in an infant born vaginally to a mother with primary genital infection is estimated to be 50%. The risk to an infant born to a mother shedding HSV as a result of reactivated infection is less than 5%. Distinguishing between primary and recurrent HSV infections in women by history is impossible. Primary and recurrent infections can be asymptomatic or associated with non-specific findings (eg, vaginal discharge, genital pain, or shallow ulcers). More than three quarters of infants who contract HSV infection

have been born to women who had no history or clinical findings suggestive of active HSV infection during pregnancy.

Children Beyond the Neonatal Period and Adolescents. Patients with primary gingivo-stomatitis or genital herpes usually shed virus for at least 1 week and occasionally for several weeks. Patients with recurrent infection shed virus for a shorter period, typically 3 to 4 days. Intermittent asymptomatic reactivation of oral and genital herpes is common and persists for life. The greatest concentration of virus is shed during symptomatic primary infections.

Infection with HSV-1 usually results from direct contact with infected oral secretions or lesions. Infections with HSV-2 usually result from direct contact with infected genital secretions or lesions through sexual activity. Genital infections caused by HSV-1 in children can result from autoinoculation of virus from the mouth, but sexual abuse always should be considered in prepubertal children with genital HSV-2 infections. Genital HSV isolates from children should be typed to differentiate between HSV-1 and HSV-2.

The incidence of HSV-2 infection correlates with the number of sexual partners and with acquisition of other STIs. After primary genital infection, some people experience frequent clinical recurrences, and others have no recurrences. Genital HSV-2 infection is more likely to recur than is genital HSV-1 infection.

Inoculation of skin occurs from direct contact with HSV-containing oral or genital secretions. This contact can result in herpes gladiatorum among wrestlers, herpes rugbiaforum among rugby players, or herpetic whitlow of the fingers in any exposed person.

Incubation Period

Ranges from 2 days to 2 weeks.

Diagnostic Tests

HSV grows readily in cell culture. Special transport media are available for specimens that cannot be inoculated immediately onto susceptible cell culture media. Cytopathogenic effects typical of HSV infection usually are observed 1 to 3 days after inoculation. PCR assay often can detect HSV DNA in CSF from patients with HSV encephalitis and is the diagnostic method of choice when performed by experienced laboratory personnel. Histologic examination and viral culture of a brain tissue specimen obtained by biopsy is the most definitive method of confirming the diagnosis of encephalitis caused by HSV. Cultures of CSF from a patient with HSV encephalitis usually are negative.

For diagnosis of neonatal HSV infection, swabs of the mouth, nasopharynx, conjunctivae, and rectum and specimens of skin vesicles, urine, stool, blood, and CSF should be obtained for culture at 24 to 48 hours after birth. Rapid diagnostic techniques also are available, such as direct fluorescent antibody staining of vesicle scrapings or enzyme immunoassay detection of HSV antigens. These techniques are as specific but slightly less sensitive than culture. Typing HSV strains differentiates between HSV-1 and HSV-2 isolates. PCR assay is a sensitive method for detecting HSV DNA and is of particular value for evaluating CSF specimens from people with suspected herpes encephalitis. Histologic examination of lesions for the presence of multinucleated giant cells is not recommended as a rapid diagnostic test.

Both type-specific and nonspecific antibodies to HSV develop during the first several weeks after infection and persist indefinitely. Although type-specific HSV-2 antibody almost always indicates anogenital infection, the presence of HSV-1 antibody does not distinguish anogenital from orolabial infection. Serologic tests can be used to diagnose people with unrecognized infection and to manage sexual partners of people with genital herpes. Serologic testing is not useful in neonates or young children.

Treatment

Neonatal. Parenteral acyclovir is the treatment of choice for neonatal HSV infections. Acyclovir should be administered to all neonates with HSV infection, regardless of manifestations and clinical findings. The best outcome in terms of morbidity and mortality is observed among infants with disease limited to the skin, eyes, and mouth. Although most neonates treated for HSV encephalitis survive, most suffer substantial neurologic sequelae.

Approximately 25% of neonates with disseminated disease die despite antiviral therapy. Relapse of diseases of the skin, eyes, mouth, and CNS can occur after cessation of treatment. The optimal management of these recurrences is not established.

Infants with ocular involvement attributable to HSV infection should receive a topical ophthalmic drug (1% trifluridine, 0.1% iododeoxyuridine, or 3% vidarabine) as well as parenteral antiviral therapy.

Genital

Primary. Many patients with first-episode herpes have mild clinical manifestations but go on to develop severe or prolonged symptoms. Therefore, most patients with initial genital herpes should receive antiviral therapy. In adults, acyclovir and valacyclovir decrease the duration of symptoms and viral shedding in primary genital herpes. Oral acyclovir therapy, initiated within 6 days of onset of disease, shortens the duration of illness and viral shedding by 3 to 5 days. Intravenous acyclovir is indicated for patients with a severe or complicated primary infection that requires hospitalization. Systemic or topical treatment of primary herpetic lesions does not affect the subsequent frequency or severity of recurrences.

Recurrent. Antiviral therapy for recurrent genital herpes can be administered either episodically to ameliorate or shorten the duration of lesions or continuously as suppressive therapy to decrease the frequency of recurrences. Oral acyclovir therapy initiated within 2 days of the onset of symptoms shortens the mean clinical course by approximately 1 day. Valacyclovir and famciclovir are licensed for treatment of adults with recurrent genital herpes; however, no data exist for treatment of pediatric disease.

In adults with frequent genital HSV recurrences (≥6 episodes per year), daily oral acyclovir suppressive therapy is effective for decreasing the frequency of symptomatic recurrences. After approximately 1 year of continuous daily therapy, acyclovir should be discontinued and the recurrence rate should be assessed. If recurrences are observed, additional suppressive therapy should be considered. Acyclovir seems to be safe for adults receiving the drug for more than 15 years, but long-term effects are unknown. Data also support suppressive therapy in adults with valacyclovir or famciclovir.

Data on use of valacyclovir or famciclovir for suppressive therapy in children are not available. Acyclovir may be administered orally to pregnant women with first-episode genital herpes or severe recurrent herpes and should be given intravenously to pregnant women with severe HSV infection.

Mucocutaneous

Immunocompromised Hosts. Intravenous acyclovir is effective for treatment and prevention of mucocutaneous HSV infections. Topical acyclovir also may accelerate healing of lesions in immunocompromised patients.

Acyclovir-resistant strains of HSV have been isolated from immunocompromised people receiving prolonged treatment with acyclovir. Under these circumstances, progressive disease can be observed despite acyclovir therapy. Foscarnet is the drug of choice for disease caused by acyclovir-resistant HSV isolates.

Immunocompetent Hosts. Limited data are available on the effects of acyclovir on the course of primary or recurrent nongenital mucocutaneous HSV infections in immunocompetent hosts. Therapeutic benefit has been noted in a limited number of children with primary gingivostomatitis treated with oral acyclovir. Minimal therapeutic benefit of oral acyclovir therapy has been demonstrated among adults with recurrent herpes labialis. Topical acyclovir is ineffective. A topical formulation of penciclovir (Denavir) and another drug, docosonal (Abreva), have limited activity for therapy of herpes labialis and are not recommended.

Other

CNS. Patients with HSV encephalitis should be treated with intravenous acyclovir. Therapy is less effective in older adults than in children. Patients who are comatose or semicomatose at initiation of therapy have a poor outcome. For people with Bell palsy, the combination of acyclovir and prednisone should be considered.

Ocular. Treatment of eye lesions should be undertaken in consultation with an ophthalmologist. Several topical drugs, such as 1% trifluridine, 0.1% iododeoxyuridine, and 3% vidarabine, have proven efficacy for superficial keratitis. Topical corticosteroids are contraindicated in suspected HSV conjunctivitis.

Image 45.1
This is a close-up of a herpes simplex lesion of the lower lip on the second day after onset.

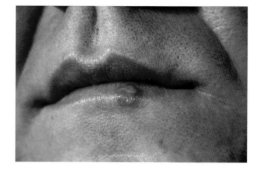

Image 45.2
Herpes simplex stomatitis, primary infection of the anterior oral mucous membranes. Tongue lesions also are common with primary herpes simplex virus infections.

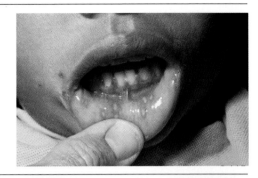

Image 45.3
Recurrent herpes simplex periorbital, ear, and facial vesicles.

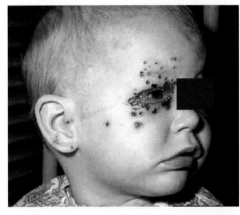

Image 45.4
Eczema herpeticum on the face of a boy with eczema and primary herpetic gingivostomatitis, day 3 to 4 after the onset. The herpetic lesions spread over 2 to 3 days to cover the skin.

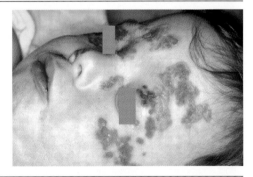

Image 45.5
A patient with extensive eczema herpeticum and primary herpetic gingivostomatitis.

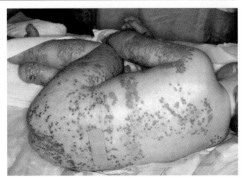

Image 45.6
A neonate born with "sucking blisters" on the hand who developed neonatal herpes simplex lesions at the site. The patient responded well while receiving treatment with acyclovir.

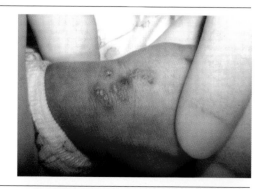

Image 45.7
Extensive herpes simplex lesions of the mouth and face in an 11-month-old immunocompromised black male.

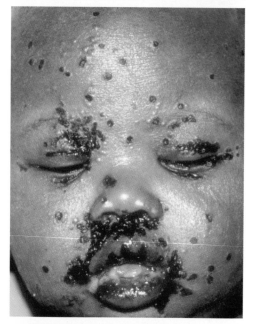

Image 45.8
This male presented with primary vesiculo-papular herpes genitalis lesions on his glans penis and penile shaft. When signs of herpes genitalis do occur, they typically appear as one or more blisters on or around the genitals or rectum. The blisters break, leaving tender ulcers (sores) that may take 2 to 4 weeks to heal the first time they occur.

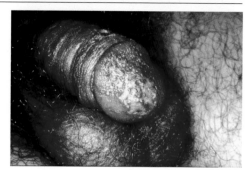

46
Histoplasmosis

Clinical Manifestations

Histoplasma capsulatum causes symptoms in fewer than 5% of infected people. Clinical manifestations can be classified according to site (pulmonary, extrapulmonary, or disseminated), duration (acute, chronic), and pattern (primary vs reactivation) of infection. Most symptomatic patients have acute pulmonary histoplasmosis, an influenza-like illness with nonpleuritic chest pain, hilar adenopathy, and mild pulmonary infiltrates; symptoms persist for 2 days to 2 weeks. Intense exposure to spores can cause severe respiratory tract symptoms and diffuse nodular pulmonary infiltrates, prolonged fever, fatigue, and weight loss. Erythema nodosum can occur in adolescents. Primary cutaneous infections after trauma are rare.

Progressive disseminated histoplasmosis (PDH) can develop in otherwise healthy infants younger than 2 years. Early manifestations include prolonged fever, failure to thrive, and hepatosplenomegaly; if untreated, malnutrition, diffuse adenopathy, pneumonia, mucosal ulceration, pancytopenia, disseminated intravascular coagulopathy, and gastrointestinal tract bleeding can ensue. CNS involvement is common. Cellular immune dysfunction caused by primary immunodeficiency disorders, HIV infection, or immunosuppressive therapy (including tumor necrosis factor–alpha inhibitors) may predispose patients with acute histoplasmosis to develop PDH. An early symptom is fever with no apparent focus. Later, diffuse pneumonitis, skin lesions, meningitis, lymphadenopathy, hepatosplenomegaly, pancytopenia, and coagulopathy occur.

Etiology

H capsulatum is a dimorphic fungus. It grows in soil as a spore-bearing mold with macroconidia but converts to yeast phase at body temperature.

Epidemiology

H capsulatum is encountered in many parts of the world and is endemic in the eastern and central United States, particularly the Mississippi, Ohio, and Missouri River valleys. Infections occur sporadically; in outbreaks when weather conditions predispose to spread of spores; or in point-source epidemics after exposure to gardening activities or playing in barns, hollow trees, caves, or bird roosts or after exposure to excavation, demolition, cleaning, or renovation of contaminated buildings. The organism grows in moist soil. Growth of the organism is facilitated by bat, bird, and chicken droppings. Spores are spread in dry and windy conditions or when occupational or recreational activities disturb contaminated sites. Infection is acquired when spores (conidia) are inhaled. Person-to-person transmission does not occur.

Incubation Period

Usually 1 to 3 weeks.

Diagnostic Tests

Culture is the definitive method of diagnosis. *H capsulatum* from bone marrow, blood, sputum, and tissue specimens grows on standard mycologic media in 1 to 6 weeks. The lysis-centrifugation method is preferred for blood cultures. A DNA probe for *H capsulatum* permits rapid identification.

Demonstration of typical intracellular yeast forms by examination with methenamine silver or other stains of tissue, blood, bone marrow, or bronchoalveolar lavage specimens strongly supports the diagnosis of histoplasmosis when clinical, epidemiologic, and other laboratory studies are compatible.

Detection of *H capsulatum* polysaccharide antigen (HPA) in serum, urine, or bronchoalveolar lavage fluid by radioimmunoassay or enzyme immunoassay is a rapid and specific diagnostic method. Antigen detection is most sensitive for progressive disseminated infections; a negative test does not exclude infection. If initially positive, the antigen test can be used to monitor treatment response and to identify relapse in HIV-infected patients. The

HPA test has low sensitivity for diagnosis of acute pulmonary histoplasmosis in immunocompetent people.

Both mycelial-phase (histoplasmin) and yeast-phase antigens are used in serologic testing for complement-fixing antibodies to *H capsulatum*. A 4-fold increase in either yeast-phase or mycelial-phase titers or a single titer of 1:32 or greater in either test is presumptive evidence of active infection. Cross-reacting antibodies can result from *Blastomyces dermatitidis* and *Coccidioides immitis* infections. In the immunodiffusion test, H bands, although infrequently encountered, are highly suggestive of acute infection; M bands also occur in acute or recent infection. The immunodiffusion test is more specific than the complement fixation test, but the complement fixation test is more sensitive.

The histoplasmin skin test is not useful for diagnostic purposes.

Treatment

Immunocompetent children with uncomplicated, primary pulmonary histoplasmosis rarely require antifungal therapy. Indications for therapy include PDH in infants, serious illness after intense exposures, and acute infection in immunocompromised patients. Other manifestations of histoplasmosis in immunocompetent children for which antifungal ther-

apy should be considered include pulmonary disease with symptoms persisting more than 4 weeks and granulomatous adenitis that obstructs critical structures (eg, bronchi or blood vessels).

Amphotericin B is recommended for disseminated disease and other serious infections. In other circumstances in which antifungal therapy is warranted, itraconazole and fluconazole also have been effective. The safety and efficacy of itraconazole for use in children have not been established, but in adults, itraconazole is preferred over fluconazole and has negligible adverse effects. Itraconazole also has proven effective in treatment of mild to moderately severe disseminated histoplasmosis in HIV-infected patients.

Mild infections in HIV-infected patients can be treated with itraconazole. Patients with HIV infection and PDH require lifelong suppressive therapy with itraconazole to prevent relapse; fluconazole can be given if itraconazole is not tolerated.

Erythema nodosum, arthritis syndromes, and pericarditis do not necessitate antifungal therapy. Pericarditis is treated with indomethacin. Dense fibrosis of mediastinal structures without an associated granulomatous inflammatory component does not respond to antifungal therapy.

Image 46.1
Methenamine silver stain reveals *Histoplasma capsulatum*.

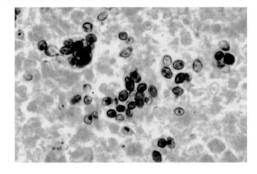

Image 46.2

Acute, primary histoplasmosis in a 13-year-old girl.

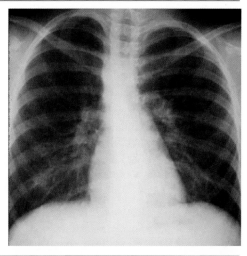

Image 46.3

CT scan of lungs showing classic snowstorm appearance of acute histoplasmosis.

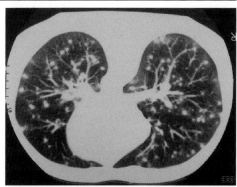

Image 46.4

A preadolescent child with calcified hilar lymph nodes bilaterally secondary to histoplasmosis.

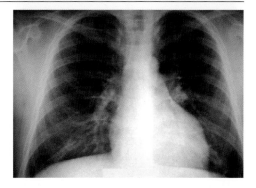

47

Hookworm Infections

(*Ancylostoma duodenale* and *Necator americanus*)

Clinical Manifestations

Patients with hookworm infection most often are asymptomatic; however, chronic hookworm infection is a common cause of hypochromic microcytic anemia in people living in tropical developing countries, and heavy infection can cause hypoproteinemia with edema. Chronic hookworm infection in children can lead to physical growth delay, deficits in cognition, and developmental delay. After contact with contaminated soil, initial skin penetration of larvae, usually involving the feet, can cause a stinging or burning sensation followed by pruritus and a papulovesicular rash that may persist for 1 to 2 weeks. Pneumonitis associated with migrating larvae is uncommon and usually mild, except in heavy infections. After oral ingestion of infectious *Ancylostoma duodenale* larvae, disease can manifest with pharyngeal itching, hoarseness, nausea, and vomiting shortly after ingestion. Colicky abdominal pain, nausea, diarrhea, and marked eosinophilia can develop 4 to 6 weeks after exposure.

Etiology

Necator americanus is the major cause of hookworm infection worldwide, although *A duodenale* also is an important hookworm in some regions. Mixed infections are common. Both are roundworms (nematodes) with similar life cycles.

Epidemiology

Humans are the only reservoir. Hookworms are prominent in rural, tropical, and subtropical areas where soil contamination with human feces is common. Although both hookworm species are equally prevalent in many areas, *A duodenale* is the predominant species in Europe, the Mediterranean region, northern Asia, and the west coast of South America. *N americanus* is predominant in the Western hemisphere, sub-Saharan Africa, Southeast Asia, and a number of Pacific islands. Larvae and eggs survive in loose, sandy, moist, shady, well-aerated, warm soil

(optimal temperature 23°C–33°C [73°F–91°F]). Hookworm eggs from stool hatch in soil in 1 to 2 days as rhabditiform larvae. These larvae develop into infective filariform larvae in soil within 5 to 7 days and can persist for weeks to months. *A duodenale* transmission can occur by oral ingestion and possibly through human milk. Untreated infected patients can harbor worms for 5 to 15 years, but a decrease in worm burden of at least 70% generally occurs within 1 to 2 years.

Incubation Period

The time from exposure to development of noncutaneous symptoms is 4 to 12 weeks.

Diagnostic Tests

Microscopic demonstration of hookworm eggs in feces is diagnostic. Adult worms or larvae rarely are seen. Approximately 5 to 10 weeks are required after infection for eggs to appear in feces. A direct stool smear with saline solution or potassium iodide is adequate for diagnosis of heavy hookworm infection; light infections require concentration techniques. Quantification techniques (eg, Kato-Katz, Beaver direct smear, or Stoll egg counting techniques) to determine the clinical significance of infection and the response to treatment may be available from state or reference laboratories.

Treatment

Albendazole, mebendazole, and pyrantel pamoate are all effective treatments. In children younger than 2 years, in whom experience with these drugs is limited, the WHO recommends one half the adult dose of albendazole or mebendazole in heavy hookworm infections. The dose of pyrantel pamoate is determined by weight. In heavy hookworm infection during pregnancy, deworming treatment is recommended by the WHO during the second or third trimester. Albendazole, mebendazole, or pyrantel pamoate can be used. A repeated stool examination, using a concentration technique, should be performed 2 weeks after treatment and, if positive, re-treatment is indicated. Nutritional supplementation, including iron, is important when anemia is present. Severely affected children may require blood transfusion.

Image 47.1
Hookworm *(Necator americanus)* ova in stool preparation.

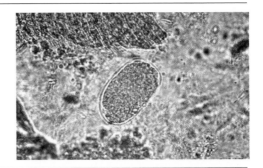

Image 47.2
A, B: Hookworm filariform larva (wet preparation).

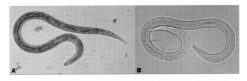

Image 47.3
This child with hookworm shows visible signs of edema and was diagnosed with anemia as well.

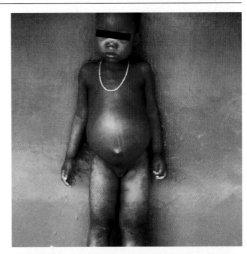

Image 47.4
Hookworms *(Ancylostoma caninum)* are shown attached to the intestinal mucosa at high magnification.

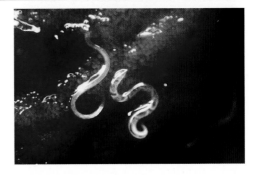

48

Human Herpesvirus 6 (Including Roseola) and 7

Clinical Manifestations

Clinical manifestations of primary infection with human herpesvirus 6 (HHV-6) include roseola (exanthem subitum, sixth disease) in approximately 20% of infected children, undifferentiated febrile illness without rash or localizing signs, and other acute febrile illnesses (febrile seizures, encephalitis and other neurologic disorders, and mononucleosis-like syndromes), often accompanied by cervical and postoccipital lymphadenopathy, gastrointestinal or respiratory tract signs, and inflamed tympanic membranes. Fever is characteristically high (>39.5°C [>103.0°F]) and persists for 3 to 7 days. In roseola, fever is followed by an erythematous maculopapular rash lasting hours to days. Seizures occur during the febrile period in approximately 10% to 15% of primary infections. A bulging anterior fontanelle and encephalopathy occur occasionally. The virus persists and may reactivate. The clinical circumstances and manifestations of reactivation in healthy people are not known. Illness associated with reactivation, primarily in immunocompromised hosts, has been described in association with manifestations such as fever, rash, hepatitis, bone marrow suppression, pneumonia, and encephalitis.

Recognition of the varied clinical manifestations of HHV-7 infection is evolving. Many, if not most, primary infections with HHV-7 can be asymptomatic or mild; some may present as typical roseola and may account for second or recurrent cases of roseola. Febrile illnesses associated with seizures also have been reported. Some investigators suggest that the association of HHV-7 with these clinical manifestations results from the ability of HHV-7 to reactivate HHV-6 from latency.

Etiology

HHV-6 and HHV-7 are lymphotropic agents that are closely related members of the Herpesviridae family. Strains of HHV-6 belong to 1 of 2 major groups, variants A and B. Almost all primary infections in children are caused by variant B strains except in some parts of Africa.

Epidemiology

Humans are the only known natural hosts for HHV-6 and HHV-7. Transmission of HHV-6 to an infant most likely results from asymptomatic shedding of persistent virus in secretions of a family member, caregiver, or other close contact. The peak rate of infection is between 6 and 24 months of age. All children are seropositive before 4 years of age. Infections occur throughout the year without a seasonal pattern. Secondary cases rarely are identified. Occasional outbreaks of roseola have been reported.

HHV-7 infection occurs somewhat later in life than HHV-6. By adulthood, the seroprevalence of HHV-7 is approximately 85%. Lifelong persistent infection with HHV-6 and HHV-7 is established after primary infection. Infectious HHV-7 is present in more than three fourths of saliva specimens obtained from healthy adults. Transmission of HHV-6 and HHV-7 to young children is likely to occur from contact with infected respiratory tract secretions of healthy contacts.

Incubation Period

For HHV-6, 9 to 10 days; HHV-7, unknown.

Diagnostic Tests

The definitive diagnosis of primary HHV-6 infection necessitates use of research techniques to isolate the virus from a peripheral blood specimen. A 4-fold increase in serum antibody concentration alone does not necessarily indicate new infection because an increase in titer also may occur with reactivation and in association with other infections. However, seroconversion from negative to positive in paired sera is good evidence of recent primary infection. Detection of specific IgM antibody also is not reliable because IgM antibodies to HHV-6 may be present in some asymptomatic previously infected people. Commercial assays for antibody detection can detect HHV-6–specific IgG, but these assays do not distinguish between primary infection and viral persistence or reactivation. Nearly all children older than 2 years have an antibody titer to HHV-6.

Diagnostic tests for HHV-7 also are limited to research laboratories, and reliable differentiation between primary infection and reactivation is problematic. Serodiagnosis of HHV-7 is confounded by serologic cross-reactivity with HHV-6 and by the potential ability of HHV-6 to be reactivated by HHV-7 and possibly other infections.

Treatment

Supportive. A few anecdotal reports suggest the use of ganciclovir may be beneficial for immunocompromised patients with serious HHV-6 disease.

Image 48.1
A 13-month-old white male developed high fever that persisted for 4 days without recognized cause. The child appeared relatively well and the fever subsided to be followed by a maculopapular rash that began on the trunk and spread to involve the face and extremities. The course was typical for roseola infantum (human hespesvirus 6).

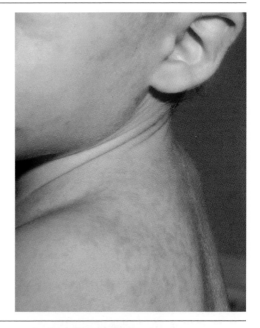

Image 48.2
The rash of human herpesvirus 6 and 7 can be identical.

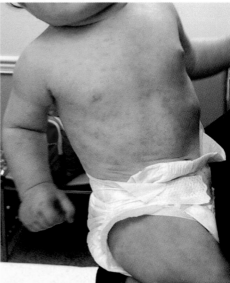

49

Human Immunodeficiency Virus Infection

Clinical Manifestations

HIV infection in children and adolescents causes a broad spectrum of disease manifestations and a varied clinical course. AIDS represents the most severe end of the clinical spectrum. The pediatric classification system emphasizes the importance of the CD4+ T-lymphocyte count as an immunologic surrogate and marker of prognosis; classification is independent of viral load as quantitated by HIV RNA PCR assay.

Manifestations of pediatric HIV infection include generalized lymphadenopathy, hepatomegaly, splenomegaly, failure to thrive, oral candidiasis, recurrent diarrhea, parotitis, cardiomyopathy, hepatitis, nephropathy, CNS disease (including microcephaly, hyperreflexia, clonus, and developmental delay), lymphoid interstitial pneumonia, recurrent invasive bacterial infections, opportunistic infections, and specific malignant neoplasms. With early and appropriate treatment, primary manifestations of HIV and development of opportunistic infections now are rare in children in the United States.

The frequency of different opportunistic pathogens among HIV-infected children in the era before highly active antiretroviral therapy (HAART) varied by age, pathogen, previous opportunistic infections, and immunologic status. In the pre-HAART era, the most common opportunistic infections among children in the United States were candidiasis, serious bacterial infections, herpes zoster, disseminated *Mycobacterium avium* complex (MAC), and *Pneumocystis jiroveci* pneumonia (PCP). Less commonly observed opportunistic infections included CMV, *Mycobacterium tuberculosis, Cryptosporidium,* and *Isospora* species, or other enteric pathogens, systemic fungal infection, and *Toxoplasma gondii* infections. In the HAART era, descriptions of infections among HIV-infected children have been limited because of substantial decreases in their occurrence.

Malignant neoplasms in children with HIV infection are uncommon, but leiomyosarcomas and certain lymphomas, including those of the CNS and non-Hodgkin B-lymphocyte lymphomas of the Burkitt type, occur more commonly in children with HIV infection than in immunocompetent children. Kaposi sarcoma is rare in children in the United States but occurs commonly among HIV-infected children in areas of the world with high rates of HIV infection.

Development of an opportunistic infection, particularly PCP, progressive neurologic disease, and severe wasting, is associated with a poor prognosis. In the absence of treatment, prognosis for survival also is poor in perinatally infected infants when viral load exceeds 100 000 copies/mL, CD4+ T-lymphocyte count and percentage is low, and clinical signs develop during the first year of life. Recent studies in the United States and Europe show that more than 95% survive to 16 years of age, with preservation of immune system integrity in at least half of those children.

Etiology

Infection is caused by human RNA retroviruses HIV-1 and, less commonly, HIV-2, a related virus that is rare in the United States but more common in West Africa.

Epidemiology

Humans are the only known reservoir of HIV. Because retroviruses integrate into the target cell genome as proviruses and the viral genome is copied during DNA replication, the virus persists in infected people for life. Data demonstrate persistence of latent virus in peripheral blood mononuclear cells, and in other cells, even when viral RNA is below the limit of detection in blood. HIV has been isolated from blood (including lymphocytes, monocytes, and plasma) and from other body fluids. Only blood, semen, cervical secretions, and human milk have been implicated in transmission of infection.

Established modes of HIV transmission in the United States are the following: (1) sexual contact (vaginal, anal, or orogenital); (2) percutaneous (from contaminated needles or other sharp instruments) or mucous membrane exposure to contaminated blood or other body fluids; and (3) mother-to-child transmission during pregnancy, around the time of labor and delivery, and postnatally through breastfeeding. Because of exclusion of infected donors, viral inactivation treatment of clotting factor concentrates, and availability of recombinant clotting factors, transfusion of blood, blood components, or clotting factor concentrates is a rare cause of HIV transmission in the United States. In the absence of documented sexual transmission or parenteral or mucous membrane contact with blood or blood-containing body fluids, transmission of HIV rarely has been demonstrated to occur in families or households or as a result of routine care in hospitals or clinics. Transmission of HIV has not been documented in schools or child care settings.

Cases of AIDS in children have accounted for approximately 1% of all reported cases in the United States. The total number of reported cases of AIDS in children decreased more than 90% as a result of a dramatic decrease in the rate of mother-to-child transmission of HIV and the availability of potent combination antiretroviral therapy for HIV-infected infants and children (resulting in fewer children progressing to symptomatic AIDS). The CDC estimates that 150 to 300 infants with HIV infection were born in 2003. Mother-to-child transmission of HIV now accounts for almost all new infections in preadolescent children.

The rate of acquisition of HIV during adolescence continues to increase and contributes to the large number of cases in young adults. Transmission of HIV among adolescents is attributable primarily to sexual exposure. Approximately 50% of HIV acquisition in the United States is estimated to occur among people 13 to 24 years of age. Among adolescents, the incidence of HIV infection in females 13 to 15 years of age exceeds that in males; for adolescents 16 to 19 years of age, the prevalence in girls and boys is equivalent. Most HIV-infected adolescents are asymptomatic and remain unaware that they are infected.

Without therapy for the HIV-seropositive mother, the absolute risk for in utero transmission is approximately 5% and for intrapartum transmission approximately 13% to 18%. Maternal viral load is a critical determinant of mother-to-child transmission of HIV, with the risk of transmission increasing from 10% for women with peripheral blood viral load less than 1000, up to 40% from women with viral load greater than 100 000. Other factors associated with an increased risk of transmission include low maternal CD4+ T-lymphocyte counts, advanced maternal illness, intrapartum events resulting in increased exposure of the fetus to maternal blood, placental membrane inflammation, mother-infant *HLA* concordance, preterm delivery, prolonged labor, vaginal delivery, and longer duration of rupture of membranes. Cesarean section seems to reduce the risk of transmission in direct proportion to the number of hours membranes were ruptured before cesarean section. (See Table 49.1 for regimen to reduce perinatal transmission of HIV.)

Postnatal transmission occurs through breastfeeding. Worldwide, an estimated one third to one half of mother-to-child HIV transmission events may occur as a result of breastfeeding. In the United States, providing safe alternative feeding for infants is possible.

Incubation Period

The median age of onset of symptoms is 12 to 18 months for untreated, perinatally infected infants, but children develop symptoms during adolescence.

Diagnostic Tests

Laboratory diagnosis of HIV infection during infancy depends on detection of virus or viral nucleic acid. Transplacental transfer of antibody complicates use of antibody-based assays (eg, HIV enzyme immunoassay [EIA] and Western blot analysis) for diagnosis of infection in infants, because all infants born to HIV-seropositive mothers have passively acquired maternal antibodies.

The preferred test for diagnosis of HIV-1 infection in infants in the United States is HIV-1 nucleic acid detection by PCR assay of DNA extracted from peripheral blood mononuclear cells (Table 49.2). Approximately 30% of infants with HIV infection will have a positive DNA PCR assay result in samples obtained before 48 hours of age. A positive result identifies infants who were infected in utero. The test routinely can detect 1 to 10 DNA copies. Approximately 93% of infected infants have detectable HIV-1 DNA by 2 weeks of age, and almost all HIV-infected infants have positive HIV DNA PCR assay results by 1 month of age. A single HIV-1 DNA PCR assay has a sensitivity of 95% and a specificity of 97% on samples collected from infants 1 to 36 months of age. Detection of the p24 antigen (including immune complex dissociated) is substantially less sensitive than HIV-1 DNA PCR assay or culture. A positive result using the plasma HIV-1 RNA PCR assay may be used to diagnose HIV infection. However, a negative test result may occur in HIV-infected people.

Infants born to HIV-infected women should be tested by HIV DNA PCR assay or HIV RNA PCR assay during the first 48 hours of life in an attempt to identify in utero transmission of HIV. Because of possible contamination with maternal blood, umbilical cord blood should not be used for this test. A second test should be performed at 1 to 2 months of age. A third test is recommended at 2 to 4 months of age. Any time an infant tests positive, testing should be repeated on a second blood sample as soon as possible to confirm the diagnosis. An infant is considered infected if 2 separate samples are positive by DNA or RNA PCR assays. Infection in nonbreastfed infants can be excluded reasonably when results of 2 HIV DNA or RNA PCR assays performed at or beyond 1 month of age and at 4 months of age or older are both negative. In infants with 2 negative HIV DNA or RNA PCR test results, HIV infection definitely can be excluded by confirming the absence of antibody to HIV on testing at 12 to 18 months of age (seroreversion). An infant with 2 blood samples obtained after 6 months of age and at an interval of at least 1 month apart that are both negative for HIV antibody also can be considered uninfected.

EIAs are used widely as the initial test for serum HIV antibody. These tests are highly sensitive and specific. Repeated EIA testing of initially reactive specimens is common practice and is followed by Western blot analysis to confirm the presence of antibody specific to HIV. A positive HIV antibody test result (EIA followed by Western Blot analysis) in a child 18 months of age or older indicates infection, although passively acquired maternal antibody rarely can persist beyond 18 months of age. An HIV antibody test can be performed on samples of blood or oral fluid. The most notable laboratory finding in perinatally infected infants is a high viral load (as measured by HIV-1 RNA PCR assay) that does not decrease rapidly during the first year of life unless combination antiretroviral therapy is initiated. As disease progresses, there is an increasing loss of cell-mediated immunity. The peripheral blood lymphocyte count at birth and during the first years of infection can be normal, but eventually lymphopenia, resulting from a decrease in the total number of circulating CD4+ lymphocytes, develops. The T-suppressor CD8+ lymphocyte count usually increases initially, and CD8+ lymphocytes are not depleted until late in the course of infection. These changes in cell populations result in a decrease in the normal CD4+ to CD8+ lymphocyte ratio. This nonspecific finding, although characteristic of HIV infection, also occurs with other acute viral infections, including infections caused by CMV and Epstein-Barr virus.

Although the B-lymphocyte count remains normal or is somewhat increased, humoral immune dysfunction can precede and accompany cellular dysfunction. Increased serum Ig concentrations, particularly IgG and IgA, are manifestations of the humoral immune dysfunction and are not necessarily directed at specific pathogens of childhood. Specific antibody responses to antigens to which the patient has not been exposed previously usually are abnormal, and later in disease recall antibody responses are slow and diminish in magnitude. A small proportion (<10%) of patients will develop panhypogammaglobulinemia.

Treatment

Physicians are encouraged to participate actively in the care of HIV-infected patients in consultation with specialists who have expertise in the care of HIV-infected infants, children, and adolescents. Current treatment recommendations for HIV-infected children are available online (**www.aidsinfo.nih.gov**). When possible, enrollment of an HIV-infected child into available clinical trials should be encouraged. Information about trials for adolescents and children can be obtained by contacting the AIDS Clinical Trials Information Service.

Antiretroviral therapy is indicated for most HIV-infected children. Initiation of antiretroviral therapy depends on virologic, immunologic, and clinical criteria. Because HIV infection is a rapidly changing area, consultation with an expert in pediatric HIV infection is suggested. Many experts recommend initiating antiretroviral therapy for all HIV-infected children younger than 6 to 12 months as soon as infection is confirmed, regardless of clinical, immunologic, or virologic parameters. For children older than 1 year who are at low risk of disease progression (eg, have viral load <100 000 copies/mL, who are asymptomatic, and who have CD4+ T-lymphocyte percentages >25%), some experts would elect not to initiate therapy. Treatment of adolescents generally follows adult guidelines. In resource-limited settings, therapy is initiated, if available, for children younger than 18 months with CD4+ lymphocyte percentage less than 20% and at CD4+ lymphocyte percentage less than 15% for older children.

Combination antiretroviral therapy has been shown to be more effective than monotherapy. Data indicate that 3 antiretroviral drugs should be given whenever possible, including 2 nucleoside analogue reverse transcriptase inhibitors plus either a protease inhibitor or a nonnucleoside reverse transcriptase inhibitor (**www.aidsinfo.nih.gov**). Suppression of virus to undetectable concentrations is the desired goal. A change in antiretroviral therapy should be considered if there is evidence of disease progression (virologic, immunologic, or clinical), toxic effects or intolerance of drugs, or new data suggest the possibility of a superior regimen.

IGIV therapy has been recommended in combination with antiretroviral agents for HIV-infected children with hypogammaglobulinemia (IgG <400 mg/dL [4.0 g/L]).

Early diagnosis and aggressive treatment of opportunistic infections may prolong survival. For infants with possible or proven HIV infection, PCP prophylaxis should be administered beginning at 4 to 6 weeks of age and continued for the first year of life unless HIV infection is excluded. The need for PCP prophylaxis for HIV-infected children 1 year of age and older is determined by the degree of immunocompromise as determined by CD4+ T-lymphocyte counts.

Guidelines for prevention and treatment of opportunistic infections in children, adolescents, and adults provide indications for administration of drugs for infection with MAC, CMV, *T gondii*, and other organisms. Successful suppression of HIV replication to undetectable levels by HAART has resulted in a dramatic decrease in the occurrence of most opportunistic infections such as PCP, disseminated CMV infection, MAC infection, and serious bacterial infections and has resulted in relatively normal CD4+ and CD8+ lymphocyte counts. Many experts recommend discontinuing primary prophylaxis for *P jiroveci* infections in children older than 1 year with CD4+ lymphocyte percentages greater than 25% who are receiving stable combination antiretroviral therapy.

Immunization Recommendations. Children with HIV infection should be immunized as soon as is age appropriate with inactivated vaccines (diphtheria and tetanus toxoids and acellular pertussis, inactivated poliovirus, *Haemophilus influenzae* type b, hepatitis B virus, hepatitis A virus, and pneumococcal conjugate vaccine) as well as annually with influenza vaccine.

Measles-mumps-rubella (MMR) vaccine should be administered to HIV-infected children at 12 months of age unless the children are severely immunocompromised. The second dose of MMR vaccine may be administered as soon as 4 weeks after the first rather than waiting until school entry. Children receiving routine IGIV prophylaxis may not respond to MMR vaccine.

Children infected with HIV may be at increased risk of morbidity from varicella-zoster virus infection. Varicella vaccine should be administered to HIV-infected children 12 months of age or older with no or mild signs or symptoms of disease, age-specific CD4+ lymphocyte percentage 15% or greater, and no evidence of varicella immunity. Two doses should be given, with a 3-month interval between doses.

Hepatitis A vaccine is recommended for all children 12 to 23 months of age. The 2 doses in this series should be administered at least 6 months apart. Hepatitis B vaccine is recommended for adolescents who were not previously immunized.

In the United States and in areas of low prevalence of tuberculosis, bacille Calmette-Guérin (BCG) vaccine is not recommended. However, in economically developing countries where the prevalence of tuberculosis is high, the WHO recommends that BCG vaccine be given to all infants at birth if they are asymptomatic, regardless of maternal HIV infection. Disseminated BCG infection has occurred rarely in HIV-infected infants immunized with BCG vaccine.

Table 49.1
Zidovudine Regimen for Decreasing the Rate of Perinatal Transmission of Human Immunodeficiency Virus (HIV)[1]

Period	Route
During pregnancy, initiate anytime after wk 14 of gestation and continue throughout pregnancy[2]	Oral
During labor and delivery[3]	Intravenous
For the newborn infant, as soon as possible after birth[4]	Oral

[1] US Public Health Service. *Public Health Service Task Force Recommendations for Use of Antiretroviral Drugs in Pregnant HIV-1-Infected Women for Maternal Health and for Interventions to Reduce Perinatal HIV-1 Transmission in the United States.* Rockville, MD: AIDSInfo, Department of Health and Human Services; 2005. Information about other antiretroviral drugs for decreasing the rate of perinatal transmission of HIV can be found online (**www.aidsinfo.nih.gov**).
[2] Most women in developed countries are treated with potent combinations of 3 antiretroviral agents (highly active antiretroviral therapy [HAART]) started after the first trimester and continuing to delivery. Oral zidovudine can be used as part of that therapy.
[3] Recommended even for women treated with other antiretroviral agents during pregnancy. Intravenous zidovudine is administered for 3 hours before cesarean section.
[4] The effectiveness of antiretroviral agents for prevention of perinatal HIV-1 transmission decreases with delay in initiation after birth. Initiation of postexposure prophylaxis after the first 48 hours of life is not likely to be efficacious in preventing transmission.

Table 49.2
Laboratory Diagnosis of HIV Infection[1]

Test	Comment
HIV DNA PCR	Preferred test to diagnose HIV-1 infection in infants and children younger than 18 months; highly sensitive and specific by 2 weeks of age and available; performed on peripheral blood mononuclear cells. False negatives can occur.
HIV p24 Ag	Less sensitive, false-positive results during first month of life, variable results; not recommended.
ICD p24 Ag	Negative test result does not rule out infection; not recommended.
HIV culture	Expensive, not easily available, requires up to 4 weeks to do test; not recommended.
HIV RNA PCR	Not recommended for routine testing of infants and children younger than 18 months because a negative result cannot be used to exclude HIV infection definitively. Preferred test to identify non-B subtype HIV-1 infections.

[1] HIV indicates human immunodeficiency virus; PCR, polymerase chain reaction; Ag, antigen; and ICD, immune complex dissociated.

Figure 49.1

Perinatal AIDS Cases in the United States by Year of Diagnosis, 1985–2000

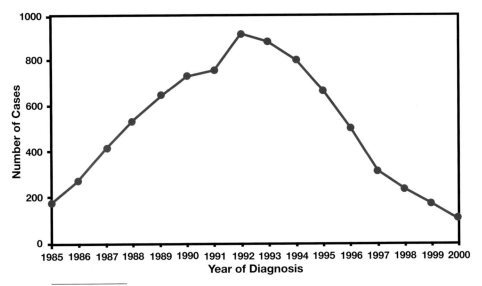

Data adjusted for reporting delays and for estimated proportional redistribution of cases reported without a risk; data reported through December 2001.

Courtesy of the Centers for Disease Control and Prevention.

Image 49.1
Bilateral parotid gland enlargement in an HIV-infected male child with lymphoid interstitial pneumonitis/pulmonary lymphoid hyperplasia. Note the presence of multiple lesions of molluscum contagiosum, which are commonly seen in patients with human immunodeficiency syndrome, particularly those with a low CD4+ lymphocyte count.

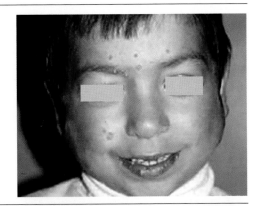

Image 49.2
Severe molluscum contagiosum in a boy with HIV infection. Some HIV-infected children develop molluscum contagiosum lesions that are unusually large or widespread. They are often seated more deeply in the epidermis.

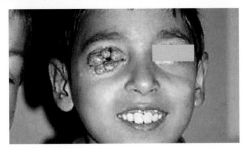

Image 49.3

This HIV-positive patient exhibited a chronic mucocutaneous herpes lesion for 1 month.

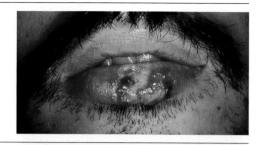

Image 49.4

Funduscopic examination of a 16-year-old female with HIV infection and CMV retinitis. There are extensive areas of hemorrhage, with white retinal exudates. Children with CMV retinitis usually present with painless visual impairment.

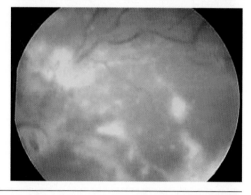

Image 49.5

Severe cutaneous warts (HPV infection) in a boy with HIV infection.

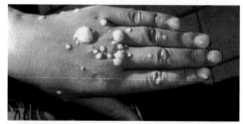

Image 49.6

CT scan of the brain of an 8-year-old boy with generalized brain atrophy. Cerebral atrophy is observed commonly among children with HIV-associated encephalopathy, but also can be observed among children who are normal neurologically and developmentally.

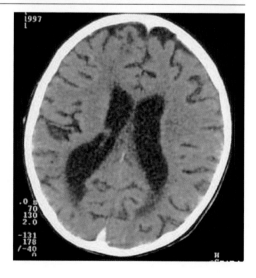

Image 49.7

A 7-year-old girl with HIV infection and a Kaposi sarcoma lesion. This tumor is rarely diagnosed among US children, with the occasional exceptions of children of Haitian descent with vertical HIV infection or older adolescents. Kaposi sarcoma has been linked to infection with a novel herpesvirus, now known as human herpesvirus 8 or Kaposi sarcoma–associated virus.

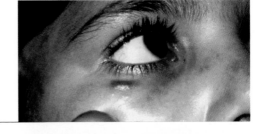

Image 49.8

Kaposi sarcoma of the ankle of a patient with HIV infection.

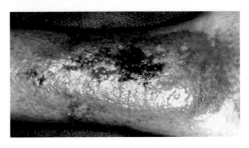

50

Influenza

Clinical Manifestations

Influenza classically is characterized by sudden onset of fever, often with chills or rigors, headache, malaise, diffuse myalgia, and nonproductive cough. Subsequently, the respiratory tract signs of sore throat, nasal congestion, rhinitis, and cough become more prominent. Conjunctival injection, abdominal pain, nausea, vomiting, and diarrhea are infrequent. In some children, influenza can appear as an upper respiratory tract infection or as a febrile illness with few respiratory tract signs. In infants, influenza can produce a sepsis-like picture or croup, bronchiolitis, or pneumonia. Acute myositis characterized by calf tenderness and refusal to walk can occur after several days of influenza illness, particularly with influenza B infection. Neurologic complications associated with influenza range from febrile seizures to severe encephalopathy and encephalitis with status epilepticus and altered consciousness that can result in neurologic sequelae and death. Myocarditis with fatal outcomes has been reported. Invasive secondary bacterial infection with respiratory tract pathogens, including group A streptococcus, *Staphylococcus aureus,* and *Streptococcus pneumoniae,* causing severe disease and death, can occur with influenza virus infection.

Etiology

Influenza viruses are orthomyxoviruses of types, A, B, and C. Epidemic disease is caused by influenza virus types A and B. Influenza A viruses are subclassified into subtypes by 2 surface antigens, hemagglutinin (HA) and neuraminidase (NA). Recent circulating human influenza A subtypes have included H1N1, H1N2, and H3N2 viruses. Specific antibodies to these various antigens, especially to HA, are important determinants of immunity.

Epidemiology

Influenza is spread from person to person primarily by droplets and also by direct contact with influenza-contaminated surfaces. During community outbreaks of influenza, the highest attack rates occur among school-aged children. Secondary spread to adults and other children within a family is common. Influenza is highly contagious, especially among semi-enclosed institutionalized populations. Patients can become infectious during the 24 hours before onset of symptoms. Viral shedding in nasal secretions usually peaks during the first 3 days of illness and ceases within 7 days but can be prolonged in young children and immunodeficient patients. Viral shedding correlates directly with height of fever. Incidence depends in part on immunity developed from recent influenza illness or immunization with the circulating influenza strain or a related strain. Minor antigenic variations within the same influenza B type or influenza A subtypes are called *antigenic drift.* Antigenic drift occurs continuously and results in new strains of influenza A and B viruses, leading to seasonal epidemics. Major changes leading to the emergence of influenza A viruses with a new HA in humans, such as H5 or H7, or new HA and new NA are called *antigenic shift.* Antigenic shift occurs only with influenza A viruses and can lead to pandemics if a strain can infect humans and efficiently be transmitted from person to person in a sustained manner; 3 pandemics occurred in the 20th century. In temperate climates, seasonal epidemics usually occur during winter months. Community outbreaks can last 4 to 8 weeks or longer. Circulation of 2 or 3 influenza virus strains in a community can be associated with a prolonged influenza season of 3 months or more and bimodal peaks in activity. Attack rates in healthy children have been estimated at 10% to 40% each year, with approximately 1% of infections resulting in hospitalization. The risk of lower respiratory tract disease complicating influenza infection in children, primarily pneumonia, croup, wheezing, and bronchiolitis, has ranged from 0.2% to 25%. Excess rates of hospitalization attributable to influenza virus infections occur in otherwise healthy children younger than 5 years, with rates in children younger than 2 years substantially higher than in children 2 years of age or older. Rates of hospitalization and morbidity attributable to complications, such as bronchiolitis and pneumonia, are even greater in children with hemoglobinopathies, bronchopulmonary dysplasia, asthma, cystic fibrosis, malignancy, diabetes mellitus, chronic renal disease, and congenital heart disease. Fatal outcomes, including sudden death, have been reported in both chronically ill and previously healthy children. In 2003 to 2004, nearly two thirds of influenza deaths occurred in children younger than 5 years and almost half had no known underlying condition.

Incubation Period

1 to 4 days (mean, 2 days).

Diagnostic Tests

Specimens for viral culture, immunofluorescent, or rapid diagnostic tests should be obtained during the first 72 hours of illness because the quantity of virus shed decreases rapidly from that point. Specimens of nasopharyngeal secretions obtained by swab, aspirate, or wash should be placed in appropriate transport media for culture. Virus usually can be isolated within 2 to 6 days. Rapid diagnostic tests for identification of influenza A and B antigens in respiratory tract specimens are available commercially, although their reported sensitivity (45%–90%) and specificity (60%–95%) compared with viral culture are variable and differ by test and specimen type. Rapid diagnostic tests should be interpreted in the context of the clinical findings and local community influenza activity because the prevalence of circulating influenza viruses influences the positive and negative predictive values of these influenza screening tests. False-positive results are more likely to occur during periods of low influenza activity; false-negative results are more likely to occur during peak influenza activity periods. Reverse transcriptase-PCR (RT-PCR) testing of respiratory tract specimens may be available at some institutions. Although RT-PCR testing has not been standardized, it offers potential for high sensitivity and specificity.

Treatment

Two classes of antiviral medications are available for therapy of influenza infections: adamantanes (ie, amantadine and rimantadine) and neuraminidase inhibitors (ie, zanamivir and oseltamivir). Amantadine and rimantadine are approved for treatment of influenza A virus infection in children 1 year of age and older and adults. Amantadine and rimantadine are also approved for chemoprophylaxis of influenza A. Studies indicate that treatment with either drug diminishes the signs and symptoms of influenza A infection and duration of illness by approximately 1 day when administered within 48 hours of onset of illness. Neither amantadine nor rimantadine is effective against influenza B infections.

However, in 2005 to 2006, the CDC reported that most influenza A (H3N2) strains tested were resistant to adamantanes and recommended against their use for treatment or prophylaxis for subsequent seasons if resistance persists. The NA inhibitors are approved for treatment of uncomplicated influenza A and B infection in patients within 2 days of onset of symptoms. The NA inhibitors are the only available antiviral agents with activity against influenza B viruses. Zanamivir is approved for treatment of influenza in people 7 years of age and older. Zanamivir is an inhaled powder formulation that is administered twice a day for 5 days. Zanamivir is not approved for chemoprophylaxis of influenza. In an efficacy trial in children 5 to 12 years of age, when therapy was instituted within 36 hours of onset, zanamivir decreased the duration of symptoms by 1 day, compared with placebo. Safety and efficacy have not been established in children with high-risk underlying medical conditions. Oseltamivir is used for treatment and chemoprophylaxis of influenza in people 1 year of age and older and is administered orally twice a day for 5 days. Oseltamivir is not approved for children younger than 12 months because of animal studies documenting neurotoxicity. Among children 1 to 12 years of age, oseltamivir treatment administered within 48 hours of illness onset decreased the duration of influenza symptoms by 1.5 days.

Therapy for influenza virus infection should be considered for (1) patients in whom shortening or amelioration of clinical symptoms can be particularly beneficial, such as children at increased risk of severe or complicated influenza infection; (2) healthy children with severe illness; and (3) people with special environmental, family, or social situations for which ongoing illness would be detrimental. Patients with any degree of renal insufficiency should be monitored for adverse events. Only zanamivir, which is administered by inhalation, does not require adjustment for people with severe renal insufficiency.

Control of fever with acetaminophen or other appropriate antipyretics may be important in young children because fever and other symptoms of influenza could exacerbate underlying chronic conditions.

Image 50.1
Influenza, like many viral infections, is spread by droplet transmission or direct contact with items recently contaminated by infected nasopharyngeal secretions.

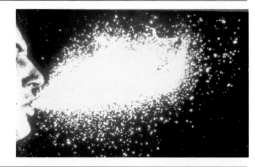

Image 50.2
This 4-year-old had high fever, poor oral intake, and lethargy; the chest radiograph shows bilateral peribronchial and right upper and middle lobe infiltrates caused by influenza A virus.

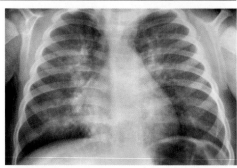

Image 50.3
Lateral view of the patient in Image 50.2 showing atelectasis of the right middle lobe and perihilar infiltrates.

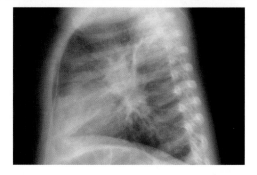

51

Kawasaki Disease
(Mucocutaneous Lymph Node Syndrome)

Clinical Manifestations

Kawasaki disease is a febrile, exanthematous, multisystem vasculitis of importance because approximately 20% of untreated children will develop coronary artery abnormalities. Most cases of Kawasaki disease occur in children between 1 and 8 years of age. The illness is characterized by fever and the following clinical features: (1) bilateral bulbar conjunctival injection without exudate; (2) erythematous mouth and pharynx, strawberry tongue, and red, cracked lips; (3) a polymorphous, generalized, erythematous rash that can be morbilliform, maculopapular, or scarlatiniform or can resemble erythema multiforme; (4) changes in the peripheral extremities consisting of induration of the hands and feet with erythematous palms and soles or periungual desquamation; and (5) acute, nonsuppurative cervical lymphadenopathy with at least one node 1.5 cm or greater in diameter. For diagnosis of classic Kawasaki disease, patients should have fever for at least 5 days and at least 4 of these 5 features and no alternative explanation for the findings. Irritability, abdominal pain, diarrhea, and vomiting commonly are associated features. Other findings include urethritis with sterile pyuria (70%), anterior uveitis (25%–50%), mild hepatic enzyme elevation (40%), arthritis or arthralgia (10%–20%), aseptic meningitis (25%), pericardial effusion (20%–40%), gallbladder hydrops (<10%), and myocarditis manifested by congestive heart failure (<5%). Fine desquamation in the groin area can occur in the acute phase of disease.

Incomplete Kawasaki disease can be diagnosed in febrile patients when fewer than 4 of 5 characteristic features are present. Incomplete Kawasaki disease is more common in infants younger than 12 months than in children older than 8 years. Infants with Kawasaki disease also have a higher risk of developing coronary artery aneurysms than do older children, making diagnosis and timely treatment especially important in infants. The laboratory findings of incomplete cases are similar to findings of classic cases. Therefore, although laboratory findings in Kawasaki disease are nonspecific, they can prove useful in increasing or decreasing the likelihood of incomplete Kawasaki disease. Early 2-dimensional echocardiographic study can be useful in evaluation of patients with suspected incomplete Kawasaki disease. A substantial number of children with Kawasaki disease and coronary artery abnormalities are not identified by the classic case definition. Incomplete Kawasaki disease should be considered in any child with unexplained fever for 5 days or more in association with 2 or more of the 5 principal features of this illness.

Without aspirin and IGIV therapy, fever can last 2 weeks or longer. After fever resolves, patients can remain anorectic or irritable for 2 to 3 weeks. During this phase, desquamation of the groin and then full-thickness desquamation of the fingers and toes and fine desquamation of other areas may occur. Recurrent disease occurring months to years later develops in less than 2% of patients.

Coronary artery abnormalities can be demonstrated by echocardiography in 20% to 25% of patients who are not treated within 10 days of onset of fever. Patients at increased risk of developing coronary artery aneurysms include males, infants younger than 12 months, children older than 8 years, fever for more than 10 days, higher baseline neutrophil and band counts or lower hemoglobin concentrations (<10 g/dL) at presentation, and children with a baseline platelet count less than 350 000/μL or fever persisting after IGIV administration. Aneurysms of the coronary arteries have been demonstrated as soon as a few days after onset of illness but more typically occur between 1 and 4 weeks after onset; their appearance later than 6 weeks is uncommon. Giant coronary artery aneurysms (≥8 mm in diameter) are likely to be associated with long-term complications. Aneurysms occurring in other medium-sized arteries (eg, iliac, femoral, renal, and axillary vessels) are uncommon and generally do not occur in the absence of coronary abnormalities. In addition to coronary artery disease, carditis can involve the pericardium, myocardium, or endocardium, and mitral and aortic regurgitation can develop. Carditis generally resolves when fever resolves.

In children with mild coronary artery dilation or ectasia, coronary artery dimensions often return to baseline within 6 to 8 weeks after onset of disease. Approximately 50% of non-giant coronary aneurysms regress to normal luminal size within 1 to 2 years, although this process can be accompanied by coronary stenosis. The current case fatality rate in the United States is less than 0.1% to 0.2%. The principal cause of death is myocardial infarction resulting from coronary artery occlusion attributable to thrombosis or progressive stenosis. Rarely, a large coronary artery aneurysm can rupture. Most fatalities occur within 6 weeks of the onset of symptoms, but myocardial infarction and sudden death can occur months to years after the acute episode. There is hypothetical concern that the vasculitis of Kawasaki disease may predispose to premature atherosclerotic disease.

Etiology

The cause is unknown. Epidemiologic and clinical features suggest an infectious cause.

Epidemiology

Peak age of occurrence in the United States is between 18 and 24 months. Fifty percent of patients are younger than 2 years, and 80% are younger than 5 years. In children younger than 6 months, the diagnosis often is delayed because of atypical symptoms. The prevalence of coronary artery abnormalities is higher when treatment is delayed beyond 10 days. The male-female ratio is approximately 1.5:1. The incidence is highest in Asian people; 3000 to 5000 cases are estimated to occur annually in the United States. A pattern of steady or increasing endemic disease with occasional sharply defined community-wide epidemics has been recognized in diverse locations in North America and Hawaii. Epidemics generally occur during winter and spring. No evidence indicates person-to-person or common-source spread, although the incidence is slightly higher in siblings of children with the disease.

Incubation Period

Unknown.

Diagnostic Tests

No specific diagnostic test is available. The diagnosis is established by fulfillment of the clinical criteria and exclusion of other possible illnesses, such as measles, parvovirus B19 infection, adenovirus or enterovirus infections, streptococcal infection (ie, scarlet fever), rickettsial exanthems, drug reactions (eg, Stevens-Johnson syndrome), staphylococcal scalded skin syndrome, toxic shock syndrome, leptospirosis, juvenile idiopathic arthritis, polyarteritis nodosa, and Reiter syndrome. An increased sedimentation rate and serum C-reactive protein concentration during the first 2 weeks of illness and an increased platelet count (>450 000/μL [>450×10^9/L]) after the first week of illness are almost universal laboratory features. These values usually normalize within 6 to 8 weeks.

Treatment

Management during the acute phase is directed at decreasing inflammation of the myocardium and coronary artery wall and providing supportive care. Therapy should be initiated when the diagnosis is established or strongly suspected. Once the acute phase has passed, therapy is directed at prevention of coronary artery thrombosis. Specific recommendations for therapy include the following measures:

IGIV. Therapy with high-dose IGIV and aspirin initiated within 10 days of the onset of fever substantially decreases progression to coronary artery dilation and aneurysms at 2 to 7 weeks, compared with treatment with aspirin alone, and results in more rapid resolution of fever and other indicators of acute inflammation. The optimal therapeutic dose of IGIV is unknown. A dose of 2 g/kg as a single dose, given over 10 to 12 hours, is recommended. Few complications occur from this regimen. Therapy with IGIV should be initiated as soon as possible; its efficacy when initiated later than the 10th day of illness or after aneurysms have been detected has not been evaluated. However, therapy with IGIV and aspirin should be provided for patients diagnosed after day 10 who have manifestations of continuing inflammation (eg, fever or other symptoms or laboratory abnormalities) or of evolving coronary artery disease. Despite prompt treatment with IGIV and aspirin, 2% to 4% of patients develop coronary artery abnormalities.

Aspirin. Aspirin is used for anti-inflammatory and antithrombotic actions. Aspirin is administered in doses of 80 to 100 mg/kg per day in 4 divided doses during the acute phase. Children with acute Kawasaki disease have decreased aspirin absorption and increased clearance, so some children may not achieve therapeutic serum concentrations. It is not necessary to monitor aspirin concentrations. After fever is controlled for 4 or 5 days (eg, day 10–14 of illness), the aspirin dose is decreased to 3 to 5 mg/kg per day to continue antithrombotic activity. Aspirin is discontinued if no coronary artery abnormalities have been detected by 6 to 8 weeks after onset of illness. Low-dose aspirin therapy should be continued indefinitely for people in whom coronary artery abnormalities are present.

Cardiac Care. The care of patients with carditis should involve a cardiologist experienced in management of patients with Kawasaki disease and in assessing echocardiographic studies of coronary arteries in children. Long-term management of Kawasaki disease should be based on the extent of coronary artery involvement. Children should be assessed during the first 2 months to detect evidence of arrhythmias, congestive heart failure, and valvular regurgitation.

Re-treatment. Approximately 5% to 10% of patients who receive IGIV and aspirin therapy have persistent fever or recurrence of fever after an initial period of being afebrile for 48 hours or less. In these situations, re-treatment with IGIV (2 g/kg) and continued high-dose aspirin therapy may be indicated. *Subsequent Immunization.* Measles and varicella immunizations should be deferred for 11 months after IGIV administration in children who have received high-dose IGIV for treatment of Kawasaki disease. The schedule for subsequent administration of other childhood immunizations should not be interrupted. Yearly influenza immunization is indicated for children 6 months of age and older who require long-term aspirin therapy because of the possible increased risk of developing Reye syndrome.

Image 51.1
Child with Kawasaki disease with conjunctivitis. Note the absence of conjunctival discharge.

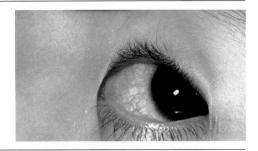

Image 51.2
Erythematous lips and injection of the oropharyngeal membranes in a patient with Kawasaki disease. Scarlet fever, toxic shock syndrome, staphylococcal scalded skin syndrome, and measles may be confused with this disease.

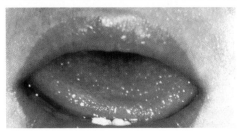

Image 51.3

Characteristic distribution of erythroderma of Kawasaki disease. The rash is accentuated in the perineal area in approximately two thirds of patients.

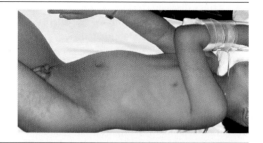

Image 51.4

Generalized erythema and early perianal and palmar desquamation.

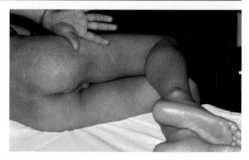

Image 51.5

Erythroderma of the palm of the hand of the child in Image 51.4 with Kawasaki disease.

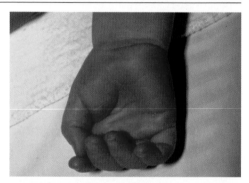

Image 51.6

A child with the characteristic desquamation of the hands in a later stage of Kawasaki disease.

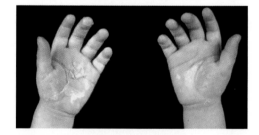

Image 51.7

Desquamation of the skin of the toes following Kawasaki disease in a 4-year-old male.

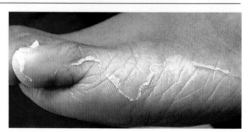

52

Leishmaniasis

Clinical Manifestations

The 3 major clinical syndromes are cutaneous, mucosal, and visceral.

Cutaneous leishmaniasis occurs after inoculation by the bite of an infected female phlebotomine sand fly (approximately 2–3 mm long) when parasites proliferate locally, leading to an erythematous papule, which typically evolves to become a nodule and then a shallow ulcerative lesion with raised borders. Lesions can persist as nodules or papules, and commonly are located on exposed body areas (eg, face and extremities) sometimes accompanied by satellite lesions, which appear as sporotrichoid-like nodules. Clinical manifestations of Old World and New World (American) cutaneous leishmaniasis are similar. Spontaneous resolution of lesions can take weeks to years and usually results in a flat atrophic (cigarette paper) scar.

Mucosal leishmaniasis (espundia) can become clinically evident from months to years after the cutaneous lesions heal; sometimes mucosal and cutaneous lesions are noted simultaneously. Parasites may disseminate to the nasooropharyngeal mucosa. In some patients, granulomatous ulceration follows, leading to facial disfigurement, secondary infection, and mucosal perforation, which may occur months to years after the initial cutaneous lesion heals.

Visceral leishmaniasis (kala-azar) occurs following cutaneous inoculation of parasites and spread throughout the mononuclear macrophage system to spleen, liver, and bone marrow. The resulting clinical illness typically manifests as fever, anorexia, weight loss, splenomegaly, hepatomegaly, lymphadenopathy (in some geographic areas), anemia, leukopenia, thrombocytopenia sometimes associated with hemorrhage, hypoalbuminemia, and hypergammaglobulinemia. Secondary gram-negative enteric and mycobacterial infections are common (eg, tuberculosis). Untreated visceral infection nearly always is fatal. Reactivation of latent visceral infection can occur in patients who become immunocompromised, including people with concurrent HIV infection and recipients of stem cell or solid organ transplants.

Etiology

In humans, *Leishmania* species are obligate intracellular parasites of mononuclear phagocytes. Cutaneous leishmaniasis typically is caused by *Leishmania tropica, Leishmania major,* and *Leishmania aethiopica* (Old World species) and by *Leishmania mexicana, Leishmania amazonensis, Leishmania braziliensis, Leishmania panamensis, Leishmania guyanensis,* and *Leishmania peruviana* (New World species). Mucosal leishmaniasis typically is caused by *L braziliensis, L panamensis,* and *L guyanensis.* Visceral leishmaniasis is caused by *Leishmania donovani, Leishmania infantum,* and *Leishmania chagasi,* which also can cause cutaneous leishmaniasis. Children with typical cutaneous leishmaniasis caused by these organisms rarely develop visceral leishmaniasis.

Epidemiology

Leishmaniasis is a zoonosis with a variety of mammalian reservoirs, including canines and rodents. The vectors are female phlebotomine sand flies. There are 88 countries worldwide with endemic leishmaniasis. Leishmaniasis is endemic from northern Argentina to southern Texas (not including Uruguay or Chile), in southern Europe, Asia (not southeast Asia), the Middle East, and Africa (particularly East and North Africa, with sporadic cases elsewhere) but not in Australia or Oceania. The estimated number of people at risk of infection is approximately 350 million with approximately 500 000 new cases annually. More than 90% of cases worldwide occur in Bangladesh, northeastern India, Nepal, and Sudan (Old World) and in northeastern Brazil (New World). The estimated annual number of new cases of cutaneous leishmaniasis is approximately 1 to 5 million; more than 90% of worldwide cases are in Afghanistan, Algeria, Iran, Iraq, Saudi Arabia, and Syria (Old World) and in Brazil and Peru (New World). Geographic distribution of cases evaluated in the developed world reflects travel and immigration patterns.

Incubation Period

Several days to months.

Diagnostic Tests

Definitive diagnosis is made by demonstration of the presence of the parasite. A common way of identifying the parasite is by microscopic identification of intracellular leishmanial organisms on Wright- or Giemsa-stained smears or histologic sections of infected tissues. In cutaneous disease, tissue can be obtained by a 3-mm punch biopsy, by lesion scrapings, or by needle aspiration of the raised non-necrotic edge of the lesion. In visceral leishmaniasis, the organisms can be identified in the spleen and, less commonly, in bone marrow and liver. In East Africa in patients with lymphadenopathy, the organisms can be identified in lymph nodes. Blood cultures, especially of buffy coat preparations, have been positive in some patients, and organisms sometimes can be observed in blood smears or observed in or cultured from buffy coat preparations in HIV-infected patients.

The diagnosis of some forms of leishmaniasis can be aided by performance of serologic testing, which is available at the CDC. Serologic test results usually are positive in cases of visceral and mucosal leishmaniasis if the patient is immunocompetent but often are negative in cutaneous leishmaniasis. False-positive results may occur in patients with other infectious diseases, especially American trypanosomiasis.

Treatment

Treatment always is indicated for patients with mucosal or visceral leishmaniasis. Treatment of cutaneous leishmaniasis should be considered, especially if skin lesions are or could become disfiguring (eg, facial lesions or disabling lesions near joints), are persistent, or are known to be or might be caused by leishmanial species that can disseminate to the naso-oropharyngeal mucosa.

Image 52.1
Leishmania organisms in a peripheral blood smear from a young man with HIV infection who had visited a jungle in Central America.

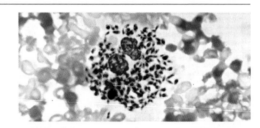

Image 52.2
Cutaneous leishmaniasis, as in this boy from India, seldom disseminates. Multiple organisms usually can be found on biopsy of the border of a lesion.

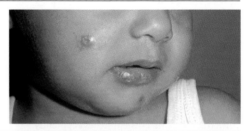

Image 52.3
Leishmaniasis of forearm with severe cutaneous involvement.

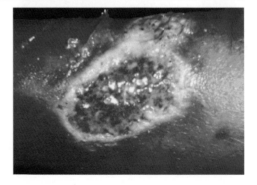

53

Leprosy

Clinical Manifestations

Leprosy (Hansen disease) infection mainly involves skin, peripheral nerves, mucosa of the upper respiratory tract, and testes. The clinical syndromes of leprosy represent a spectrum that reflects the cellular immune response to *Mycobacterium leprae* and its unique tropism for peripheral nerves. The 2 leprosy syndromes are tuberculoid and lepromatous forms. Characteristic features include the following:

- *Tuberculoid:* One or a few well-demarcated, hypopigmented or erythematous, hypoesthetic or anesthetic skin lesions, often with raised, active, spreading edges and central clearing. Cell-mediated immune responses are intact.

- *Lepromatous:* Initial numerous, ill-defined, hypopigmented, or erythematous maculae that progress to papules, nodules, or plaques; and late-occurring hypoesthesia. Dermal infiltration of the face, hands, and feet in bilateral, symmetric distribution can occur without preceding maculopapular lesions. *M leprae*–specific, cell-mediated immunity is diminished greatly, but serum antibody responses to *M leprae*–derived antigens can occur, or titers of nonspecific antibodies (such as rheumatoid factor or syphilis [on nontreponemal tests]) can be increased.

The cell-mediated immunity of most patients, and their clinical presentation, occurs between these 2 extremes. Leprosy rashes usually do not itch or hurt; they lack sensation to heat, touch, and pain. The classic presentation of the "leonine facies" and loss of lateral eyebrows (medarosis) occurs in patients with end-stage lepromatous leprosy. A simplified scheme introduced by the WHO classifies leprosy involving 1 to 5 patches of skin as paucibacillary and leprosy involving more than 5 patches as multibacillary.

Serious consequences of leprosy occur from immune reactions and nerve involvement with resulting anesthesia, which can lead to repeated unrecognized trauma, ulcerations, fractures, and bone resorption. Leprosy should be considered in any patient with a hypoesthetic or anesthetic skin rash.

Etiology

Leprosy is caused by *M leprae,* an obligate intracellular, acid-fast bacillus that can be Gram-stain variable.

Epidemiology

Leprosy primarily is a disease of poverty and rural residency. Approximately 95% of people are immune genetically to infection with *M leprae.* Accordingly, spouses of leprosy patients are not likely to develop leprosy, but biological parents, children, and siblings who are household contacts of untreated patients with leprosy are at increased risk. The major source of infectious material probably is nasal secretions from patients with untreated or drug-resistant infection. Little shedding of *M leprae* from involved intact skin occurs. In 2004, 105 new cases of leprosy were reported in the United States. Native-born US citizens with leprosy predominantly were from Texas, Louisiana, New York, and California. Foreign-born patients with leprosy (>80% of reported cases) emigrated predominantly from Mexico, India, the Dominican Republic, Brazil, and the Philippines. The infectivity of lepromatous patients probably ceases after treatment is instituted, often within a few days or weeks of initiating rifampin or approximately 3 months after initiating dapsone or clofazimine. Contaminated soil or insect vectors may play a role in disease transmission.

Incubation Period

1 to many years (usually 3–5 years); tuberculoid tends to be shorter.

Diagnostic Tests

Histopathologic examination is the best method of establishing the diagnosis and is the basis for classification of leprosy. Skin biopsies should be stained with hematoxylin-eosin and Fite-Faraco stains. Acid-fast bacilli can be found in slit-smears or biopsy specimens of skin lesions but rarely from patients with the tuberculoid and indeterminate forms of disease. Organisms have not been cultured successfully in vitro.

A PCR test for *M leprae* is available on a limited basis. No serologic test is available for routine diagnosis of leprosy.

Treatment

Therapy for patients with leprosy should be undertaken in consultation with an expert in leprosy. The National Hansen's Disease Programs (call 225/756-3701 for clinical information) provides consultation on clinical and pathologic issues and can provide information.

The primary goal of therapy is prevention of permanent nerve damage, which can be accomplished by early diagnosis and treatment. Combination antimicrobial therapy called multidrug therapy (MDT) can be obtained free of charge in the United States from the National Hansen's Disease Programs. It is important to treat *M leprae* infections with more than 1 antimicrobial agent to minimize development of antimicrobial-resistant organisms. Adults with multibacillary leprosy are treated with dapsone, rifampin, and clofazimine. As of November 1, 2005, clofazimine

is available in the United States only under an investigational new drug protocol. Clofazimine is not available for administration to children and pregnant women. Paucibacillary leprosy should be treated with dapsone and rifampin.

Before beginning antimicrobial therapy, patients should be tested for glucose-6-phosphate dehydrogenase deficiency, have baseline complete blood cell counts and liver function tests documented, and be evaluated for any evidence of tuberculosis infection, especially if the patient is infected with HIV. This consideration is important to avoid monotherapy of active tuberculosis with rifampin while treating active leprosy.

Relapse of disease after completing MDT is rare (0.01%–0.14% of patients with Hansen disease) and may present as new skin patches with loss of skin sensation. Relapse usually is attributable to reactivation of drug-susceptible organisms. People with relapses of disease require another course of MDT.

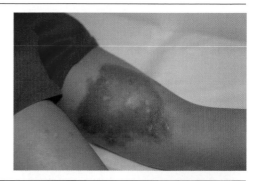

Image 53.1
Hansen disease. A young Vietnamese boy who spent 2 years in a refugee camp in the Philippines presented with the nodular violaceous skin lesion shown. The results of a biopsy of the lesion showed acid-fast organisms surrounding blood vessels. A diagnosis of lepromatous leprosy was made and the child was treated with a multidrug regimen.

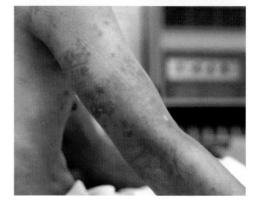

Image 53.2
Erythema nodosum leprosum in a 29-year-old Asian man.

Image 53.3
Erythema nodosum in the same patient as in Image 53.2.

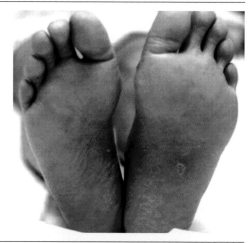

Image 53.4
Lepromatous leprosy in an Asian man. Newly diagnosed cases are considered contagious until treatment is established and should be reported to local and state public health departments.

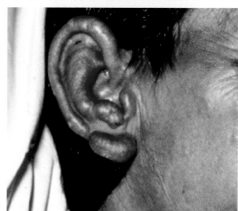

Image 53.5
An adult male with lepromatous leprosy.

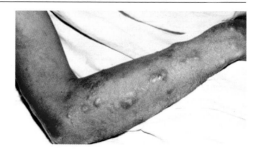

54

Leptospirosis

Clinical Manifestations

Leptospirosis is an acute febrile disease with varied manifestations resulting from generalized vasculitis. The severity of disease ranges from self-limited systemic illness (approximately 90% of patients) to life-threatening illness with jaundice, renal failure, and hemorrhagic pneumonitis. Regardless of its severity, onset usually is characterized by nonspecific symptoms, including fever, chills, headache, nausea, vomiting, and a transient rash. The most distinct clinical findings are conjunctival suffusion without purulent discharge (30%–40%) and myalgias of the calf and lumbar regions (80%). This initial "septicemic" phase usually lasts for 3 to 7 days and can be followed by a second "immune-mediated" phase. In some patients, these 2 phases are separated by a short-lived abatement of fever (1–3 days). Findings commonly associated with the immune-mediated phase include fever, aseptic meningitis, conjunctival suffusion, uveitis, muscle tenderness, adenopathy, and purpuric rash. Approximately 10% of patients have severe illness, including jaundice and renal dysfunction (Weil syndrome), hemorrhagic pneumonitis, cardiac arrhythmias, or circulatory collapse associated with a case fatality rate of 5% to 40%. The overall duration of symptoms for both phases of disease varies from less than 1 week to several months.

Etiology

Leptospirosis is caused by spirochetes of the genus *Leptospira*. Leptospires are classified into a number of species defined by their degree of genetic relatedness as determined by DNA reassociation. There are 13 named pathogenic and nonpathogenic species.

Epidemiology

The reservoirs for *Leptospira* species include a wide range of wild and domestic animals that may remain asymptomatic shedders for years. *Leptospira* organisms excreted in animal urine, amniotic fluid, or placental tissue are viable in soil or water for weeks to months. Humans become infected through contact of mucosal surfaces or abraded skin with contaminated soil, water, or animal tissues. People who are predisposed by occupation include abattoir and sewer workers, veterinarians, farmers, and military personnel. Recreational exposures and clusters of disease have been associated with wading, swimming (especially swallowing water), or boating in contaminated water, particularly during flooding. Person-to-person transmission is rare.

Incubation Period

5 to 14 days (range, 2–30 days).

Diagnostic Tests

Leptospira organisms can be isolated from blood or CSF specimens during the early septicemic phase of illness and from urine specimens after 7 to 10 days of illness. Isolation of the organism can be very difficult. Serum specimens always should be obtained to facilitate serologic diagnosis. Antibodies usually develop during the second week of illness and can be measured by commercially available immunoassays; increases in antibody titer can be delayed or absent in some patients. Microscopic agglutination, the confirmatory serologic test, is performed only in reference laboratories. Immunohistochemical techniques can detect leptospiral antigens in infected tissues.

Treatment

Intravenous penicillin is the drug of choice for patients requiring hospitalization. Penicillin G decreases the duration of systemic symptoms and the persistence of associated laboratory abnormalities. As with other spirochete infections, a Jarisch-Herxheimer reaction (an acute febrile reaction accompanied by headache, myalgia, and an aggravated clinical picture lasting <24 hours) can develop after initiation of penicillin therapy. For patients with mild disease, oral doxycycline has been shown to shorten the course of illness. Doxycycline should not be used in pregnant women or children younger than 8 years because of the risk of dental staining. Ceftriaxone is an alternative therapy.

Image 54.1

Leptospirosis rash in an adolescent male that shows the generalized vasculitis caused by this infection.

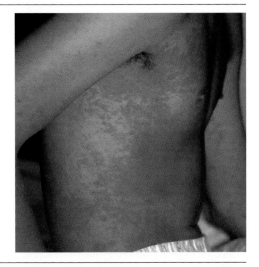

Image 54.2

A: Renal biopsy shows inflammatory cell infiltrate in the interstitium and focal denudation of tubular epithelial cells (hematoxylin-eosin, 100x). B: Immunostaining of fragmented leptospire (arrowhead) and granular form of bacterial antigens (arrows) (158x).

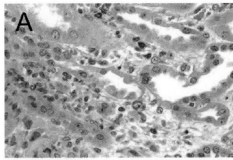

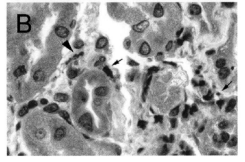

55

Listeria monocytogenes Infections

(Listeriosis)

Clinical Manifestations

Listeriosis is a severe but relatively uncommon infection that is primarily food-borne and occurs most frequently among people who are older, pregnant, or immunocompromised. Infections are categorized as maternal, neonatal, or childhood with or without associated predisposing conditions. Maternal infections can be associated with an influenza-like illness, fever, malaise, headache, gastrointestinal tract symptoms, and back pain. Approximately 65% of women experience a symptomatic prodromal illness before the diagnosis of listeriosis in their fetus or newborn infant. Amnionitis during labor, brown staining of amniotic fluid, or asymptomatic perinatal infection can occur. Neonatal illnesses have early-onset and late-onset syndromes similar to those of group B streptococcal infections. Prematurity, pneumonia, and septicemia are common in early-onset disease. An erythematous rash with small, pale nodules characterized histologically by granulomas can occur in severe newborn infection and is termed "granulomatosis infantisepticum." Late-onset infections occur after the first week of life and usually result in meningitis. Infection occurs most commonly in the perinatal period. Clinical features for which listeriosis should be considered outside the neonatal period or pregnancy are (1) meningitis or parenchymal brain infection in immunocompromised hosts, patients with hepatic or renal disease, or people older than 50 years; (2) meningitis and parenchymal brain infection together; and (3) subcortical brain abscess. *Listeria monocytogenes* rarely causes diffuse encephalitis, rhombencephalitis (brain stem encephalitis), brain abscess, and endocarditis. Outbreaks caused by contaminated food usually are characterized clinically by fever and diarrhea.

Etiology

L monocytogenes is an aerobic, nonspore–forming, motile, gram-positive bacillus that produces a narrow zone of hemolysis on blood agar medium.

Epidemiology

L monocytogenes is distributed widely in the environment and is an important cause of zoonoses, especially in herd animals. Food-borne transmission causes outbreaks and sporadic infections. Incriminated foods include unpasteurized milk and soft cheeses; prepared ready-to-eat meats, such as hot dogs, deli meat, and pâté; undercooked poultry; and unwashed raw vegetables. Fecal or vaginal carriage in pregnant women can result in sporadic neonatal disease from transplacental or ascending routes of infection or from exposure during delivery. Maternal infection is associated with abortion, preterm delivery, and fetal death. Late-onset neonatal infection can result from acquisition of the organism during passage through the birth canal or from environmental sources, followed by hematogenous invasion of the organism from the intestine.

Incubation Period

1 day to more than 3 weeks.

Diagnostic Tests

The organism can be recovered on blood agar media from cultures of blood, CSF, meconium, gastric washings, placental tissue, amniotic fluid, and other infected tissue specimens, including joint, pleural, or pericardial fluid. Gram stain of gastric aspirate material, placental tissue, biopsy specimens of the rash of early-onset infection, or CSF from an infected patient can demonstrate the organism. *L monocytogenes* can be mistaken for a contaminant or saprophyte because of its morphologic similarity to diphtheroids and streptococci.

Treatment

Initial therapy with intravenous ampicillin and an aminoglycoside, usually gentamicin, is recommended for severe infections. This combination is more effective than ampicillin alone in vitro and in animal models of *L mono-cytogenes* infection. In immunocompetent hosts, ampicillin alone can be given once a favorable clinical response has occurred or for patients with mild infections. For the penicillin-allergic patient, the alternative regimen is trimethoprim-sulfamethoxazole. Cephalosporins are not active against *L monocytogenes*.

Image 55.1
CSF shows characteristic gram-positive rods (Gram stain). Listeriosis is much more common among patients with HIV infection or AIDS compared with the general population.

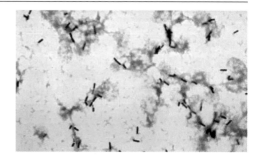

56

Lyme Disease
(Lyme borreliosis, *Borrelia burgdorferi* Infection)

Clinical Manifestations

The clinical manifestations of Lyme disease are divided into 3 stages: early localized, early disseminated, and late disease. Early localized disease is characterized by a distinctive rash, *erythema migrans,* at the site of a recent tick bite. Erythema migrans begins as a red macule or papule that usually expands over days to weeks to form a large, annular, erythematous lesion that may increase in size to 5 cm or more in diameter, sometimes with partial central clearing. The lesion usually is painless and not pruritic. Localized erythema migrans can vary greatly in size and shape and can have vesicular or necrotic areas in its center and can be confused with cellulitis. Fever, malaise, headache, mild neck stiffness, myalgia, and arthralgia often accompany the rash of early localized disease.

Early disseminated disease manifests most commonly as multiple erythema migrans in approximately 15% of patients. This rash usually occurs several weeks after an infective tick bite and consists of secondary annular, erythematous lesions similar to, but usually smaller than, the primary lesion. These lesions reflect spirochetemia with cutaneous dissemination. Other common manifestations of early disseminated illness (that may occur with or without rash) are palsies of the cranial nerves (especially cranial nerve VII), lymphocytic meningitis, and conjunctivitis. Systemic symptoms, such as arthralgia, myalgia, headache, and fatigue, also are common during the early disseminated stage. Carditis, which usually is characterized by various degrees of heart block, occurs rarely in children. Among infected children who do not receive antimicrobial therapy, approximately 50% develop arthritis, approximately 10% develop CNS disease, and fewer than 5% develop cardiac involvement. Some individuals with early Lyme disease can have concurrent human granulocytic ehrlichiosis or babesiosis, transmitted by the same tick, which may contribute to symptomatology.

Late disease is characterized most commonly by recurrent arthritis that usually is pauciarticular and affects large joints, particularly knees. Arthritis can occur without a history of earlier stages of illness (including erythema migrans). Peripheral neuropathy and CNS manifestations also can occur rarely during late disease. Late disease is uncommon in children who are treated with antimicrobial agents in the early stage of disease.

Because congenital infection occurs with other spirochetal infections, there has been concern that an infected pregnant woman could transmit *Borrelia burgdorferi* to her fetus. No causal relationship between maternal Lyme disease and abnormalities of pregnancy or congenital disease caused by *B burgdorferi* has been documented conclusively. No evidence exists that Lyme disease can be transmitted via human milk.

Etiology

In the United States, infection is caused by the spirochete *B burgdorferi*.

Epidemiology

Lyme disease occurs primarily in 3 distinct geographic regions of the United States. Most cases occur in southern New England and in the eastern mid-Atlantic states. The disease also occurs, but with lower frequency, in the upper Midwest, especially Wisconsin and Minnesota, and less commonly on the West Coast, especially northern California. The occurrence of cases in the United States correlates with the distribution and frequency of infected tick vectors—*Ixodes scapularis* in the East and Midwest and *Ixodes pacificus* in the West. Reported cases from states without known enzootic risks may have been acquired in states with endemic infection or may be misdiagnoses resulting from false-positive serologic test results. Rash similar to erythema migrans has been reported in states without endemic infection, possibly attributable to other *Borrelia* species harbored in the Lone Star tick. Most cases occur between April and October; more than 50% of cases occur during June and July. People of all ages may be affected, but incidence in the United States is highest among children 5 to 9 years of age and adults 45 to 54 years of age.

Incubation Period

1 to 55 days (median, 11 days); late manifestations occur months to years later.

Diagnostic Tests

During the early stages of Lyme disease, the diagnosis is best made clinically by recognizing the characteristic rash, a singular lesion of erythema migrans, because antibodies against *B burgdorferi* are not detectable in most individuals within the first few weeks after infection. Diagnosis in patients who possibly have early disseminated or late Lyme disease should be based on clinical findings and serologic tests. Some patients treated with antimicrobial agents for early Lyme disease never develop antibodies against *B burgdorferi*. However, most patients with early disseminated disease and virtually all patients with late disease have antibodies against *B burgdorferi*. Once such antibodies develop, they persist for many years and perhaps for life. Consequently, tests for antibodies should not be used to assess the success of treatment. The results of serologic tests for Lyme disease should be interpreted with careful consideration of the clinical setting and the quality of the testing laboratory.

A 2-step approach is recommended for serologic diagnosis of *B burgdorferi*. First, a screening test for serum antibodies should be performed using a sensitive enzyme immunoassay (EIA) or immunofluorescent antibody assay (IFA). Serum specimens that give positive or equivocal results should then be tested by a standardized Western immunoblot for presence of antibodies to *B burgdorferi*; serum specimens that yield negative results by EIA or IFA do not require immunoblot testing. When testing to confirm early disease, IgG and IgM immunoblot assays should be performed. To confirm late disease, only an IgG immunoblot assay should be performed, because false-positive results may occur with the IgM immunoblot. A positive result of an IgG immunoblot test requires detection of antibody ("bands") to 5 or more of the following: 18, 23/24, 28, 30, 39, 41, 45, 60, 66, and

93 kDa polypeptides. A positive test result of IgM immunoblot requires detection of antibody to at least 2 of the 23/24, 39, and 41 kDa polypeptides. Two-step testing is needed because EIA and IFA can yield false-positive results because of the presence of antibodies directed against spirochetes in normal oral flora that cross-react with antigens of *B burgdorferi* or to cross-reactive antibodies in patients with other spirochetal infections (eg, syphilis, leptospirosis, relapsing fever), certain viral infections (eg, varicella, Epstein-Barr virus), or certain autoimmune diseases (eg, systemic lupus erythematosus).

Suspected CNS Lyme disease can be confirmed by demonstration of intrathecal production of antibodies against *B burgdorferi*. However, interpretation of results of antibody tests of CSF is complex, and advice from a specialist experienced in the management of patients with Lyme disease should assist in interpreting results.

The widespread practice of ordering serologic tests for patients with nonspecific symptoms, such as fatigue or arthralgia, who have a low probability of having Lyme disease is not recommended. Almost all positive serologic test results in these patients are false-positive results.

Treatment

Early Localized Disease. Doxycycline is the drug of choice for children 8 years of age and older and, unlike amoxicillin, also treats patients with ehrlichiosis. For children younger than 8 years, amoxicillin is recommended. For patients who are allergic to penicillin, the alternative drug is cefuroxime. Erythromycin and azithromycin are less effective. Treatment of erythema migrans almost always prevents development of later stages of Lyme disease. Erythema migrans usually resolves within several days of initiating treatment, but other signs and symptoms may persist for several weeks, even in successfully treated patients.

Early Disseminated and Late Disease. Orally administered antimicrobial agents are recommended for treating multiple erythema migrans and uncomplicated Lyme arthritis. Most experts also recommend oral agents for treatment of facial nerve palsy and do not recommend a lumbar puncture unless other CNS involvement, such as signs or symptoms of meningitis or raised intracranial pressure, are present. If CSF pleocytosis is found, parenterally administered antimicrobial therapy is indicated. Recurrent or persistent arthritis after treatment with a course of oral antibiotic therapy and CNS infection should be treated with parenterally administered antimicrobial agents. The optimal duration of therapy for manifestations of early disseminated or late disease is not well established, but there is no evidence that children with any manifestation of Lyme disease benefit from prolonged courses of orally or parenterally administered antimicrobial agents.

The Jarisch-Herxheimer reaction (an acute febrile reaction accompanied by headache, myalgia, and an aggravated clinical picture lasting <24 hours) can occur when therapy is initiated. Nonsteroidal anti-inflammatory agents may be beneficial, and the antimicrobial agent should be continued.

Image 56.1
Erythema migrans lesion at the site of a tick bite characteristic of early, localized Lyme disease. It is annular with central clearing (ie, a target lesion). Systemic symptoms, such as fever, myalgia, headache, or malaise, can occur with infection.

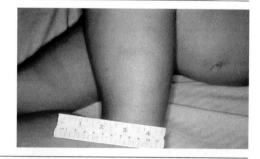

Image 56.2
The rash at the site of a tick bite on the lower leg is indicative of the variation in the initial rash of Lyme disease. Central clearing is incomplete, and a central necrotic area is apparent at the presumed site of the tick bite.

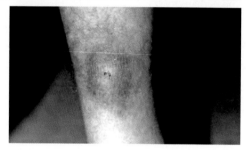

Image 56.3

A 14-year-old white female with multiple erythema migrans lesions of disseminated Lyme
disease following a known tick bite approximately
3 weeks prior to the clinical onset of fever, myalgias, and headache. A more typical erythema
migrans lesion preceded these skin lesions.

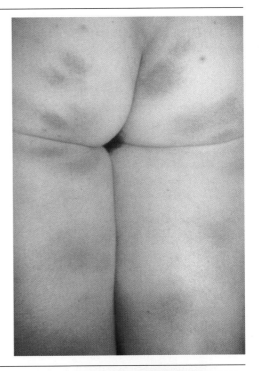

Image 56.4

A 15-month-old girl with left facial nerve palsy
complicating Lyme disease.

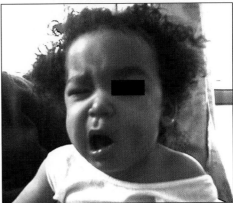

57

Lymphatic Filariasis
(Bancroftian, Malayan, and Timorian)

Clinical Manifestations

Most filarial infections are asymptomatic. Even in asymptomatic people, adult filarial worms commonly cause subclinical lymphatic dilatation and dysfunction. Lymphadenopathy is the most common clinical sign of lymphatic filariasis in children, most frequently of the inguinal, crural, and epitrochlear lymph nodes, in association with living adult worms. Death of the adult worm triggers an acute inflammatory response, which progresses distally (retrograde) along the affected lymphatic vessel, usually in the limbs. If present, systemic symptoms, such as headache or fever, usually are mild. In postpubertal males, adult *Wuchereria bancrofti* organisms are found most commonly in the intrascrotal lymphatic vessels; thus inflammation resulting from adult worm death may present as funiculitis, epididymitis, or orchitis. A tender granulomatous nodule is palpable at the site of the dead adult worms. The chronic manifestations of lymphedema and hydrocele rarely occur in children. Recurrent secondary bacterial infections hasten the progression of lymphedema to its advanced stage, known as elephantiasis. Chyluria can occur as a manifestation of bancroftian filariasis. Cough, fever, marked eosinophilia, and high serum IgE concentrations are manifestations of the tropical pulmonary eosinophilia syndrome.

Etiology

Filariasis is caused by 3 filarial nematodes: *W bancrofti, Brugia malayi,* and *Brugia timori.*

Epidemiology

The parasite is transmitted by the bite of infected species of various genera of mosquitoes, including *Culex, Aedes, Anopheles,* and *Mansonia. W bancrofti* is found in Haiti, the Dominican Republic, Guyana, Brazil, sub-Saharan and North Africa, and Asia, extending into a broad zone from India through the Indonesian archipelago into Oceania. Humans are the only definitive host. *B malayi* is found mostly in Southeast Asia and parts of India. *B timori* is restricted to certain islands at the eastern end of the Indonesian archipelago. Because adult worms are long lived (5–8 years on average) and reinfection is common, microfilariae infective for mosquitoes may remain in the patient's blood for decades; individual microfilaria have a life span up to 1.5 years. The adult worm is not transmissible from person to person or by blood transfusion, but microfilariae may be transmitted by transfusion.

Incubation Period

From acquisition to the appearance of microfilariae in blood can be 3 to 12 months.

Diagnostic Tests

Microfilariae can be detected microscopically on blood smears obtained at night (10 pm–4 am). Adult worms or microfilariae can be identified in tissue specimens obtained at biopsy. Serologic enzyme immunoassay tests are available, but interpretation of results is affected by cross-reactions of filarial antibodies with antibodies against other helminths. Lymphatic filariasis often must be diagnosed clinically because dependable serologic assays are not available uniformly, and in patients with lymphedema, the microfilariae no longer may be present.

Treatment

The main goal of treatment of an infected person is to kill the adult worm. Diethylcarbamazine citrate (DEC) is the drug of choice for lymphatic filariasis. The late phase of chronic disease is not affected by chemotherapy. Ivermectin is effective against the microfilariae of *W bancrofti* but has no effect on the adult parasite. In some studies, combination therapy with single-dose DEC-albendazole or ivermectin-albendazole has been shown to be more effective than any one drug alone in suppressing microfilaremia.

Complex decongestive physiotherapy may be effective for treating lymphedema. Chyluria originating in the bladder responds to fulguration; chyluria originating in the kidney usually cannot be corrected. Prompt identification and treatment of superinfections, particularly streptococcal and staphylococcal infections, and careful treatment of intertriginous and ungual infections are important aspects of therapy for lymphedema.

Image 57.1

Microfilaria of *Wuchereria bancrofti,* from a patient in Haiti (thick blood smear; hematoxylin-eosin stain). The microfilaria is sheathed, its body is gently curved, and the tail is tapered to a point. The nuclear column (ie, the cells that constitute the body of the microfilaria) is loosely packed, the cells can be visualized individually and do not extend to the tip of the tail. The sheath is slightly stained by hematoxylin-eosin.

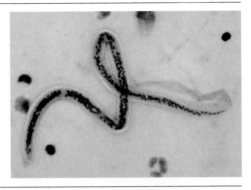

Image 57.2

Elephantiasis of both legs due to filariasis (Luzon, Philippines).

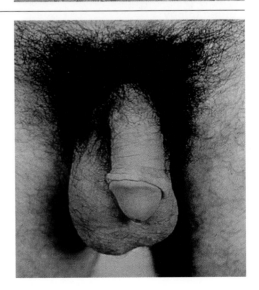

Image 57.3

Scrotal lymphangitis due to filariasis.

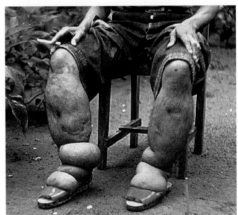

58

Lymphocytic Choriomeningitis

Clinical Manifestations

Postnatal infection is asymptomatic in approximately one third of cases. Symptomatic infection may result in a mild to severe influenza-like illness, which includes fever, malaise, myalgia, retro-orbital headache, photophobia, anorexia, and nausea. Fever usually lasts 1 to 3 weeks, and rash is rare. A biphasic febrile course is common. Up to half of symptomatic patients will develop neurologic manifestations varying from aseptic meningitis to severe encephalitis. Arthralgia or arthritis, respiratory tract symptoms, orchitis, and leukopenia occasionally develop. Recovery without sequelae is the usual outcome. Infection during pregnancy has been associated with abortion. Congenital infection can cause hydrocephalus, chorioretinitis, intracranial calcifications, microcephaly, and mental retardation. Congenital lymphocytic choriomeningitis may be difficult to differentiate from congenital infection attributable to CMV, toxoplasmosis, or rubella.

Etiology

Lymphocytic choriomeningitis virus is an arenavirus.

Epidemiology

Lymphocytic choriomeningitis is a chronic infection of the common house mouse and pet hamsters, which often are infected asymptomatically and chronically shed virus in urine and other excretions. In addition, laboratory mice, guinea pigs, and colonized golden hamsters can have chronic infection and can be sources of human infection. Humans are infected by aerosol or by ingestion of dust or food contaminated with the virus from the urine, feces, blood, or nasopharyngeal secretions of infected rodents. The disease is most prevalent in young adults. Human-to-human spread by transplacental passage of the virus and via organ transplantation from an acutely infected, undiagnosed, lymphocytic choriomeningitis virus-infected organ donor has been reported. The source of the virus in one organ donor was traced to a pet hamster purchased by the donor.

Incubation Period

6 to 13 days, occasionally 3 weeks.

Diagnostic Tests

In patients with CNS disease, mononuclear pleocytosis occasionally exceeding several thousand cells is present in the CSF. Hypoglycorrhachia also can occur. Lymphocytic choriomeningitis virus can be isolated from blood, CSF, urine and, rarely, nasopharyngeal secretion specimens. Acute and convalescent serum specimens can be tested for increases in antibody titers by immunofluorescent or enzyme immunoassay. Demonstration of virus-specific IgM antibodies in serum or CSF specimens is useful. In congenital infections, diagnosis usually is suspected at the sequela phase, and diagnosis usually is made by serologic testing.

Treatment

Supportive.

Image 58.1
Fundus photograph of a 9-month-old girl with congenital lymphocytic choriomeningitis virus infection. Extensive chorioretinal scarring is visible. Hydrocephalus and periventricular calcification were visible on CT scan and MRI.

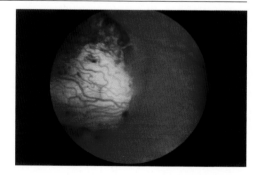

59

Malaria

Clinical Manifestations

The classic symptoms of malaria are high fever with chills, rigor, sweats, and headache, which can be paroxysmal. If appropriate treatment is not administered, fever and paroxysms can occur in a cyclic pattern. Depending on the infecting species, fever appears every other or every third day. Other manifestations can include nausea, vomiting, diarrhea, cough, arthralgia, and abdominal and back pain. Anemia and thrombocytopenia are common, and pallor and jaundice caused by hemolysis can occur. Hepatosplenomegaly may be present. More severe disease occurs in people without previous exposure and people who are pregnant or immunocompromised.

Infection with *Plasmodium falciparum* potentially is fatal and most commonly manifests as a febrile nonspecific influenza-like illness without localizing signs. With more severe disease, *P falciparum* infection can manifest as one of the following clinical syndromes:

- *Cerebral malaria* can have variable neurologic manifestations, including seizures, signs of increased intracranial pressure, confusion, and progression to stupor, coma, and death.
- *Hypoglycemia* sometimes is associated with quinine treatment and requires urgent correction.
- *Noncardiogenic pulmonary edema* is difficult to manage and can be fatal (rare in children).
- *Renal failure* is caused by acute tubular necrosis (rare in young children).
- *Respiratory failure and metabolic acidosis,* without pulmonary edema, can occur.
- *Severe anemia* attributable to high parasitemia and consequent hemolysis can occur.
- *Vascular collapse and shock* is associated with hypothermia and adrenal insufficiency.

Individuals with asplenia can be at increased risk of more severe illness and death.

Syndromes primarily associated with *Plasmodium vivax* and *Plasmodium ovale* infection are as follows:

- *Anemia* is attributable to acute parasitemia.
- *Hypersplenism* with danger of late splenic rupture can occur.
- *Relapse,* for as long as 3 to 5 years after the primary infection, is attributable to latent hepatic stages.

Syndromes associated with *Plasmodium malariae* infection include

- *Chronic asymptomatic parasitemia* can last as long as several years.
- *Nephrotic syndrome* from deposition of immune complexes in the kidney can occur.

Congenital malaria secondary to perinatal transmission rarely can occur. Most congenital cases have been caused by *P vivax* and *P falciparum; P malariae* and *P ovale* account for fewer than 20% of such cases. Manifestations can resemble those of neonatal sepsis, including fever and nonspecific symptoms of poor appetite, irritability, and lethargy.

Etiology

The genus *Plasmodium* includes species of intraerythrocytic parasites that infect a wide range of mammals, birds, and reptiles. The 4 species that infect humans are *P falciparum, P vivax, P ovale,* and *P malariae.*

Epidemiology

Malaria is endemic throughout the tropical areas of the world and is acquired from the bite of the female nocturnal-feeding *Anopheles* species of mosquito. One half of the world's population lives in areas where transmission occurs. Worldwide, there are 300 to 500 million cases annually and 1.5 to 2.7 million deaths. Most deaths occur in young children. Malarial infection poses substantial risks to pregnant women and their fetuses and can result in spontaneous abortion and stillbirth. The risk of malaria is highest, but variable, for travelers to sub-Saharan Africa, Papua New Guinea, the Solomon Islands, and Vanuatu; the risk is intermediate in the Indian subcontinent and is low in most of Southeast Asia and Latin America. Transmission is possible in more temperate climates, including areas of the United States where *Anopheles* species mosquitoes are present. Mosquitoes in airplanes flying from tropical climates have been the source of occasional cases in people working or residing near international airports. However, nearly all of the approximately 1400 annual reported cases in the United States result from infection acquired abroad. Other less common modes of malaria transmission are congenital, through transfusions, or through the use of contaminated needles or syringes.

P vivax and *P falciparum* are the most common species worldwide. *P vivax* malaria is prevalent on the Indian subcontinent and in Central America. *P falciparum* malaria is prevalent in Africa and Papua New Guinea. Malaria attributable to *P vivax* and *P falciparum* is common in southern and Southeast Asia, Oceania, and South America. *P malariae,* although much less common, has a wide distribution. *P ovale* malaria occurs most often in West Africa but has been reported in other areas.

Relapses may occur in *P vivax* and *P ovale* malaria because of a persistent hepatic (hypnozoite) stage of infection. Recrudescence of *P falciparum* and *P malariae* infection occurs when a persistent low-concentration parasitemia causes recurrence of symptoms. In areas of Africa and Asia with hyperendemic infection, reinfection in people with partial immunity results in a high prevalence of asymptomatic parasitemia.

The spread of chloroquine-resistant *P falciparum* strains throughout the world is of increasing importance. Resistance to other antimalarial drugs now is occurring in many areas where the drugs are used widely. Chloroquine-resistant *P vivax* has been reported in Indonesia, Papua New Guinea, the Solomon Islands, Myanmar, India, and Guyana.

Diagnostic Tests

Definitive diagnosis relies on identification of the parasite on stained blood films. Both thick and thin blood films should be examined. The thick film allows for concentration of the blood to find parasites present in small numbers, whereas the thin film is most useful for species identification and determination of the degree of parasitemia (the percentage of erythrocytes harboring parasites). If initial blood smears are negative for *Plasmodium* species but malaria remains a possibility, the smear should be repeated every 12 to 24 hours during a 72-hour period.

In areas with hyperendemic infection, the presence of malaria on a blood smear is not conclusive evidence of malaria as a cause of the manifesting illness because other infections often are superimposed on low-concentration parasitemia in children and adults with partial immunity.

Confirmation and identification of the species of malaria parasites on the blood smear is important in guiding therapy. Serologic testing generally is not helpful. Other diagnostic tests, including PCR assay, DNA probes, and malarial ribosomal RNA testing, currently are used in experimental studies only. Antigen detection tests using dipstick techniques for diagnosis are being evaluated. Most of these tests detect trophozoites of *P falciparum* infections.

Treatment

The choice of malaria chemotherapy is based on the infecting species, possible drug resistance, and the severity of disease. Severe malaria is defined as a parasitemia greater than 5% of red blood cells, signs of CNS or other end-organ involvement, shock, acidosis, or hypoglycemia. Patients with severe malaria require intensive care and parenteral treatment until the parasite density decreases to less than 1% and patients are able to tolerate oral therapy. Exchange transfusion may be warranted when parasitemia exceeds 10% or if there is evidence of complications (eg, cerebral malaria) at lower parasite densities. New antimalarial drugs are undergoing clinical trials for treatment and chemoprophylaxis of malaria. For patients with *P falciparum* malaria, sequential blood smears for percentage of parasitemia are indicated to monitor treatment.

Figure 59.1
Malaria Endemic Countries, 2000

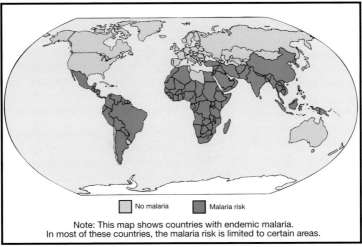

No malaria   Malaria risk

Note: This map shows countries with endemic malaria.
In most of these countries, the malaria risk is limited to certain areas.

Malaria generally occurs in areas where environmental conditions allow parasite multiplication in the vector. Thus malaria usually is restricted to tropical and subtropical areas (see map) and altitudes below 1500 m. However, this distribution might be affected by climatic changes, especially global warming, and population movements. Both *Plasmodium falciparum* and *Plasmodium malariae* are encountered in all shaded areas of the map (with *P falciparum* the most prevalent). *Plasmodium vivax* and *Plasmodium ovale* are traditionally thought to occupy complementary niches, with *P ovale* predominating in sub-Saharan Africa and *P vivax* in the other areas; however, these species are not always distinguishable on the basis of morphologic characteristics alone; the use of molecular tools will help clarify their exact distribution.

Courtesy of the Centers for Disease Control and Prevention.

Image 59.1

This thin film Giemsa-stained micrograph reveals *Plasmodium vivax, Plasmodium malariae,* and *Plasmodium ovale* trophozoites.

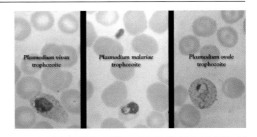

Image 59.2

Plasmodium falciparum: schizonts smears from patients. Schizonts are seldom seen in peripheral blood. Mature schizonts have 8 to 24 small merozoites with dark pigment and clumped in one mass. A: Immature schizont in a thin blood smear. B: Mature schizont. C, D: Ruptured schizonts in a thin blood smear.

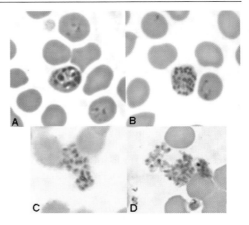

60
Measles

Clinical Manifestations

Measles is an acute disease characterized by fever, cough, coryza, conjunctivitis, an erythematous maculopapular rash, and a pathognomonic enanthema (Koplik spots). Complications including otitis media, bronchopneumonia, laryngotracheobronchitis (croup), and diarrhea occur commonly in young children. Acute encephalitis often results in brain damage and occurs in approximately 1 of every 1000 cases. Death, predominantly resulting from respiratory or neurologic complications, occurs in 1 to 3 of every 1000 cases reported in the United States. Case fatality rates are increased in children younger than 5 years and immunocompromised children, including children with leukemia, HIV infection, and severe malnutrition. The characteristic rash may not develop in immunocompromised patients.

Subacute sclerosing panencephalitis (SSPE) is a rare degenerative CNS characterized by behavioral and intellectual deterioration and seizures. Widespread measles immunization has led to the virtual disappearance of SSPE in the United States.

Etiology

Measles virus is an RNA virus with 1 serotype, classified as a member of the genus Morbillivirus in the Paramyxoviridae family.

Epidemiology

The only natural hosts of measles virus are humans. Measles is transmitted by direct contact with infectious droplets or, less commonly, by airborne spread. In temperate areas, the peak incidence of infection usually occurs during late winter and spring. In the prevaccine era, most cases of measles in the United States occurred in preschool and young school-aged children, and few people remained susceptible by 20 years of age. The childhood and adolescent immunization program in the United States has resulted in a greater than 99% decrease in the reported incidence of measles since measles vaccine was first licensed in 1963.

From 1989 to 1991, the incidence of measles in the United States increased because of low immunization rates in preschool-aged children, especially in urban areas. From 1997 to 2004, the incidence of measles in the United States has been low (37–116 cases reported per year), consistent with an absence of endemic transmission. Cases of measles continue to occur as a result of importation of the virus from other countries. Cases are considered international importations if the rash onset occurs within 18 days after entering the United States. Almost half of the imported cases occur in US residents returning from foreign travel.

Vaccine failure occurs in as many as 5% of people who have received a single dose of vaccine at 12 months of age or older. Although waning immunity after immunization can be a factor in some cases, most cases of measles in previously immunized children seem to occur in people in whom response to the vaccine was inadequate (ie, primary vaccine failures).

Patients are contagious from 1 to 2 days before onset of symptoms (3–5 days before the rash) to 4 days after appearance of the rash. Immunocompromised patients who may have prolonged excretion of the virus in respiratory tract secretions can be contagious for the duration of the illness. Patients with SSPE are not contagious.

Incubation Period

8 to 12 days (range, 7–18 days); in SSPE, mean, 10.8 years.

Diagnostic Tests

Measles virus infection can be diagnosed by a positive serologic test result for measles IgM antibody, a significant increase in measles IgG antibody concentration in paired acute and convalescent serum specimens by any standard serologic assay, or isolation of measles virus from clinical specimens, such as urine, blood, throat, or nasopharyngeal secretions. The simplest method of establishing the diagnosis of measles is testing for IgM antibody on a single serum specimen. The sensitivity of measles IgM assays varies and may be diminished during the first 72 hours after rash onset. If the result is negative for measles IgM and the patient has a generalized rash lasting more than 72 hours, the measles IgM test should be repeated. Measles IgM is detectable for at least 1 month after rash onset. People with febrile rash illness who are seronegative for measles IgM should be tested for rubella. Genotyping of viral isolates allows determination of patterns of importation and transmission, and genome sequencing can be used to differentiate between wild-type and vaccine virus infection.

Treatment

No specific antiviral therapy is available. The WHO and the United Nations International Children's Emergency Fund recommend administering vitamin A to all children diagnosed with measles in communities where vitamin A deficiency is a recognized problem or the measles case fatality rate is 1% or greater. Vitamin A treatment of children with measles

in developing countries has been associated with decreased morbidity and mortality rates. Vitamin A supplementation should be considered for hospitalized children 6 months to 2 years of age with measles and its complications (eg, croup, pneumonia, and diarrhea), and children older than 6 months with measles who have immunodeficiency, clinical evidence of vitamin A deficiency, impaired intestinal absorption, moderate to severe malnutrition, or recent emigration from areas of high mortality rates.

Parenteral and oral formulations of vitamin A are available.

Transmission precautions are indicated for 4 days after the onset of rash in otherwise healthy children and for the duration of illness in immunocompromised patients.

Image 60.1
Child with measles (rubeola) who appears to feel miserable.

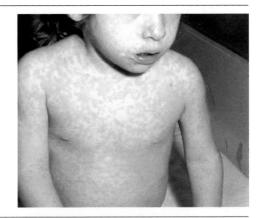

Image 60.2
Measles (rubeola) rash and conjunctivitis. Conjunctivitis results in clear tearing. Photophobia is common.

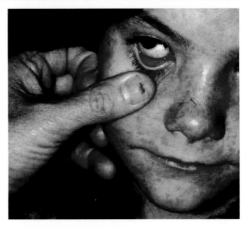

Image 60.3
Measles (rubeola) with Koplik spots on fifth
day of the rash.

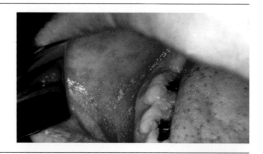

Image 60.4
Face of a boy with measles, characteristic of
the third day of the rash.

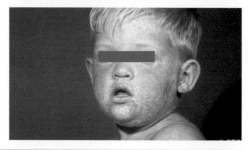

Image 60.5
This child with measles is showing the characteristic red blotchy rash on his buttocks and back
during the third day of the rash.

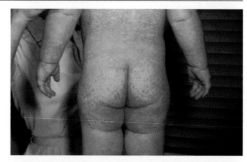

Image 60.6
Coronal T2-weighted MR image shows
swelling and hyperintensity of the right parietal
occipital cortex (arrows) in a patient with
measles encephalitis.

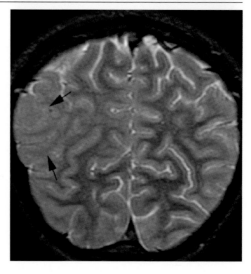

61

Meningococcal Infections

Clinical Manifestations

Invasive infection usually results in meningococcemia, meningitis, or both. Onset often is abrupt in meningococcemia, with fever, chills, malaise, prostration, and a rash that initially can be macular, maculopapular, or petechial. The progression of disease often is rapid. In fulminant cases (Waterhouse-Friderichsen syndrome), purpura, disseminated intravascular coagulation, shock, coma, and death can ensue despite appropriate therapy. The signs and symptoms of meningococcal meningitis are indistinguishable from signs and symptoms of acute meningitis caused by *Streptococcus pneumoniae* or other meningeal pathogens. The case fatality rate for meningococcal disease in all ages remains at 10%; mortality in adolescents approaches 25%. Less common manifestations include pneumonia, febrile occult bacteremia, conjunctivitis, and chronic meningococcemia. Invasive meningococcal infections can be complicated by arthritis, myocarditis, pericarditis, and endophthalmitis. Sequelae associated with meningococcal disease occur in 11% to 19% of patients and include hearing loss, neurologic disability, digit or limb amputations, and skin scarring, sometimes requiring skin grafts.

Etiology

Neisseria meningitidis is a gram-negative diplococcus with at least 13 serogroups.

Epidemiology

Strains belonging to groups A, B, C, Y, and W-135 cause most invasive disease worldwide. The distribution of meningococcal serogroups in the United States has shifted in recent years. Serogroups B, C, and Y each account for approximately 30% of reported cases, but serogroup distribution varies by age, location, and time. Approximately two thirds of cases among adolescents and young adults are caused by serogroups C, Y, or W-135 and potentially are preventable with available vaccines. In infants, nearly 50% of cases are caused by serogroup B and are not preventable with vaccines available in the United States.

Serogroup A has been associated frequently with epidemics elsewhere in the world, primarily in sub-Saharan Africa. An increase in cases of serogroup W-135 meningococcal disease was associated with the Hajj pilgrimage in Saudi Arabia in 2002. Since then, serogroup W-135 meningococcal disease has been reported in sub-Saharan African countries during epidemic seasons.

Asymptomatic colonization of the upper respiratory tract provides the source from which the organism is spread. Transmission occurs from person to person through droplets from the respiratory tract. Disease most often occurs in children younger than 5 years; the peak attack rate occurs in children younger than 1 year. Another peak occurs in adolescents 15 to 18 years of age. Freshman college students who live in dormitories have a higher rate of disease compared with individuals who are the same age and are not attending college. Close contacts of patients with meningococcal disease are at increased risk of becoming infected. Patients with deficiency of a terminal complement component (C5–C9), C3 or properdin deficiencies, or anatomical or functional asplenia are at increased risk of invasive and recurrent meningococcal disease. Patients are considered capable of transmitting the organism for up to 24 hours after initiation of effective antimicrobial treatment.

Outbreaks have occurred in communities and institutions, including child care centers, schools, colleges, and military recruit camps. An increased number of meningococcal serogroup C outbreaks in the United States were first reported during the 1990s. However, most cases of meningococcal disease are sporadic, with fewer than 5% associated with outbreaks. Outbreaks often are heralded by a shift in the distribution of cases to an older age group.

Incubation Period

1 to 10 days, usually less than 4 days.

Diagnostic Tests

Blood and CSF cultures yielding *N meningitidis* are diagnostic. Cultures of a petechial or purpuric lesion, synovial fluid, sputum, and other body fluid specimens yield the organism in some patients. A Gram stain of a petechial or purpuric scraping, CSF, and buffy coat smear of blood can be helpful. Bacterial antigen detection in CSF supports the diagnosis of a probable case if the clinical illness is consistent with meningococcal disease. A serogroup-specific PCR test to detect N meningitidis from clinical specimens is used routinely in the United Kingdom, where up to 56% of cases are confirmed by PCR assay alone. This test is useful in patients who receive antimicrobial therapy before cultures are obtained.

Routine susceptibility testing of meningococcal isolates is not recommended. However, N meningitidis strains with decreased suscep-tibility to penicillin have been identified sporadically from several regions of the United States and widely from Spain, Italy, and parts of Africa.

Treatment

Penicillin G should be administered intravenously for patients with invasive meningococcal disease, including meningitis. Cefotaxime, ceftriaxone, and ampicillin are acceptable alternatives. In a patient with penicillin allergy characterized by anaphylaxis, chloramphenicol is recommended. For travelers from areas such as Spain, where penicillin resistance has been reported, cefotaxime, ceftriaxone, or chloramphenicol is recommended.

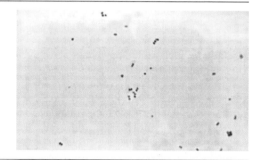

Image 61.1
This micrograph depicts the presence of aerobic gram-negative *Neisseria meningitidis* diplococcal bacteria (150x). Meningococci live in the throat of 5% to 10% of healthy people.

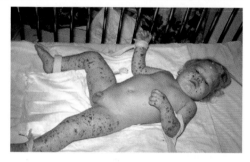

Image 61.2
Young boy with meningococcemia that demonstrates striking involvement of the extremities with sparing of the trunk.

Image 61.3

Meningococcemia in an adolescent.

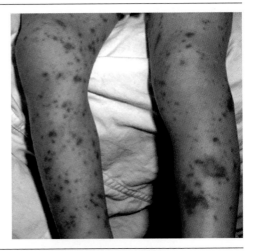

Image 61.4

Papular skin lesions of early meningococcemia.

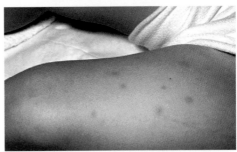

Image 61.5

Patient with marked purpura of the left foot.

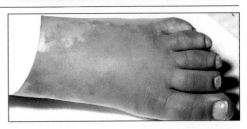

Image 61.6

Meningococcemia with gangrene of the toes, several days after hospital admission.

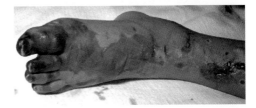

Image 61.7

Meningococcemia with cutaneous necrosis.

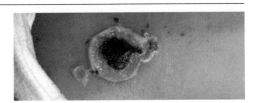

Image 61.8
Adrenal hemorrhage in a patient with meningococcemia (Waterhouse-Friderichsen syndrome).

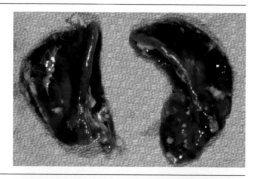

Image 61.9
Fatal meningococcal meningitis with purulent
exudate in the subarachnoid space covering
the cerebral convexities.

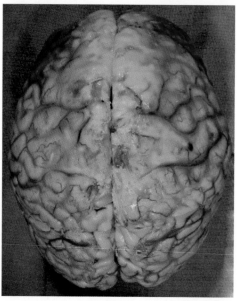

Image 61.10
This 6-month-old male presented with fever,
erythema, and tenderness over the ankle.
Blood culture and needle aspirate of the
cellulitis grew *Neisseria meningitidis.*

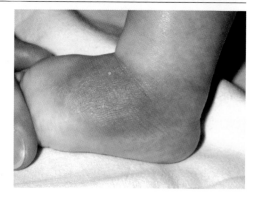

62

Molluscum Contagiosum

Clinical Manifestations

Molluscum contagiosum is a benign, usually asymptomatic viral infection of the skin with no systemic manifestations. It usually is characterized by 2 to 20 discrete, 1- to 5-mm diameter, flesh-colored to translucent, dome-shaped papules, some with central umbilication. Lesions commonly occur on the trunk, face, and extremities but rarely are generalized. An eczematous reaction encircles lesions in approximately 10% of patients. People with eczema, immunocompromising conditions, and HIV infection tend to have more widespread and prolonged eruptions.

Etiology

The cause is a poxvirus, which is the sole member of the genus *Molluscipoxvirus.*

Epidemiology

Humans are the only known source of the virus, which is spread by direct contact, including sexual contact, or by fomites. Lesions can be disseminated by autoinoculation. Infectivity generally is low, but occasional outbreaks have been reported, including outbreaks in child care centers. The period of communicability is unknown.

Incubation Period

Varies between 2 and 7 weeks; can be as long as 6 months.

Diagnostic Tests

The diagnosis usually can be made clinically from the characteristic appearance of the lesions. Wright or Giemsa staining of cells expressed from the central core of a lesion reveals characteristic intracytoplasmic inclusions. Electron microscopic examination of these cells identifies typical poxvirus particles.

Treatment

Lesions usually regress spontaneously, but mechanical removal (curettage) of the central core of each lesion may result in more rapid resolution. A topical anesthetic is applied 30 minutes to 2 hours before curettage. Children with single or widely scattered lesions should not be treated. Although lesions can regress spontaneously, treatment may prevent autoinoculation and spread to other people. Scarring is a rare occurrence. Cidofovir intravenous treatment of immunocompromised adults with severe lesions has been reported to be curative.

Image 62.1
Molluscum contagiosum lesions adjacent to nasal bridge.

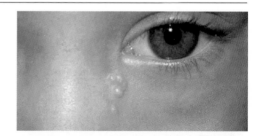

Image 62.2
Pearly papules on the nasal bridge and eyelid in a black child with molluscum contagiosum lesions, which commonly occur on the face.

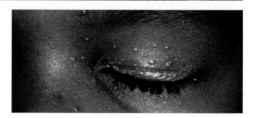

Image 62.3
A central dimple or umbilication is the hallmark of molluscum contagiosum. The lesions of molluscum contagiosum vary in size from 1 to 6 mm and, unlike venereal warts, are smooth and pearly and have an umbilicated center.

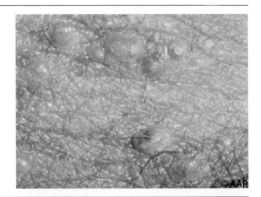

Image 62.4
Molluscum contagiosum is characterized by one or more translucent or white papules. Intracytoplasmic inclusions may be seen with Wright or Giemsa staining of material expressed from the core of the lesion.

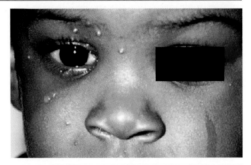

Image 62.5
Histopathology of skin showing characteristic findings of molluscum contagiosum.

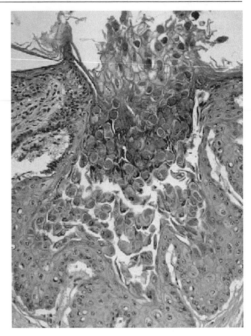

63

Mumps

Clinical Manifestations

Mumps is a systemic disease characterized by swelling of one or more of the salivary glands, usually the parotid glands. Approximately one third of infections do not cause clinically apparent salivary gland swelling and can manifest primarily as respiratory tract infection. More than 50% of people with mumps have CSF pleocytosis, but fewer than 10% have symptoms of CNS infection. Orchitis is a common complication after puberty, but sterility rarely occurs. Other rare complications include arthritis, thyroiditis, mastitis, glomerulonephritis, myocarditis, endocardial fibroelastosis, thrombocytopenia, cerebellar ataxia, transverse myelitis, ascending polyradiculitis, pancreatitis, oophoritis, and hearing impairment. In the absence of immunization, mumps typically occurs during childhood. Infection occurring among adults is more likely to be severe, and death resulting from mumps complications, although rare, can occur. Mumps during the first trimester of pregnancy is associated with an increased rate of spontaneous abortion. Although mumps can cross the placenta, no evidence exists that this results in congenital malformation.

Etiology

Mumps is caused by an RNA virus classified as a Rubulavirus in the Paramyxoviridae family. Other causes of parotitis include infection with CMV, parainfluenza virus types 1 and 3, influenza A virus, coxsackieviruses and other enteroviruses, lymphocytic choriomeningitis virus, HIV, *Staphylococcus aureus*, nontuberculous mycobacterium and, less often, other gram-positive and gram-negative bacteria; salivary duct calculi; starch ingestion; drug reactions (eg, phenylbutazone, thiouracil, iodides); and metabolic disorders (diabetes mellitus, cirrhosis, and malnutrition).

Epidemiology

Mumps occurs worldwide, and humans are the only known natural hosts. The virus is spread by contact with infected respiratory tract secretions. The incidence in the United States, which has decreased markedly since introduction of the mumps vaccine, is fewer than 300 reported cases per year. Most cases now are reported among individuals older than 14 years. In immunized children, most cases of parotitis are not caused by mumps infection. Outbreaks can occur in highly immunized populations. The period of maximum communicability is from 1 to 2 days before to 5 days after onset of parotid swelling. Virus has been isolated from saliva from 7 days before through 9 days after onset of swelling.

Incubation Period

16 to 18 days; occasionally 12 to 25 days.

Diagnostic Tests

In the United States, mumps now is an uncommon infection, and parotitis has many other causes. People with parotitis lasting 2 days or more without other apparent cause should undergo diagnostic testing to confirm mumps virus as the cause. Mumps can be confirmed by isolating the virus in cell culture inoculated with throat washing, saliva, urine, or spinal fluid specimens; by detection of mumps-specific IgM antibody; by detection of mumps virus by reverse transcriptase-PCR; or by a significant increase between acute and convalescent titers in serum mumps IgG antibody titer determined by standard serologic assay (eg, complement fixation, neutralization, hemagglutination inhibition test, or enzyme immunoassay).

Treatment

Supportive.

Image 63.1
This is a photograph of a patient with bilateral swelling in the submaxillary regions due to mumps.

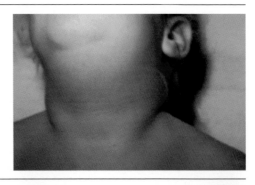

Image 63.2
Mumps parotitis with cervical and presternal edema and erythema that resolved spontaneously.

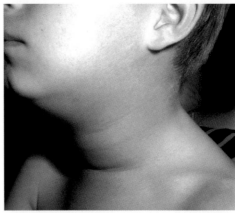

Image 63.3
Swelling and erythema of Stenson's duct in the 10-year-old white male with mumps parotitis in Image 63.2.

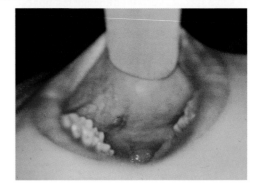

64

Mycoplasma pneumoniae Infections

Clinical Manifestations

The most common clinical syndromes are pneumonia and upper respiratory tract infections, including pharyngitis and, occasionally, otitis media or myringitis, which may be bullous. Coryza, sinusitis, and croup are rare. Malaise, fever and, occasionally, headache are nonspecific manifestations of infection. In approximately 10% of patients, pneumonia with cough develops within a few days and lasts for 3 to 4 weeks. The cough is nonproductive initially but later may become productive, particularly in older children and adolescents. Approximately 10% of children with pneumonia exhibit a rash, most often maculopapular. Abnormalities detected on radiography vary, but bilateral, diffuse infiltrates are common, and focal abnormalities, such as consolidation, effusion, and hilar adenopathy, can occur.

Unusual manifestations include nervous system disease (eg, aseptic meningitis, encephalitis, demyelinating disease, cerebellar ataxia, transverse myelitis, peripheral neuropathy) as well as myocarditis, pericarditis, polymorphous mucocutaneous eruptions (including Stevens-Johnson syndrome), hemolytic anemia, and arthritis. In patients with sickle cell disease, Down syndrome, immunodeficiencies, and chronic cardiorespiratory disease, severe pneumonia with pleural effusion can develop. A substantial proportion of acute chest syndrome and pneumonia associated with sickle cell disease seems to be attributable to *Mycoplasma pneumoniae*.

Etiology

Mycoplasmas, including *M pneumoniae,* are the smallest free-living microorganisms; they lack a cell wall and are pleomorphic.

Epidemiology

Mycoplasmas are ubiquitous in animals and plants, but *M pneumoniae* causes disease only in humans. *M pneumoniae* is transmissible by respiratory droplets during close contact with a symptomatic person. Outbreaks have been described in hospitals, military bases, colleges, and summer camps. People of any age can be infected, but specific disease syndromes are age-related. *M pneumoniae* is an uncommon cause of pneumonia in children younger than 5 years but is a leading cause of pneumonia in school-aged children and young adults. Infections occur throughout the world, in any season, and in all geographic settings. Community-wide epidemics occur every 4 to 7 years. Because of a long incubation period, familial spread can continue for many months. Clinical illness within a group or family ranges from mild upper respiratory tract infection to tracheobronchitis or pharyngitis to pneumonia. Asymptomatic carriage after infection can occur for weeks to months. Immunity after infection is not long lasting.

Incubation Period

2 to 3 weeks.

Diagnostic Tests

M pneumoniae can be grown in artificial media, but growth requires special enriched media, and takes up to 21 days. Sensitive and specific PCR tests for *M pneumoniae* have been developed and seem to be superior to serology for diagnosis. First-line use awaits standardization and availability.

Commercially available immunofluorescent tests and enzyme immunoassay detect *M pneumoniae*–specific IgM and IgG antibodies. Although the presence of IgM antibodies confirms recent *M pneumoniae* infection, these antibodies persist in serum for several months and may not necessarily indicate current infection; false-positive test results also occur. Serologic diagnosis can be made by demonstrating a 4-fold or greater increase in antibody titer between acute and convalescent serum specimens when the complement fixation assay is used. The antibody titer peaks at approximately 3 to 6 weeks and persists for 2 to 3 months after infection. Because *M pneumoniae* antibodies may cross-react with some other antigens, results of these tests should be interpreted cautiously when evaluating febrile illnesses of unknown origin.

With the wide availability of specific antibody tests, use of cold hemagglutinin titers has been deemphasized.

Treatment

Acute upper respiratory tract illness caused by *M pneumoniae* generally is mild and resolves without antimicrobial therapy. Macrolides, including erythromycin, azithromycin, and clarithromycin, are the preferred antimicrobial agents for treatment of pneumonia in children younger than 8 years. Tetracycline and doxycycline also are effective and may be used for children 8 years of age and older. Fluoroquinolones are effective but are not recommended for children. There is no evidence that treatment of nonrespiratory tract disease alters the course of illness.

Image 64.1
Preadolescent boy with bilateral perihilar infiltrates and right lower lobe pneumonia and pleural effusion due to *Mycoplasma pneumoniae.*

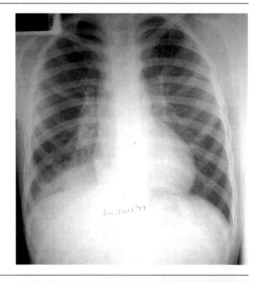

Image 64.2
This 10-year-old boy presented with fever; macular lesions on the face, chest, arms, and back; and facial swelling. He had a 4-day period of increasing cough and low-grade fever before the onset of the skin lesions and facial swelling. Chest x-ray revealed infiltrates in the right lung. Cold agglutinins were markedly elevated, and he had a >4-fold rise in complement fixation antibody to *Mycoplasma pneumoniae.*

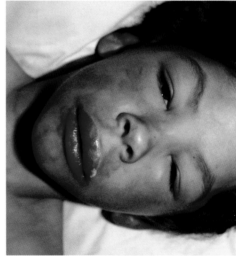

65

Nocardiosis

Clinical Manifestations

Immunocompetent children typically have cutaneous or lymphocutaneous disease with pustular or ulcerative lesions that remain localized after soil contamination of a skin injury. Invasive disease occurs most commonly in immunocompromised patients, particularly people with chronic granulomatous disease, organ transplantation, HIV infection, or disease requiring long-term systemic corticosteroid therapy. In these children, infection characteristically begins in the lungs, and the illness can be acute, subacute, or chronic. Pulmonary disease commonly manifests as rounded nodular infiltrates that can undergo cavitation. Hematogenous spread may occur from the lungs to the brain (single or multiple abscesses), in skin (pustules, pyoderma, abscesses, mycetoma), and occasionally in other organs. *Nocardia* organisms can be recovered from patients with cystic fibrosis, but their role as a lung pathogen is not clear.

Etiology

Nocardia species are aerobic actinomycetes, a large and diverse group of gram-positive bacteria, which include *Actinomyces israelii, Rhodococcus equi,* and *Tropheryma whippelii* (Whipple disease). Pulmonary or disseminated disease is caused most commonly by the *Nocardia asteroides* complex, which includes *Nocardia farcinica* and *Nocardia nova.* Primary cutaneous disease most commonly is caused by *Nocardia brasiliensis. Nocardia pseudobrasiliensis* is associated with pulmonary, CNS, and systemic nocardiosis. Other pathogenic species include *Nocardia abscessus, Nocardia otitidiscaviarum, Nocardia transvalensis, Nocardia veterana, Nocardia cyriacigeorgica,* and *Nocardia paucivorans.*

Epidemiology

Found worldwide, *Nocardia* species are ubiquitous environmental saprophytes living in soil, organic matter, and water. The lungs are the probable portals of entry for pulmonary or disseminated disease. Direct skin inoculation occurs, often as the result of contact with contaminated soil after minor trauma. Person-to-person and animal-to-human transmission does not occur.

Incubation Period

Unknown.

Diagnostic Tests

Isolation of *Nocardia* organisms from body fluid, abscess material, or tissue specimens provides a definitive diagnosis. Stained smears of sputum, body fluids, or pus demonstrating beaded, branched, weakly gram-positive, variably acid-fast rods suggest the diagnosis. The Brown and Brenn and methenamine silver stains are recommended to demonstrate microorganisms in tissue specimens. *Nocardia* organisms are slow growing but grow readily on blood and chocolate agar in 3 to 5 days. Cultures from normally sterile sites should be maintained for 3 weeks in an appropriate liquid medium. Serologic tests for *Nocardia* species are not useful.

Treatment

Trimethoprim-sulfamethoxazole or a sulfonamide alone (eg, sulfisoxazole or sulfamethoxazole) is the drug of choice. Immunocompetent patients with primary lymphocutaneous disease usually respond after 6 to 12 weeks of therapy. Immunocompromised patients and patients with invasive disease should be treated longer because of the tendency for relapse. For patients with CNS disease, disseminated disease, or overwhelming infection, amikacin plus ceftriaxone should be given initially. Patients with meningitis or brain abscess should be monitored with serial neuroimaging studies. If response to trimethoprim-sulfamethoxazole does not occur, other agents, such as clarithromycin *(N nova)*, amoxicillin-clavulanate *(N brasiliensis* and *N abscessus)*, imipenem, or meropenem may be beneficial. Linezolid is highly active against all *Nocardia* species in vitro, and it may be effective for the treatment of invasive infections. Drainage of abscesses is beneficial.

Image 65.1
Nocardia organisms (Gram stain).

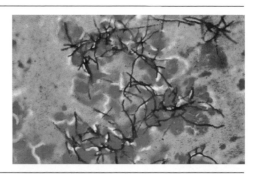

Image 65.2
Nocardia mediastinitis following surgical repair of ventricular septal defect (nosocomial infection).

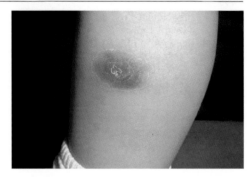

Image 65.3
Cutaneous nocardiosis of lower leg of immunocompetent preschool-aged female.

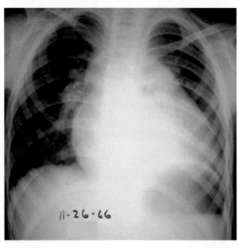

Image 65.4

Nocardia pneumonia, bilateral, in an immuno-compromised child. Invasive nocardiosis is unusual in immunocompetent children.

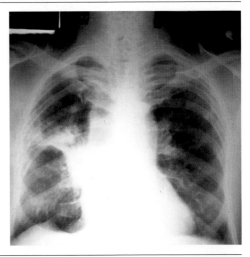

Image 65.5

Cutaneous *Nocardia braziliensis* lesion in a 10-year-old boy with no evidence of disseminated disease.

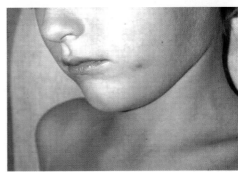

Image 65.6

Cutaneous nocardiosis of forearm in an immunocompetent preschool-aged boy.

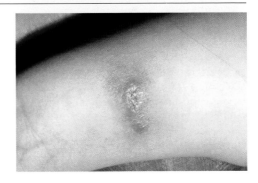

66

Onchocerciasis
(River Blindness, Filariasis)

Clinical Manifestations

The disease involves skin, subcutaneous tissues, lymphatic vessels, and eyes. Subcutaneous nodules of varying sizes containing adult worms develop 6 to 12 months after initial infection. In patients in Africa, the nodules tend to be found on the lower torso, pelvis, and lower extremities, whereas in patients in Central and South America, the nodules more often are located on the upper body (the head and trunk) but may occur on the extremities. After the worms mature, microfilariae are produced and migrate to the tissues and can cause a chronic, pruritic, papular dermatitis. After a period of years, the skin can become lichenified and hypopigmented or hyperpigmented. The presence of living or dead microfilariae in the ocular structures leads to photophobia and inflammation of the cornea, iris, ciliary body, retina, choroid, and optic nerve. Blindness can result if the disease is untreated.

Etiology

Onchocerca volvulus is a filarial nematode.

Epidemiology

Larvae are transmitted by the bite of an infected *Simulium* species black fly that breeds in fast-flowing streams and rivers (hence the colloquial name of the disease, river blindness). The disease occurs primarily in equatorial Africa, but small foci are found in southern Mexico, Guatemala, northern South America, and Yemen. Prevalence is greatest among people who live near vector breeding sites. *O volvulus* is an exclusively human para-site and has no animal reservoir host. Adult worms continue to produce microfilariae capable of infecting flies for more than a decade. The infection is not transmissible by person-to-person contact or blood transfusion.

Incubation Period

Usually 6 to 12 months; can be as long as 3 years.

Diagnostic Tests

Direct examination of a 1- to 2-mg shaving or biopsy specimen of the epidermis and upper dermis (taken from the scapular or iliac crest area) can reveal microfilariae. Microfilariae are not found in blood. Adult worms may be demonstrated in excised nodules that have been sectioned and stained. A slit-lamp examination of the anterior chamber of an involved eye can reveal motile microfilariae or corneal lesions typical of onchocerciasis. Eosinophilia is common.

Treatment

Ivermectin, a microfilaricidal agent, is the drug of choice for treatment of onchocerciasis. Treatment decreases dermatitis and the risk of developing severe ocular disease, but treatment does not kill the adult worms and, thus, is not curative. One single oral dose of ivermectin is given every 6 to 12 months until asymptomatic. Adverse reactions caused by the death of microfilariae can include rash, edema, fever, myalgia, asthma exacerbation, and hypotension (which rarely is severe). Safety and effectiveness in pediatric patients weighing less than 15 kg have not been established. A 6-week course of doxycycline may be considered as adjunctive therapy for children 8 years of age or older and nonpregnant adults.

Image 66.1

As an adult, this *Simulium* species larva, or black fly, is a vector of the disease onchocerciasis, or river blindness. The black fly larva is usually a filter-feeder, feeding on nutrients extracted from passing currents. Before entering the pupal stage, a *Simulium* species larva passes through 6 larval stages, then encases itself in a silken, submerged cocoon.

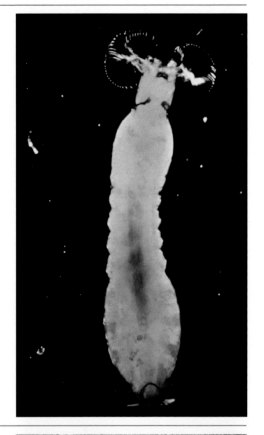

Image 66.2

Histopathologic features of *Onchocerca* nodule in onchocerciasis.

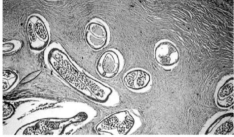

Image 66.3
An African boy with chronic onchocerciasis (filiariasis) with lichenified and hypopigmented skin.

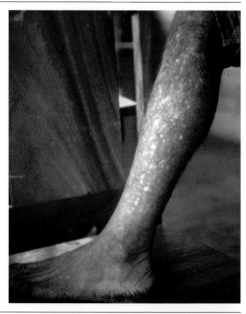

Image 66.4
The abdomen of the patient in Image 66.3.

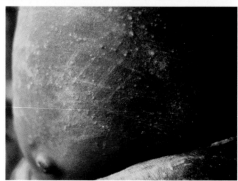

Image 66.5
A Guatemalan girl with nodules on her hand from onchocerciasis.

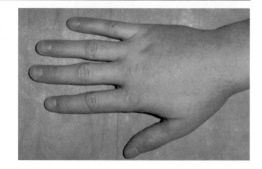

67

Human Papillomaviruses

Clinical Manifestations

Most HPV infections produce no lesions and are inapparent clinically. However, HPVs can produce benign epithelial proliferation (warts) of the skin and mucous membranes and are associated with anogenital dysplasias and cancers. Cutaneous nongenital warts include common skin warts, plantar warts, flat warts, thread-like (filiform) warts, and epidermodysplasia verruciformis. Warts also occur on the mucous membranes, including the anogenital, oral, nasal, and conjunctival areas and the respiratory tract, where respiratory papillomatosis occurs.

Common **skin warts** are dome-shaped with conical projections that give the surface a rough appearance. They usually are painless and multiple, occurring commonly on the hands and around or under the nails. When small dermal vessels become thrombosed, black dots appear in the warts. Plantar warts on the foot can be painful and are characterized by marked hyperkeratosis, sometimes with black dots.

Flat warts (juvenile warts) commonly are found on the face and extremities of children and adolescents. They usually are small, multiple, and flat topped; seldom exhibit papillomatosis; and rarely cause pain. Filiform warts occur on the face and neck. Cutaneous warts are benign.

Anogenital warts, also called **condylomata acuminata,** are skin-colored warts with a cauliflower-like surface that range in size from a few millimeters to several centimeters. In males, these warts may be found on the penis, scrotum, or anal and perianal area. In females, these lesions may occur on the vulva or perianal areas and less commonly in the vagina or on the cervix. Anogenital warts often are multiple and attract attention because of their appearance. Warts usually are painless, although they may cause itching, burning, local pain, or bleeding.

Anogenital HPV infection may be associated with clinically inapparent dysplastic lesions,

particularly in women (cervix and vagina). These lesions may be made more apparent by applying 3% to 5% acetic acid to the mucosal surface and examining it by magnification. The HPV types associated with these dysplasias also are associated with cancers that occur in the anogenital tract. HPV causes more than 99% of cervical cancers and a substantial proportion of vulvar, anal, and penile cancers.

Respiratory tract papillomatosis is a rare condition characterized by recurring papillomas in the larynx or other areas of the upper respiratory tract. This condition is diagnosed most commonly in children between 2 and 5 years of age and manifests as a voice change, stridor, or abnormal cry. Respiratory papillomas have been associated with respiratory tract obstruction in young children. Adult onset also has been described.

Epidermodysplasia verruciformis is a rare, lifelong, severe papillomavirus infection believed to be a consequence of an inherited deficiency of cell-mediated immunity. The lesions can resemble flat warts but often are similar to tinea versicolor, covering the torso and upper extremities. Most appear during the first decade of life, but malignant transformation, which occurs in approximately one third of affected people, usually is delayed until adulthood.

Etiology

HPVs are members of the *Papillomavirus* genus of the Papillomaviridae family and are DNA viruses. More than 100 types have been identified. These viruses are grouped into cutaneous and mucosal types. Based on their detection in cancers, mucosal HPVs are divided into low-risk and high-risk types. More than 18 high-risk types are recognized, the most common being types 16, 18, 31, and 45. Types 6 and 11 frequently are associated with condylomata acuminata, recurrent respiratory papillomatosis, and conjunctival papillomas and carcinomas.

Epidemiology

Papillomaviruses are distributed widely among mammals and are species-specific. Cutaneous warts occur commonly among school-aged children; the prevalence rate is as high as

50%. HPV infections are transmitted from person to person by close contact. Nongenital warts are acquired through minor trauma to the skin. An increase in the incidence of plantar warts has been associated with swimming in public pools. The intense and often widespread appearance of warts in patients with compromised cellular immunity (particularly patients who have undergone transplantation and people with HIV infection) suggests that alterations in immunity predispose to reactivation of latent intraepithelial infection.

Anogenital HPV infection is the most common STI in the United States, occurring in more than 40% of sexually active adolescent females. Most infections are transient and clear spontaneously. Anogenital HPV infections are transmitted primarily by sexual contact and most are subclinical. Rarely, infection is transmitted to a child through the birth canal during delivery or transmitted from nongenital sites. When anogenital warts are found in a child who is beyond infancy but prepubertal, sexual abuse must be considered.

Respiratory papillomatosis is believed to be acquired by aspiration of infectious secretions during passage through an infected birth canal.

Incubation Period

Unknown; estimated to range from 3 months to several years. Neoplasias are long-term (>10 years) sequelae of chronic persistent infection.

Diagnostic Tests

Most cutaneous and anogenital warts are diagnosed clinically. Respiratory papillomatosis is diagnosed using endoscopy and biopsy. Cervical dysplasias are detected by cytologic examination of a Pap smear, or liquid-based cytology and biopsy specimens of any tissue.

A definitive diagnosis of HPV infection is based on detection of viral nucleic acid (DNA or RNA) or capsid protein. Tests that detect high-risk or low-risk types of HPV DNA in cells obtained from the cervix are available. Testing for HPV types is used in combination with Pap test to determine whether patients need to be sent for colposcopy; otherwise,

screening for clinically inapparent HPV infection or evaluating anogenital warts using HPV DNA or RNA tests is not recommended.

Treatment

Treatment of HPV infection is directed toward eliminating the lesions that result from the infection rather than HPV itself. Most nongenital warts eventually regress spontaneously but can persist for months or years. The optimal treatment for warts that do not resolve spontaneously has not been identified. Most methods of treatment rely on chemical or physical destruction of the infected epithelium, such as application of salicylic acid products, cryotherapy with liquid nitrogen, or application of duct tape. Daily treatment with tretinoin has been useful for widespread flat warts in children. Care must be taken to avoid a deleterious cosmetic result with therapy.

The optimal treatment for anogenital warts has not been identified. Spontaneous regression occurs within months in some cases. The application of podophyllum resin or patient-applied podofilox solution or gel (the major cytotoxic ingredient of podophyllum resin) often is the initial therapy of choice. These agents have not been tested for safety and efficacy in children, and their use is contraindicated in pregnancy. Other treatment modalities are cryotherapy, trichloroacetic acid or bichloroacetic acid, imiquimod (patient-applied), electrocautery, laser surgery, and surgical excision. Treatment may not eradicate HPV infection from the surrounding normal tissue and recurrences are common.

Cytologic screening of cervical cells should be initiated within 3 years of the onset of consensual and nonconsensual sexual activity. Approximately 40% of people with HPV will develop abnormal Pap smears. Of those with abnormal Pap smears associated with low-risk HPV, 100% will resolve in 3 years and 80% of those associated with high-risk HPV will resolve in 3 years. Suggestions for evaluation and management are available at www.asccp.org/pdfs/consensus/algorithms.pdf.

Respiratory papillomatosis is difficult to treat and is best managed by an otolaryngologist. Local recurrence is common, and repeated surgical procedures for removal are often necessary. Extension or dissemination of respiratory papillomas from the larynx into the trachea, bronchi, or lung parenchyma is a rare complication that can result in increased morbidity and mortality. Intralesional interferon, indole-3-carbinole, photodynamic therapy,

and intralesional cidofovir have been used as investigational treatments and may be of benefit for patients with frequent recurrences.

Oral warts can be removed through cryotherapy, electrocautery, or surgical excision.

Image 67.1
Digitate HPV wart with finger-like projections on a child's index finger.

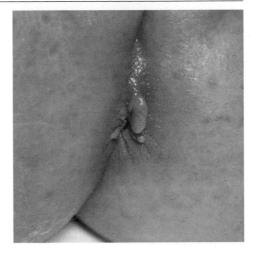

Image 67.2
Laryngeal papillomas may cause hoarseness. Though rare, they occur in infants of mothers infected with HPV.

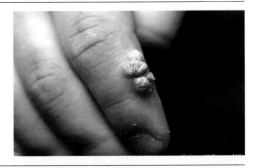

Image 67.3
A 13-month-old girl with condylomata acuminata around the anus from sexual abuse.

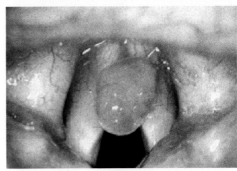

68

Paracoccidioidomycosis
(South American Blastomycosis)

Clinical Manifestations

Disease occurs primarily in adults and is rare in children. The site of initial infection is the lungs. Clinical patterns in childhood include the acute-subacute and chronic forms. In both forms, constitutional symptoms, such as fever, malaise, and weight loss, are common. In the more common acute-subacute form, symptoms are related to the extensive involvement of the reticuloendothelial system with enlarged lymph nodes and involvement of the liver, spleen, bone marrow, and bones as well as joints, skin, and mucous membranes. Occasionally, enlarged lymph nodes coalesce and form abscesses or fistulas. The chronic form of the illness can be localized to the lungs or can disseminate. Chronic granulomatous lesions of the mucous membranes, especially of the mouth and palate, occur more often in children in association with enlarged, draining lymph nodes.

Etiology

Paracoccidioides brasiliensis is a dimorphic fungus with a yeast phase and a mycelial phase.

Epidemiology

The infection occurs in Latin America, from Mexico to Argentina. The natural reservoir is unknown, although soil is suspected. The mode of transmission is unknown; person-to-person transmission does not occur.

Incubation Period

1 month to many years.

Diagnostic Tests

Round, multiple-budding cells with a distinguishing pilot's wheel appearance can be seen in 10% potassium hydroxide preparations of sputum specimens, bronchoalveolar lavage specimens, scrapings from ulcers, and material from lesions or in tissue biopsy specimens. The organism can be cultured easily on most enriched media. Complement fixation, enzyme immunoassay, and immunodiffusion methods are useful for detecting specific antibodies.

Treatment

Amphotericin B is preferred by many experts for treatment of people with severe paracoccidioidomycosis, but amphotericin B is not curative. Itraconazole is the drug of choice for less severe or localized infection and to complete treatment when amphotericin B is used initially. Prolonged therapy for at least 6 months is necessary to minimize the relapse rate. A sulfonamide can be used in resource-limited countries, but maintenance treatment must be continued for 3 to 5 years to avoid relapse, which occurs in 20% to 25% of patients.

Image 68.1
Histopathologic features of paracoccidioidomycosis, liver. Minute buds on several cells of *Paracoccidioides brasiliensis* (methenamine silver stain).

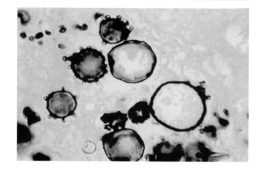

Image 68.2

Histopathologic features of paracoccidioidomycosis of skin sample (silver stain). Budding cell of *Paracoccidioides brasiliensis*.

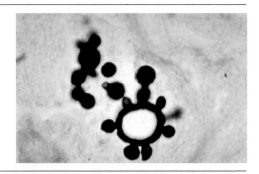

Image 68.3

This is a slant culture growing the fungus *Paracoccidioides brasiliensis* during its yeast phase. Inhalation of *P brasiliensis* conidia is presumably the route of acquisition. The primary infection is asymptomatic in most cases and can remain dormant for years within lymph nodes, reappearing later usually because of immunodeficiency.

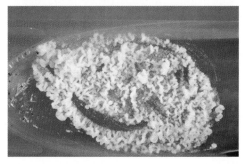

69

Paragonimiasis

Clinical Manifestations

The disease has an insidious onset and a chronic course. The 2 major forms of paragonimiasis described are (1) pulmonary and (2) extrapulmonary, which results in a larval migrans syndrome. Pulmonary disease is associated with chronic cough and dyspnea, but most infections probably are inapparent or result in mild symptoms. Heavy infestations cause paroxysms of coughing, which often produce blood-tinged sputum that is brown because of the presence of *Paragonimus* species eggs. Hemoptysis can be severe. Pleural effusion, pneumothorax, bronchiectasis, and pulmonary fibrosis with clubbing can develop. Extrapulmonary manifestations also can involve the liver, spleen, abdominal cavity, intestinal wall, intra-abdominal lymph nodes, skin, and CNS, with meningoencephalitis, seizures, and space-occupying tumors attributable to invasion of the brain by adult flukes, usually occurring within a year of pulmonary infection. Symptoms tend to subside after approximately 5 years but can persist for as many as 20 years.

Extrapulmonary paragonimiasis is associated with migratory allergic subcutaneous nodules containing juvenile worms. Pleural effusion is common, as is invasion of the brain.

Etiology

In Asia, classical paragonimiasis is caused by *Paragonimus westermani* and *Paragonimus heterotremus* adult flukes and their eggs. The adult flukes of *P westermani* are up to 12 mm long and 7 mm wide and occur throughout the Far East. A triploid parthenogenetic form of *P westermani*, which is larger, produces more eggs, and elicits greater disease, has been described in Japan, Korea, Taiwan, and parts of eastern China. *P heterotremus* occurs in Southeast Asia and adjacent parts of China. Extrapulmonary paragonimiasis is caused by larval stages of *Paragonimus skrjabini* and *Paragonimus miyazakii*. *P skrjabini* occurs in China, and *P miyazakii* occurs in Japan.

African forms causing extrapulmonary paragonimiasis include *Paragonimus africanus* (Nigeria, Cameroon) and *Paragonimus uterobilateralis* (Liberia, Guinea, Nigeria, Gabon). *Paragonimus mexicanus* and *Paragonimus ecuadoriensis* occur in Mexico, Costa Rica, Ecuador, and Peru. *Paragonimus kellicotti,* a lung fluke of mink and opossums in the United States, also can cause a zoonotic infection in humans.

Epidemiology

Transmission occurs when raw or undercooked freshwater crabs or crayfish containing larvae (metacercariae) are ingested. The metacercariae excyst in the small intestine and penetrate the abdominal cavity, where they remain for a few days before migrating to the lungs. *P westermani* and *P heterotremus* mature within the lungs over 6 to 10 weeks, when they then begin egg production. Eggs escape from pulmonary capsules into the bronchi and exit from the human host in sputum or feces. Eggs hatch in freshwater within 3 weeks, giving rise to miracidia. Miracidia penetrate freshwater snails and emerge several weeks later as cercariae, which encyst within the muscles and viscera of freshwater crustaceans before maturing into infective metacercariae. Transmission also occurs when humans ingest raw pork, usually from wild pigs, containing the juvenile stages of *Paragonimus* species (described as occurring in Japan).

Humans are accidental ("dead-end") hosts for *P skrjabini* and *P miyazakii.* These flukes cannot mature in humans and, hence, do not produce eggs.

Paragonimus species also infect a variety of other mammals, such as canids, mustelids, felids, and rodents, which can serve as animal reservoir hosts.

Incubation Period

Variable.

Diagnostic Tests

Microscopic examination of stool, sputum, pleural effusion, CSF, and other tissue specimens can reveal eggs. A Western blot serologic antibody test, available at the CDC, is sensitive and specific but does not distinguish active from past infection. Charcot-Leyden crystals and eosinophils in sputum are useful diagnostic elements. Chest radiographs can appear normal or resemble radiographs from patients with tuberculosis.

Treatment

Praziquantel in a 2-day course is the treatment of choice and is associated with high cure rates as demonstrated by the disappearance of egg production and radiographic lesions in the lungs. The drug also is effective for some extrapulmonary manifestations. Bithionol is an alternate drug.

Figure 69.1
Life Cycle of *Paragonimus westermani*, One of the Causal Agents of Paragonimiasis

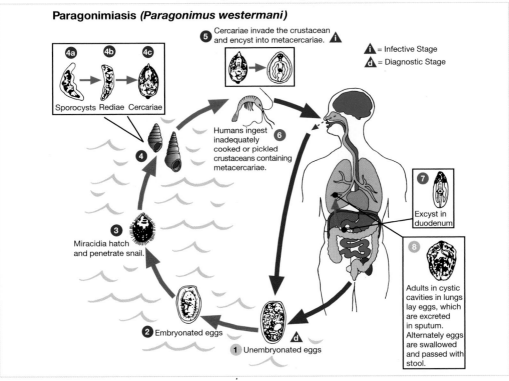

Courtesy of the Centers for Disease Control and Prevention.

Image 69.1
Paragonimus westermani ova in stool preparation (400x).

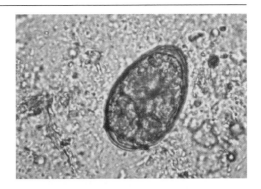

70

Parainfluenza Viral Infections

Clinical Manifestations

Parainfluenza viruses are the major cause of laryngotracheobronchitis (croup), but they also commonly cause upper respiratory tract infection, pneumonia, or bronchiolitis. Types 1 and 2 viruses are the most common pathogens associated with croup, and type 3 virus is associated with bronchiolitis and pneumonia. Rarely, parotitis, aseptic meningitis, and encephalitis have been associated with type 3 infections. Parainfluenza virus infections can exacerbate symptoms of asthma and chronic lung disease in children and adults. Infections can be particularly severe and persistent in immunodeficient children. Because type 4 virus is not detected as often as the other serotypes, infections with type 4 virus are not as well characterized. Parainfluenza infections do not confer complete protective immunity; therefore, reinfections can occur with all serotypes and at any age, but reinfections usually cause a mild illness limited to the upper respiratory tract.

Etiology

Parainfluenza viruses are enveloped RNA viruses classified as paramyxoviruses. Four antigenically distinct types—1, 2, 3, and 4 (with 2 subtypes, 4A and 4B)—have been identified.

Epidemiology

Parainfluenza viruses are transmitted from person to person by direct contact and exposure to contaminated nasopharyngeal secretions through respiratory tract droplets and fomites. Parainfluenza viral infections produce sporadic infections as well as epidemics of disease. Seasonal patterns of infection are distinctive, predictable, and cyclic. Different serotypes have distinct epidemiologic patterns. Type 1 virus tends to produce outbreaks of respiratory tract illness, usually croup, in the autumn of every other year. Type 2 virus also can cause outbreaks of respiratory tract illness in the autumn, often in conjunction with type 1 outbreaks, but type 2 outbreaks tend to be less severe, irregular, and less common. Parainflu-

enza type 3 virus usually is prominent during spring and summer in temperate climates but often continues into autumn, especially in years when autumn outbreaks of parainfluenza types 1 or 2 are absent. Infections with type 4 virus are recognized less commonly, sporadic, and generally associated with mild illnesses.

The age of primary infection varies with serotype. Primary infection with all types usually occurs by 5 years of age. Infection with type 3 virus more often occurs in infants and is a prominent cause of lower respiratory tract illnesses. By 12 months of age, 50% of infants have acquired type 3 infection. Infections between 1 and 5 years of age are associated most commonly with type 1 virus and less so with type 2 virus.

Immunocompetent children with primary parainfluenza infection can shed virus for up to 1 week before the onset of clinical symptoms until 1 to 3 weeks after symptoms have disappeared, depending on serotype. Severe lower respiratory tract disease with prolonged shedding of the virus can develop in immunodeficient people. In these patients, infection may spread beyond the respiratory tract to the liver and lymph nodes.

Incubation Period

2 to 6 days.

Diagnostic Tests

Virus may be isolated from nasopharyngeal secretions usually within 4 to 7 days of culture inoculation or earlier by using centrifugation of a specimen onto a monolayer of susceptible cells with subsequent staining for viral antigen (shell viral assay). Confirmation is made by rapid antigen detection, usually immunofluorescent. Rapid antigen identification techniques, including immunofluorescent assays, enzyme immunoassays, and fluoroimmunoassays, can be used to detect the virus in nasopharyngeal secretions, but the sensitivities of the tests vary. Multiplex reverse transcriptase-PCR assay, with high sensitivity and specificity, is available for detection and differentiation of parainfluenza viruses. Serologic diagnosis, made retrospectively by a significant increase in antibody titer between serum specimens obtained during acute infection and convalescence, is less useful because infection may not always be accompanied by a significant homotypic antibody response.

Treatment

Specific antiviral therapy is not available. Most infections are self-limited and require no treatment. Monitoring for oxygenation and hypercapnia for more severely affected chil-

dren with lower respiratory tract disease may be helpful. Epinephrine aerosol commonly is given to severely affected, hospitalized patients with laryngotracheobronchitis to decrease airway obstruction. Parenteral dexamethasone in high doses, oral dexamethasone, and nebulized corticosteroids have been demonstrated to lessen the severity and duration of symptoms and hospitalization in patients with moderate to severe laryngotracheobronchitis. Management otherwise is supportive.

Image 70.1
Croup in a 2-year-old due to parainfluenza virus infection with classic tenting of the tracheal lumen.

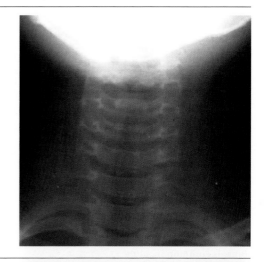

Image 70.2
Fatal croup. Edema, congestion, and inflammation of larynx and pharynx.

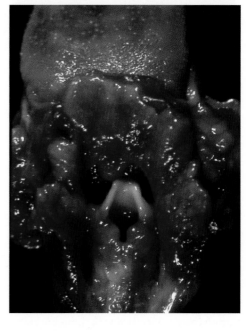

71

Parvovirus B19
(Erythema Infectiosum, Fifth Disease)

Clinical Manifestations

Infection with parvovirus B19 is recognized most often as erythema infectiosum (EI), which is characterized by a distinctive rash that can be preceded by mild systemic symptoms, including fever in 15% to 30% of patients. The facial rash can be intensely red with a "slapped cheek" appearance that often is accompanied by circumoral pallor. A symmetric, maculopapular, lace-like, and often pruritic rash also occurs on the trunk, moving peripherally to involve the arms, buttocks, and thighs. The rash can fluctuate in intensity and recur with environmental changes, such as temperature and exposure to sunlight, for weeks to months. A brief, mild, nonspecific illness consisting of fever, malaise, myalgias, and headache often precedes the characteristic exanthema by approximately 7 to 10 days. Arthralgia and arthritis occur in less than 10% of infected children but commonly among adults, especially women. Knees are involved most commonly in children, but a symmetric polyarthropathy of knees, fingers, and other joints is common in adults.

Human parvovirus B19 also can cause other manifestations (Table 71.1), including asymptomatic infection, a mild respiratory tract illness with no rash, a rash atypical for EI that may be rubelliform or petechial, papulopurpuric gloves-and-socks syndrome (painful and pruritic papules, petechiae, and purpura of hands and feet, often with fever and enanthem), polyarthropathy syndrome (arthralgia and arthritis in adults in the absence of other manifestations of EI), chronic erythroid hypoplasia in immunodeficient patients, and transient aplastic crisis lasting 7 to 10 days in patients with hemolytic anemias (eg, sickle cell disease and autoimmune hemolytic anemia) and other conditions associated with low hemoglobin concentrations, including hemorrhage, severe anemia, and thalassemia. Chronic parvovirus B19 infection can cause severe anemia in patients infected with HIV. In addition, parvovirus B19 infection sometimes has been associated with thrombocyto-penia and neutropenia. Patients with aplastic crisis can have a prodromal illness with fever, malaise, and myalgia, but rash usually is absent. Red blood cell aplasia is related to lytic infection in erythrocyte precursors.

Parvovirus B19 infection occurring during pregnancy can cause fetal hydrops, intrauterine growth retardation, isolated pleural and pericardial effusions, and death but is not a proven cause of congenital anomalies. The risk of fetal death is between 2% and 6%, with the greatest risk occurring during the first half of pregnancy.

Etiology

Human parvovirus B19 is a nonenveloped, single-stranded DNA virus that replicates only in human erythrocyte precursors.

Epidemiology

Parvovirus B19 is distributed worldwide and is a common cause of infection in humans, who are the only known hosts. Modes of transmission include contact with respiratory tract secretions, percutaneous exposure to blood or blood products, and vertical transmission from mother to fetus. Since 2002, plasma derivatives have been screened using quantitative DNA measurement to reduce the risk of parvovirus B19 transmission. Parvovirus B19 infections are ubiquitous, and cases of EI can occur sporadically or in outbreaks in elementary or junior high schools during late winter and early spring. Secondary spread among susceptible household members is common and occurs in approximately 50% of susceptible contacts. The transmission rate in schools is less, but infection can be an occupational risk for school and child care personnel, with approximately 20% of susceptible people becoming infected. In young children, antibody seroprevalence generally is 5% to 10%. In most communities, approximately 50% of young adults and often more than 90% of elderly people are seropositive. The annual seroconversion rate in women of childbearing age has been reported to be approximately 1.5%. The timing of the presence of parvovirus B19 DNA in serum and respiratory tract secretions indicates that people with EI are most infectious before onset of the rash and are unlikely to be infectious after onset of the rash. In contrast, patients with aplastic crises are contagious from before the onset of symptoms through at least the week after onset. Symptoms of the papulopurpuric gloves-and-socks syndrome occur in association with viremia and before development of antibody response, and affected patients should be considered infectious. Transmission from patients with aplastic crisis to hospital personnel can occur.

Incubation

Usually 4 to 14 days; can be as long as 21 days.

Diagnostic Tests

In the immunocompetent host, detection of serum parvovirus B19–specific IgM antibody is the preferred diagnostic test. A positive IgM test result indicates that infection probably occurred within the previous 2 to 4 months. On the basis of radioimmunoassay or enzyme immunoassay results, antibody can be detected in 90% or more of patients at the time of the EI rash and by the third day of illness in patients with transient aplastic crisis. Serum IgG antibody appears by approximately day 7 of EI and persists for life; it is not necessarily indicative of acute infection. These assays are available through commercial laboratories and through some state health department laboratories.

However, their sensitivity and specificity may vary, particularly for IgM antibody. The optimal method for detecting chronic infection in the immunocompromised patient is demonstration of virus by nucleic acid hybridization or PCR assays because parvovirus B19 antibody is variably present in persistent infection. Because parvovirus B19 DNA can be detected at low levels by PCR assay in serum for up to 9 months after the acute viremic phase, detection of parvovirus B19 DNA by PCR assay does not necessarily indicate acute infection. The less sensitive nucleic acid hybridization assays usually are positive for only 2 to 4 days after onset of illness. For HIV-infected patients with severe anemia associated with chronic infection, dot blot hybridization of serum specimens may have adequate sensitivity. Parvovirus B19 has not been grown in standard cell culture.

Treatment

For most patients, only supportive care is indicated. Patients with aplastic crises can require transfusion. For treatment of chronic infection in immunodeficient patients, IGIV therapy often is effective. Some cases of parvovirus B19 infection concurrent with hydrops fetalis have been treated successfully with intrauterine blood transfusions.

Table 71.1
Clinical Manifestations of Human Parvovirus B19 Infection

Conditions	Usual Hosts
Erythema infectiosum (fifth disease)	Immunocompetent children
Polyarthropathy syndrome	Immunocompetent adults (more common in women)
Chronic anemia/pure red cell aplasia	Immunocompromised hosts
Transient aplastic crisis	People with hemolytic anemia (ie, sickle cell anemia)
Hydrops fetalis/congenital anemia	Fetus (first 20 weeks of pregnancy)
Persistent anemia	Immunocompromised people

Image 71.1

Characteristic slapped cheek appearance of the face in a child who has fifth disease. The characteristic rash also is present on the arms.

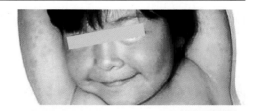

Image 71.2

Parvovirus B19 infection (erythema infectiosum, fifth disease) in a 5-year-old girl.

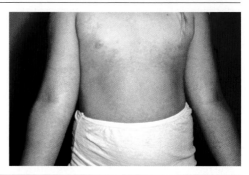

Image 71.3

Close-up view of the lace-like pattern of fifth disease in a 6-year-old female.

Image 71.4

Parvovirus infection in pregnancy. Villus capillary containing nucleated red blood cells with viral inclusion.

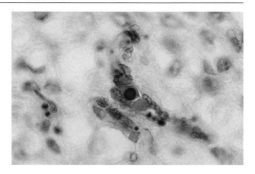

72

Pasteurella Infections

Clinical Manifestations

The most common manifestation in children is cellulitis at the site of a scratch or bite of a cat, dog, or other animal. Cellulitis usually develops within 24 hours of the injury and includes swelling, erythema, tenderness, and serous or sanguinopurulent discharge at the site. Regional lymphadenopathy, chills, and fever can occur. Local complications, such as septic arthritis, osteomyelitis, and teno-synovitis, can occur. Less common mani-festations of infection include septicemia, meningitis, respiratory tract infections (eg, pneumonia, pulmonary abscesses, pleural empyema), appendicitis, hepatic abscess, peritonitis, urinary tract infection, and ocular infections (eg, conjunctivitis, corneal ulcer endophthalmitis). People with liver disease or underlying host defense abnormalities are predisposed to bacteremia attributable to *Pasteurella multocida* infection.

Etiology

Species of the genus *Pasteurella* are nonmotile, facultative anaerobic, saccharolytic, gram-negative coccobacilli or rods that are primary pathogens in animals. The most common human pathogen is *P multocida*.

Epidemiology

Pasteurella species are found in the oral flora of 70% to 90% of cats, 25% to 50% of dogs, and many other animals. Transmission can occur from the bite or scratch of a cat or dog or, less commonly, from another animal. Respiratory tract spread from animals to humans also occurs. In a significant proportion of cases, no animal exposure can be identified. Human-to-human spread has not been documented.

Incubation Period

Usually less than 24 hours.

Diagnostic Tests

The isolation of *Pasteurella* species from skin lesion drainage or other sites of infection (eg, blood, joint fluid, CSF, sputum, pleural fluid, or suppurative lymph nodes) is diagnos-tic. Although *Pasteurella* species resemble sev-eral other organisms morphologically and grow on many culture media at 37°C (98°F), laboratory differentiation is not difficult.

Treatment

The drug of choice is penicillin. Other effective oral agents include ampicillin, amoxicillin-clavulanate, cefuroxime, cefpodoxime, doxycy-cline, and fluoroquinolones. Erythromycin, clindamycin, cephalexin, cefadroxil, cefaclor, and dicloxacillin should not be used. For patients allergic to beta-lactam agents, azithro-mycin and trimethoprim-sulfamethoxazole are alternative choices. Doxycycline is effective but should not be given to children younger than 8 years. For suspected polymicrobial infection, oral amoxicillin-clavulanate or, for severe infection, intravenous ampicillin-sulbactam or ticarcillin-clavulanate can be given. Wound drainage or debridement may be necessary.

Image 72.1
Right forearm of 1-year-old boy bitten by a stray cat. The infant developed fever, redness, and swelling 10 hours after the bite.

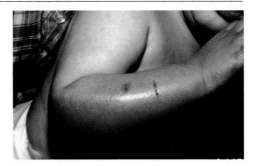

73

Pediculosis Capitis
(Head Lice)

Clinical Manifestations

Itching is the most common symptom of head lice infestation, but many children are asymptomatic. Adult lice or eggs (nits) are found in the hair, usually behind the ears and near the nape of the neck. Excoriations and crusting caused by secondary bacterial infection may occur and often are associated with regional lymphadenopathy. In temperate climates, head lice deposit their eggs on a hair shaft 3 to 4 mm from the scalp. Because hair grows at a rate of approximately 1 cm per month, the duration of infestation can be estimated by the distance of the nit from the scalp.

Etiology

Pediculus humanus capitis is the head louse. Both nymphs and adult lice feed on human blood.

Epidemiology

Head lice infestation in children attending child care and school is common in the United States. Head lice are not a sign of poor hygiene, and all socioeconomic groups are affected. Infestations are less common in African American children than in children of other races in the United States. Head lice infestation is not influenced by hair length or frequency of shampooing or brushing. Head lice are not a health hazard because they are not responsible for the spread of any disease. Transmission occurs by direct contact with hair of infested people and, uncommonly, by contact with personal belongings, such as combs, hair brushes, and hats. Head lice may survive up to 2 days away from the scalp, and their eggs cannot hatch at a lower ambient temperature than that close to the scalp.

Incubation Period

From laying of eggs to hatching, 10 to 14 days (shorter in hot climates and longer in cold climates).

Diagnostic Tests

Identification of eggs (nits), nymphs, and lice with the naked eye is possible; the diagnosis can be confirmed by using a hand lens or microscope. Adult lice seldom are seen because they move rapidly and conceal themselves effectively. It is important to differentiate nits from dandruff, benign hair casts (a layer of follicular cells that easily slides off the hair shaft), plugs of desquamated cells, and external hair debris.

Treatment

Therapy could be started with over-the-counter 1% permethrin, but resistance is common. For treatment failures, malathion should be used. When lice are resistant to all topical agents, ivermectin can be used. No drug is truly ovicidal. Drugs that leave a residual can kill nymphs as they emerge from eggs. Safety is a major concern with pediculicides because the infestation itself does not present a risk to the host. Pediculicides should be used only as directed and with care. Instructions on proper use of any product should be explained carefully.

- *Permethrin (1%).* Permethrin is available without a prescription in a 1% cream rinse that is applied to the scalp and hair for 10 minutes after washing and towel drying the hair.
- *Permethrin (5%).* Not approved by the FDA as a pediculicide, 5% permethrin is available by prescription as a cream usually applied overnight for scabies (down to 2 months of age). It is applied to the scalp and left on for several hours or overnight, then rinsed off.
- *Malathion (0.5%).* This organophosphate pesticide is available only by prescription as a lotion and is highly effective. However, this drug has been approved only for use in children 6 years and older. It is applied to dry hair as an 8- to 12-hour application. Malathion is contraindicated in children younger than 2 years.
- *Lindane (1%).* Lindane shampoo is an organochloride available only by prescription. It should be used as second-line treatment on the basis of safety concerns.

It must be rinsed out no longer than 4 minutes after application and should not be used more than once to treat a lice infestation.

- **Crotamiton (10%).** Not approved by the FDA as a pediculicide, crotamiton (10%) lotion is used to treat scabies, and limited studies have shown it to be effective against head lice when applied to the scalp and left on for 24 hours before rinsing out. Safety and absorption in children, adults, and pregnant women have not been evaluated.
- **Oral trimethoprim-sulfamethoxazole.** Not approved by the FDA as a pediculicide, a 10-day course of this antibiotic has been cited as effective against head lice. Oral trimethoprim-sulfamethoxazole plus topical

1% permethrin cream rinse may be more effective but should be reserved for treatment failures.

- **Oral ivermectin.** Not approved by the FDA as a pediculicide, ivermectin is an anthelmintic agent that may be effective against head lice. It has been given as a single oral dose with a second dose given after 7 to 10 days. Ivermectin should not be used in children weighing less than 15 kg.

Topical corticosteroid and oral antihistamine agents may be beneficial to relieve itching or burning of the scalp. Removal of nits after successful treatment with a pediculicide is not necessary to prevent spread.

Image 73.1
Nits on the hair shafts.

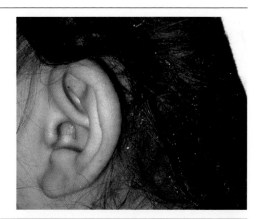

Image 73.2
Pediculosis with nits and excoriations of the scalp.

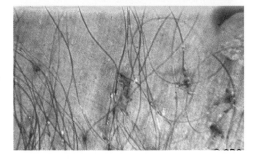

74

Pediculosis Corporis
(Body Lice)

Clinical Manifestations

Intense itching, particularly at night, is common with body lice infestations that manifest as small erythematous macules, papules, and excoriations primarily on the trunk. Body lice and their eggs live in the seams of clothing. Secondary bacterial infection of the skin caused by scratching is common.

Etiology

Pediculus humanus corporis (or *humanus*) is the body louse. Nymphs and adult lice feed on human blood.

Epidemiology

Body lice generally are found on people with poor hygiene. Fomites have a role in transmission. Body lice cannot survive away from a blood source for longer than 10 days. In contrast with head lice, body lice are well-recognized vectors of disease (eg, epidemic typhus, trench fever, and relapsing fever).

Incubation Period

6 to 10 days to nymph hatching; 2 to 3 weeks to adult lice.

Diagnostic Tests

Identification of eggs, nymphs, and lice with the naked eye is possible; the diagnosis can be confirmed by using a hand lens or microscope. Adult lice seldom are seen because they move rapidly and conceal themselves effectively.

Treatment

Treatment consists of improving hygiene and cleaning clothes and bedding. Infested materials can be washed and dried at hot temperatures to kill lice. Pediculicides are not necessary if materials are laundered at least weekly.

Image 74.1
Pediculosis corporis (body lice) feeding on the arm of an adolescent girl.

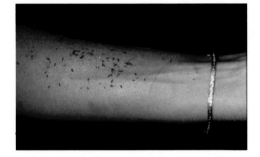

75

Pediculosis Pubis

(Pubic Lice)

Clinical Manifestations

Pruritus of the anogenital area is a common symptom in pubic lice infestations ("crabs"). Many hairy areas of the body can be infested, including the eyelashes, eyebrows, beard, axilla, perianal area and, rarely, the scalp. A characteristic sign of heavy pubic lice infestation is the presence of bluish or slate-colored maculae on the chest, abdomen, or thighs, known as maculae ceruleae.

Etiology

Phthirus pubis is the pubic or crab louse. Nymphs and adult lice feed on human blood.

Epidemiology

Pubic lice infestations are common in adolescents and young adults and usually are transmitted through sexual contact. The pubic louse also can be transferred by contaminated items, such as towels. Pubic lice can be found on the eyelashes of younger children. Infested people should be examined for other STIs, including syphilis and infection with *Neisseria gonorrhoeae, Chlamydia trachomatis,* hepatitis B virus, and HIV.

Incubation Period

6 to 10 days to nymph hatching; 2 to 3 weeks to adult lice.

Diagnostic Tests

Identification of eggs (nits), nymphs, and lice with the naked eye is possible; the diagnosis can be confirmed by using a hand lens or microscope. Adult lice seldom are seen because they move rapidly and conceal themselves effectively.

Treatment

The pediculicides used to treat pediculosis capitis are effective for treatment of pubic lice. Re-treatment is recommended 7 to 10 days later. Pediculicides should not be used for infestation of eyelashes by pubic lice; petrolatum ointment applied 2 to 4 times daily for 8 to 10 days or oral trimethoprim-sulfamethoxazole for 10 days has been reported to be effective. Nits should be removed by hand from the eyelashes.

Image 75.1
Phthirus pubis in the eyelashes of a 3-year-old boy. The diagnosis can be confirmed by the use of a hand lens or microscope.

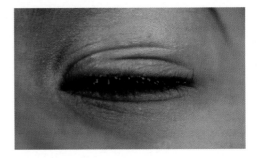

76

Pertussis
(Whooping Cough)

Clinical Manifestations

Pertussis begins with mild upper respiratory tract symptoms similar to the common cold (catarrhal stage) and progresses to cough and then usually to paroxysms of cough (paroxysmal stage) characterized by inspiratory whoop and commonly followed by vomiting. Fever is absent or minimal. Symptoms wane gradually over weeks to months (convalescent stage). Disease in infants younger than 6 months can be atypical with a short catarrhal stage, gagging, gasping, or apnea as prominent early manifestations; absence of whoop; and prolonged convalescence. Sudden unexpected death can be caused by pertussis. Disease in older children and adults also can have atypical manifestations when the cough is not accompanied by paroxysms or whoop. The duration of classic pertussis is 6 to 10 weeks in children. Approximately one-half of adolescents with pertussis cough for 10 weeks or longer. Complications among adolescents and adults include syncope, sleep disturbance, incontinence, rib fractures, and pneumonia. Pertussis is most severe when it occurs during the first 6 months of life, particularly in preterm and unimmunized infants. Complications among infants include pneumonia (22%), seizures (2%), encephalopathy (<0.5%), and death. Rare pertussis deaths at older ages occur in people with underlying conditions, especially neuromuscular disorders.

Etiology

Pertussis is caused by a fastidious, gram-negative, pleomorphic bacillus, *Bordetella pertussis*.

Epidemiology

Humans are the only known hosts of *B pertussis*. Transmission occurs by close contact with cases via aerosolized droplets. Neither infection nor immunization provides lifelong immunity. Lack of natural booster events and waning immunity since childhood immunization are responsible for the growing number of cases of pertussis in people older than 10 years.

Pertussis occurs endemically with 3- to 5-year cycles of increased disease. Since 1976, when an all-time low number of cases was reported in the United States, the annual number of reported cases has increased to 25 827 in 2004, with less year-to-year cycling. Incidence is highest in infants younger than 6 months, followed by people 10 to 14 years of age. In 2003 the number of reported cases in middle school ages exceeded the number of cases in infants. Regardless of immunization status, as many as 80% of household contacts acquire infection with varying degrees of cough illness. Older siblings (including adolescents) and adults can have mild or atypical unrecognized disease but are important sources of pertussis for infants and young children. Infected individuals are most contagious during the catarrhal stage and the first 2 weeks after cough onset. Factors affecting the length of communicability include age, immunization status or previous episode of pertussis, and appropriate antimicrobial therapy. For example, a young unimmunized and untreated infant may be infectious for 6 or more weeks after cough onset; an untreated immunized adolescent may be infectious for 2 weeks or more after cough onset. Nasopharyngeal cultures usually test negative for *B pertussis* within 5 days after initiating macrolide therapy.

Incubation Period

7 to 10 days (range, 5–21 days).

Diagnostic Tests

Culture still is considered the gold standard for laboratory diagnosis of pertussis. Although culture is 100% specific, *B pertussis* is a fastidious organism. Culture requires collection of an appropriate nasopharyngeal specimen, obtained either by aspiration or with Dacron (polyethylene terephthalate) or calcium alginate swabs. Because culture requires a specialized medium, laboratory personnel should be contacted when *B pertussis* is suspected. A negative culture does not exclude the diagnosis of pertussis.

PCR assay is being used increasingly for detection of *B pertussis* because of its improved sensitivity and rapid result. The PCR test requires collection of an adequate nasopharyngeal specimen using a Dacron swab or nasal wash. Calcium alginate swabs should not be used for PCR tests. The PCR test lacks sensitivity in previously immunized individuals. Unacceptably high rates of false-positive results are reported from some laboratories.

Direct fluorescent antibody (DFA) testing takes only a few hours to perform and is available commercially, but is performed reliably only by experienced technologists. Although use of monoclonal reagents has increased the specificity of DFA testing, sensitivity is still low and DFA testing generally is not recommended for laboratory confirmation of pertussis. A single-specimen serologic test would be ideal for diagnosis in adolescents and adults whose culture or PCR test result usually is negative. In the absence of immunization within 2 years, a single serum serologic test result with elevated IgG antibody to pertussis toxin is suggestive of recent *B pertussis* infection. Although commercial serologic tests for pertussis infection exist, none currently is licensed by the FDA for diagnostic use.

An increased absolute white blood cell count with an absolute lymphocytosis often is present in infants and young children but not in adolescents with pertussis.

Treatment

Infants younger than 6 months and older individuals with underlying conditions commonly require hospitalization for supportive care, to assess ability for self-rescue after paroxysms during accelerating phase of disease, or to manage apnea, hypoxia, feeding difficulties, and other complications. Intensive care facilities may be required.

Antimicrobial agents given during the catarrhal stage may ameliorate the disease. After the cough is established, antimicrobial agents have no discernible effect on the course of illness but are recommended to limit the spread of organisms to others. Azithromycin and clarithromycin have microbiologic effectiveness comparable with erythromycin for treatment of pertussis in previously immunized people who are 6 months of age or older.

Antimicrobial agents for infants younger than 6 months require special consideration. Until additional information is available, azithromycin is the drug of choice for treatment or prophylaxis of pertussis in infants younger than 1 month. All infants younger than 1 month who receive any macrolide should be monitored for development of infantile hypertrophic pyloric stenosis for 1 month after completing the course.

Trimethoprim-sulfamethoxazole is an alternative for patients who cannot tolerate macrolides or who are infected with a macrolide-resistant strain.

Image 76.1
A preschool-aged male with pertussis. Thick respiratory secretions were produced by a paroxysmal coughing spell.

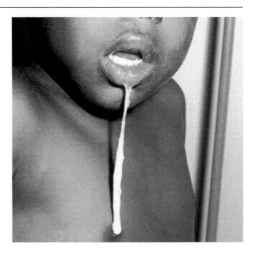

Image 76.2
Bilateral subconjunctival hemorrhages and thick
nasal mucus in an infant with pertussis.

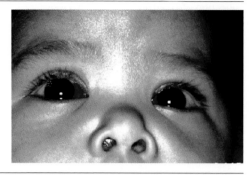

Image 76.3
Bronchiolar plugging in a neonate who died
of pertussis pneumonia. Infants and children
often acquire pertussis from an infected adult
or sibling contact.

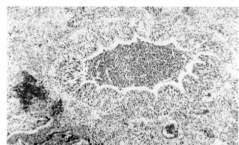

Image 76.4
Subdural bleeding secondary to whooping
cough in a 4-week-old neonate.

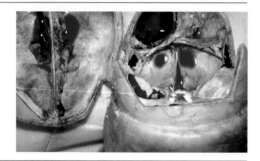

Image 76.5
Pertussis pneumonia in a 2-month-old at hospital
admission. His mother had been coughing since
shortly after delivery.

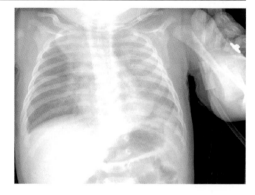

Image 76.6

The infant in Image 76.5 2 days
after hospitalization.

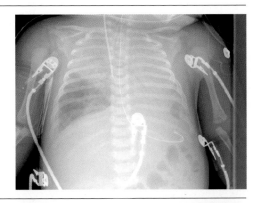

Image 76.7

The infant pictured in Image 76.5 and 76.6
who required mechanical ventilation because
of respiratory failure.

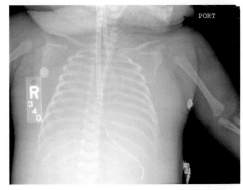

77

Pinworm Infection
(Enterobius vermicularis)

Clinical Manifestations

Although some people are asymptomatic, pinworm infection (enterobiasis) can cause pruritus ani and, rarely, pruritus vulvae. Pinworms have been found in the lumen of the appendix, but most evidence indicates that they are not related causally to acute appendicitis. Many clinical findings, such as grinding of the teeth at night, weight loss, and enuresis, have been attributed to pinworm infections, but proof of a causal relationship has not been established. Urethritis, vaginitis, salpingitis, or pelvic peritonitis can occur from aberrant migration of an adult worm from the perineum.

Etiology

Enterobius vermicularis is a nematode or roundworm.

Epidemiology

Enterobiasis occurs worldwide and commonly clusters within families. Prevalence rates are higher in preschool- and school-aged children, in primary caregivers for infected children, and in institutionalized people; up to 50% of these populations may be infected.

Egg transmission occurs by the fecal-oral route directly, indirectly, or inadvertently by contaminated hands or fomites, such as shared toys, bedding, clothing, toilet seats, and baths. Female pinworms usually die after depositing eggs on the perianal skin. Reinfection occurs by reingestion of eggs (ie, autoinfection) or acquisition from a new source. A person remains infectious as long as female nematodes are discharging eggs on perianal skin. Eggs remain infective in an indoor environment, usually for 2 to 3 weeks. Humans are the only known natural hosts; dogs and cats do not harbor *E vermicularis*.

Incubation Period

From ingestion to the perianal region is 1 to 2 months or longer.

Diagnostic Tests

Diagnosis usually is made when adult worms are visualized in the perianal region, which is best examined 2 to 3 hours after the child is asleep. Very few ova are present in stool. Alternatively, transparent (not translucent) adhesive tape can be applied to the perianal skin to collect any eggs that may be present; the tape then is applied to a glass slide and examined under a low-power microscopic lens. Three consecutive specimens should be obtained when the patient first awakens in the morning. Eosinophilia is unusual in cases of pinworm infection. Serologic testing is not available.

Treatment

The drugs of choice are mebendazole, pyrantel pamoate, and albendazole, each of which is given in a single dose and repeated in 2 weeks. Pyrantel pamoate is available without prescription. Reinfection with pinworms occurs easily. Infected people should bathe in the morning; bathing removes a large proportion of eggs. Frequently changing the infected person's underclothes, bedclothes, and bedsheets can decrease the egg contamination of the local environment and decrease risk of reinfection. Specific personal hygiene measures (eg, exercising hand hygiene before eating or preparing food, keeping fingernails short, avoiding scratching of the perianal region, and avoiding nail biting) may decrease risk of autoinfection and continued transmission. All family members should be treated as a group in situations in which multiple or repeated symptomatic infections occur. Vaginitis is self-limited and does not require separate treatment.

Image 77.1

A, B: Enterobius egg(s). C: Enterobius eggs on cellulose tape prep.

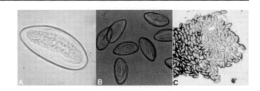

Image 77.2

Adult pinworm *(Enterobius vermicularis)* in the perianal area of a 14-year-old boy. Perianal inspection 2 to 3 hours after the child goes to sleep may reveal pinworms that have migrated outside of the intestinal tract.

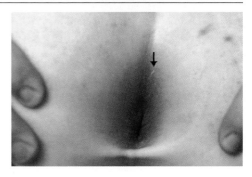

78

Pityriasis Versicolor
(Tinea Versicolor)

Clinical Manifestations

Pityriasis versicolor (formerly tinea versicolor) is a common superficial yeast infection of the skin characterized by multiple, scaling, oval, and patchy macular lesions usually distributed over upper portions of the trunk, proximal areas of the arms, and neck. Facial involvement particularly is common in children. Lesions may be hypopigmented or hyperpigmented (fawn colored or brown). Lesions fail to tan during the summer and during the winter are relatively darker, hence the term *versicolor*. Common conditions confused with this disorder include pityriasis alba, postinflammatory hypopigmentation, vitiligo, melasma, seborrheic dermatitis, pityriasis rosea, and dermatologic manifestations of secondary syphilis.

Etiology

The cause of pityriasis versicolor is *Malassezia* species, a group of dimorphic lipid-dependent yeasts that exist on healthy skin in yeast phase and cause clinical lesions only when substantial growth of hyphae occurs. Moist heat and lipid-containing sebaceous secretions encourage rapid overgrowth.

Epidemiology

Pityriasis versicolor occurs worldwide but is more prevalent in tropical and subtropical areas. Although primarily a disorder of adolescents and young adults, pityriasis versicolor also may occur in prepubertal children and infants. *Malassezia* species commonly colonize the skin in the first year of life and usually are harmless commensals.

Incubation Period

Unknown.

Diagnosis

The clinical appearance usually is diagnostic. Involved areas are fluorescent yellow under Wood light examination. Skin scrapings examined microscopically in a potassium hydroxide wet mount preparation or stained with methylene blue or May-Grünwald-Giemsa stain disclose the pathognomonic clusters of yeast cells and hyphae ("spaghetti and meatball" appearance). Growth of this yeast on culture requires a source of long-chain fatty acids, which may be provided by overlaying Sabouraud dextrose agar medium with sterile olive oil.

Treatment

Topical treatment with selenium sulfide as 2.5% lotion or 1% shampoo has been the traditional treatment of choice. These preparations are applied in a thin layer covering the body surface from the face to the knees for 30 minutes daily for a week, then monthly applications for 3 months to help prevent recurrences. Other topical preparations with therapeutic efficacy include sodium hyposulfite or thiosulfate in 15% to 25% concentrations (eg, Tinver lotion) applied twice a day for 2 to 4 weeks. Because *Malassezia* species are part of normal flora, relapses are common. Multiple topical treatments may be necessary.

Oral antifungal therapy has advantages over topical therapy, including ease of administration and shorter duration of treatment, but oral therapy is more expensive and associated with a greater risk of adverse reactions. Ketoconazole, fluconazole, or itraconazole has been effective in adults. These drugs have not been studied extensively in children and are not approved by the FDA for this purpose. Exercise to increase sweating and skin concentrations of medication may enhance the effectiveness of systemic therapy. Patients should be advised that repigmentation may not occur for several months after successful treatment.

Image 78.1

The spores and pseudohyphae of *Malassezia furfur* (a yeast that can cause pityriasis versicolor) resemble "spaghetti and meatballs" on a potassium hydroxide slide.

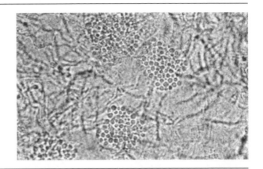

Image 78.2

Pityriasis versicolor.

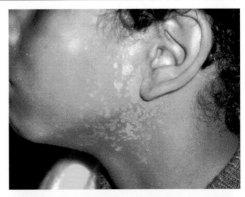

Image 78.3

Tinea versicolor in a 14-year-old boy.

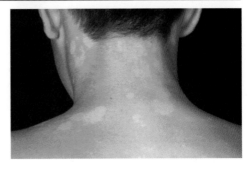

Image 78.4
Pityriasis versicolor in a 16-year-old boy.

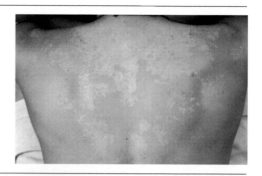

Image 78.5
Pityriasis rosea with herald patch in the inguinal area of a child. Because the herald patch precedes the widespread eruption, it may be mistaken for tinea corporis, though a potassium hydroxide preparation would be negative.

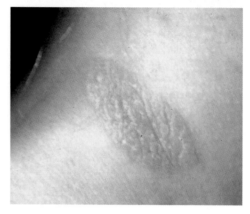

79

Plague

Clinical Manifestations

Naturally acquired plague most commonly manifests in the bubonic form, with acute onset of fever and painful swollen regional lymph nodes (buboes), whereas bioterrorism-related plague would manifest chiefly as pneumonic plague. Buboes occur most often in the inguinal region but also occur in axillary or cervical areas. Less commonly, plague manifests in the septicemic form (hypotension, acute respiratory distress, intravascular coagulopathy) or as pneumonic plague (cough, fever, dyspnea, and hemoptysis) and, rarely, as meningeal, pharyngeal, ocular, or gastrointestinal plague. Abrupt onset of fever, chills, headache, and malaise are characteristic in all forms. Occasionally, patients have symptoms of mild lymphadenitis or prominent gastrointestinal tract symptoms, which can obscure the correct diagnosis. When left untreated, plague often will progress to overwhelming sepsis with renal failure, acute respiratory distress syndrome, hemodynamic instability, diffuse intravascular coagulation, and necrosis of distal extremities. Plague has been referred to as black death or blackwater fever.

Etiology

Plague is caused by *Yersinia pestis,* a pleomorphic, bipolar-staining, gram-negative coccobacillus.

Epidemiology

Plague is a zoonotic infection of rodents, carnivores, and their fleas that occurs in many areas of the world, especially Africa. Plague has been reported throughout the western United States, but most human cases (approximately 85%) occur in New Mexico, Arizona, California, and Colorado as isolated cases or in small clusters. More cases occur during summers that follow mild winters and wet springs. In the United States, human plague is a rural disease, usually associated with epizootic infections in ground squirrels, prairie dogs, and other wild rodents. Bubonic plague usually is transmitted by bites of infected rodent fleas or by direct contact with tissues and fluids of infected rodents or other mammals, including domestic cats.

Septicemic plague can result from direct contact with infectious materials or the bite of an infected flea. Primary pneumonic plague is acquired by inhalation of respiratory tract droplets from a human or animal with pneumonic plague or from exposure to laboratory aerosols. If aerosolized organisms were spread intentionally, plague pneumonia would be the most common manifestation and the greatest risk. Secondary pneumonic plague arises from hematogenous seeding of the lungs with *Y pestis* in patients with bubonic or septicemic plague.

Incubation Period

2 to 8 days for bubonic plague; 1 to 6 days for primary pneumonic plague.

Diagnostic Tests

The diagnosis of plague usually is confirmed by culture of *Y pestis* from blood, bubo aspirate, or other clinical specimen. The organism has a bipolar (safety-pin) appearance when viewed with Wayson or Gram stains. The microbiology laboratory examining specimens should be informed when plague is suspected to minimize risks of transmission to laboratory personnel. A positive fluorescent antibody test result for the presence of *Y pestis* in direct smears or cultures of a bubo aspirate, sputum, CSF, or blood specimen provides presumptive evidence of *Y pestis* infection. The organism can be detected in fixed tissues by monoclonal antibody–based histochemical methods at the CDC. A single positive serologic test result by passive hemagglutination assay or enzyme immunoassay in an unimmunized patient who has not had plague previously also provides presumptive evidence of infection. A 4-fold difference in antibody titer between 2 serum specimens obtained 4 weeks to 3 months apart also confirms the diagnosis of plague. PCR assay and immunohistochemical staining for rapid diagnosis of *Y pestis* are available in some reference or public health laboratories.

Treatment

For children, streptomycin is the treatment of choice in most cases. Gentamicin in standard doses for age given intramuscularly or intravenously seems to be an equally effective alternative to streptomycin. Tetracycline, doxycycline, chloramphenicol, trimethoprim-sulfamethoxazole, and ciprofloxacin are alternative drugs. Doxycycline or tetracycline should not be given to children younger than 8 years unless the benefits of its use outweigh the risks of dental staining. Chloramphenicol is the preferred treatment for plague meningitis. Fluoroquino-lones also have been found to be effective in some cases of plague but currently are not approved by the FDA for this indication.

Drainage of abscessed buboes may be necessary; drainage material is infectious until effective antimicrobial therapy has been given.

Image 79.1
Yersinia pestis (direct fluorescent antibody stain [DFA], 200x). Positive identification of the bacillus may be facilitated through the application of DFA stain and its affinity for the *Y pestis* capsular antigen.

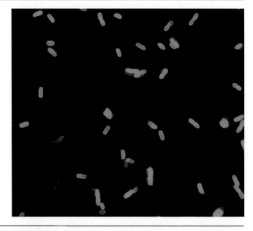

Image 79.2
Dark-stained bipolar ends of *Yersinia pestis* can clearly be seen in this Wright stain of blood from a plague victim. The actual cause of the disease is the plague bacillus *Y pestis*. It is a nonmotile, non-spore–forming, gram-negative, non-lactose–fermenting, bipolar, ovoid, safety pin–shaped bacterium.

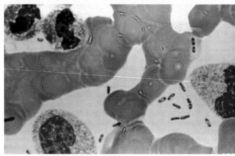

Image 79.3
Inguinal plague buboes in an 8-year-old boy. If left untreated, bubonic plague often becomes septicemic, with meningitis occurring in 6% of cases.

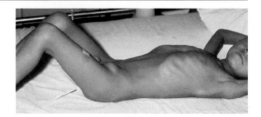

Image 79.4

Small hemorrhages on the skin of a plague victim. Capillary fragility is one of the manifestations of a plague infection, evident here on the leg of an infected patient.

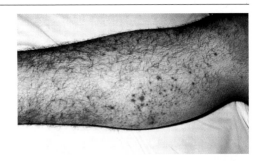

Image 79.5

Right hand of a plague patient displaying acral gangrene. Gangrene is one of the manifestations of plague, and is the origin of the term black death given to plague throughout the ages. (Disseminated intravascular coagulation is not uncommon in septicemic plague.)

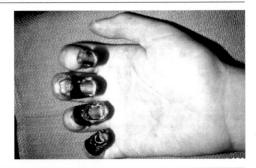

Image 79.6

This photomicrograph depicts the histopathologic changes in lung tissue in a case of fatal human plague pneumonia (160x). Note the moderate suppurative pneumonia, including the presence of many polymorphonuclear leukocytes, capillary engorgement, and intraalveolar debris, all indicative of an acute infection. Hematoxylin-eosin stain was used to process this slide.

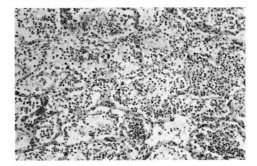

Image 79.7

Histopathology of spleen in fatal human plague. Vasculitis and thrombosis with hemorrhage.

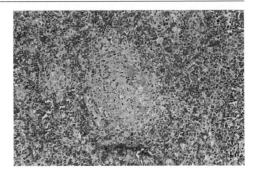

80

Pneumococcal Infections

Clinical Manifestations

Before routine use of heptavalent pneumococcal conjugate vaccine (PCV7), *Streptococcus pneumoniae* was the most common bacterial cause of acute otitis media and of invasive bacterial infections in children. Pneumococci also are a common cause of sinusitis, community-acquired pneumonia, meningitis, and conjunctivitis. Pneumococcus occasionally causes periorbital cellulitis, endocarditis, osteomyelitis, pericarditis, peritonitis, pyogenic arthritis, soft tissue infection, and neonatal septicemia.

Etiology

S pneumoniae (pneumococci) are lancet-shaped, gram-positive diplococci. At least 90 pneumococcal serotypes have been identified. Serotypes 4, 6B, 9V, 14, 18C, 19F, and 23F (Danish serotyping system) cause most invasive childhood pneumococcal infections in the United States and are the 7 types contained in the licensed heptavalent pneumococcal conjugate vaccine. Serotypes 6B, 9V, 14, 19A, 19F, and 23F are the most common isolates associated with resistance to penicillin.

Epidemiology

Pneumococci are ubiquitous, with many people having colonization of their upper respiratory tract. Transmission is from person to person, presumably by respiratory droplet contact. The period of communicability is unknown. Among young children who acquire a new pneumococcal serotype in the nasopharynx, illness (eg, otitis media) occurs in approximately 15%, usually within 1 month of acquisition. Viral upper respiratory tract infections, including influenza, may predispose to pneumococcal infections. Pneumococcal infections are most prevalent during winter months. Rates of infection are highest in infants, young children, the elderly, and black, Alaska Native, and some Native American populations. Other categories of children at presumed high risk or at moderate risk of developing invasive pneumococcal disease are outlined in Table 80.1.

Since 2000, when PCV7 was recommended for routine use in infants, the incidence of all invasive pneumococcal infections has decreased by 80% for children younger than 2 years and by approximately 90% for infections caused by vaccine-related serotypes and also has decreased in unimmunized older children and adults. The proportion of invasive isolates nonsusceptible to penicillin also has decreased in some areas. In some areas, an increase in the frequency of acute otitis media and invasive disease caused by serotypes not contained in PCV7 (serotype replacement) has been noted.

Incubation Period

Varies by site of infection and can be as short as 1 to 3 days.

Diagnostic Tests

Recovery of *S pneumoniae* from a normally sterile site is diagnostic. Blood cultures should be obtained from all patients with suspected invasive pneumococcal disease; cultures of CSF and other specimens (eg, pleural fluid) also may be indicated. Recovery of pneumococci from an upper respiratory tract culture is not indicative of the etiologic diagnosis of pneumococcal disease in the middle ear, lower respiratory tract, or sinus. Rapid methods to detect pneumococcal capsular antigen in CSF, pleural and joint fluid, and concentrated urine lack sufficient sensitivity or specificity to be of value.

All *S pneumoniae* isolates from normally sterile body fluids (eg, CSF, blood, middle ear fluid, or pleural or joint fluid) should be tested for in vitro antimicrobial susceptibility to determine the minimum inhibitory concentration of penicillin and cefotaxime or ceftriaxone. *Nonsusceptible* is defined to include both *intermediate* and *resistant* isolates. Accordingly, current definitions by the Clinical and Laboratory Standards Institute of in vitro susceptibility and nonsusceptibility for nonmeningeal and meningeal isolates are listed in Table 80.2.

Table 80.1
Children at High or Moderate Risk of Invasive Pneumococcal Infection

High Risk (incidence of invasive pneumococcal disease ≥150 cases/100 000 people per year)
Children with • Sickle cell disease, congenital or acquired asplenia, or splenic dysfunction • Human immunodeficiency virus infection • Cochlear implants
Presumed High Risk (insufficient data to calculate rates)
Children with • Congenital immune deficiency; some B- (humoral) or T-lymphocyte deficiencies, complement deficiencies (particularly C1, C2, C3, and C4), or phagocytic disorders (excluding chronic granulomatous disease) • Chronic cardiac disease (particularly cyanotic congenital heart disease and cardiac failure) • Chronic pulmonary disease (including asthma treated with high-dose oral corticosteroid therapy) • Cerebrospinal leaks from a congenital malformation, skull fracture, or neurologic procedure • Chronic renal insufficiency, including nephrotic syndrome • Diseases associated with immunosuppressive therapy or radiation therapy (including malignant neoplasms, leukemias, lymphomas, and Hodgkin disease) and solid organ transplantation • Diabetes mellitus
Moderate Risk (incidence of invasive pneumococcal disease ≥20 cases/100 000 people per year)
• All children 24–35 mo of age • Children 36–59 mo of age attending out-of-home child care • Children 36–59 mo of age who are black or of American Indian/Alaska Native descent

Table 80.2
Definition of In Vitro Susceptibility and Nonsusceptibility

Drug and Isolate Location	Susceptible, µg/mL	Nonsusceptible, µg/mL	
		Intermediate	Resistant
Penicillin	≤0.06	0.1–1.0	≥2.0
Cefotaxime **OR** ceftriaxone			
Nonmeningeal	≤1.0	2.0	≥4.0
Meningeal	≤0.5	1.0	≥2.0

Treatment

S pneumoniae strains that are nonsusceptible to penicillin G, cefotaxime, ceftriaxone, and other antimicrobial agents have been identified throughout the United States and worldwide. Vancomycin resistance has not been reported in the United States.

Bacterial Meningitis. Combination therapy with vancomycin and cefotaxime or ceftriax- one should be administered initially to all children 1 month of age or older with definite or probable bacterial meningitis. For children with life-threatening hypersensitivity to beta-lactam antimicrobial agents (ie, penicillins and cephalosporins), the combination of van- comycin and rifampin should be considered. Other possible antimicrobial agents for treat- ment of pneumococcal meningitis include meropenem or chloramphenicol.

On the basis of available results of susceptibility testing of the pneumococcal isolate, therapy should be modified according to the guidelines in Table 80.3.

For infants and children 6 weeks of age and older, adjunctive therapy with dexamethasone may be considered after weighing the potential benefits and possible risks. Experts do not agree on a recommendation to use corticosteroids in pneumococcal meningitis; data are not sufficient to demonstrate a clear benefit in children. If used, dexamethasone should be given before or concurrently with the first dose of the antimicrobial agent.

Nonmeningeal Invasive Pneumococcal Infections Requiring Hospitalization. For nonmeningeal invasive infections in previously well children who are not critically ill, antimicrobial agents currently in use to treat *S pneumoniae* and other potential pathogens should be initiated at the usually recommended dosages. For critically ill infants and children with invasive infections potentially attributable to *S pneumoniae*, additional initial antimicrobial therapy may be considered for strains that possibly are nonsusceptible to penicillin, cefotaxime, or ceftriaxone. Such patients include those with myopericarditis or severe multilobar pneumonia with hypoxia or hypotension. For children with severe hypersensitivity to the beta-lactam antimicrobial agents (ie, penicillins and cephalosporins), initial management for a potential pneumococcal infection should include clindamycin or vancomycin, in addition to antimicrobial agents for other potential pathogens as indicated. Consultation with an infectious diseases specialist should be considered.

Nonmeningeal Invasive Pneumococcal Infections in the Immunocompromised Host. The preceding recommendations for management of possible pneumococcal infections requiring hospitalization also apply to immunocompromised children, provided they are not critically ill. For critically ill patients, consideration should be given to initiating therapy with vancomycin and cefotaxime or ceftriaxone.

Table 80.3
Antimicrobial Therapy for Infants and Children With Meningitis Caused by *Streptococcus pneumoniae* on the Basis of Susceptibility Test Results

Susceptibility Test Results	Antimicrobial Management
Susceptible to penicillin	**Discontinue vancomycin** **AND** Begin penicillin (and discontinue cephalosporin) **OR** Continue cefotaxime or ceftriaxone alone
Nonsusceptible to penicillin (*intermediate* or *resistant*) **AND** *Susceptible* to cefotaxime and ceftriaxone	**Discontinue vancomycin** **AND** Continue cefotaxime or ceftriaxone
Nonsusceptible to penicillin (*intermediate* or *resistant*) **AND** *Nonsusceptible* to cefotaxime and ceftriaxone (*intermediate* or *resistant*) **AND** *Susceptible* to rifampin	Continue vancomycin and cefotaxime or ceftriaxone. Rifampin may be added to vancomycin in selected circumstances (see text).

Otitis Media. Most experts recommend empiric initial treatment of acute otitis media with high-dose oral amoxicillin (80 mg/kg per day). Standard duration of therapy is 10 days, but children older than 2 years with uncomplicated cases can be treated for 5 days. On the basis of concentrations in middle ear fluid and in vitro activity, no currently available oral antimicrobial agent has better activity than amoxicillin against penicillin-nonsusceptible *S pneumoniae.*

For patients with clinically defined treatment failures when assessed after 3 to 5 days of initial therapy, suitable alternative agents should be active against penicillin-nonsusceptible pneumococci as well as beta-lactamase–producing *Haemophilus influenzae* and *Moraxella catarrhalis.* Such agents include high-dose oral amoxicillin-clavulanate; oral cefdinir, cefpodoxime, or cefuroxime; or intramuscular ceftriaxone. Myringotomy or tympanocentesis should be considered for cases failing to respond to second-line therapy and for severe cases to obtain cultures to guide therapy. For multidrug-resistant strains of *S pneumoniae,* the use of clindamycin, rifampin, or other agents should be considered in consultation with an expert in infectious diseases.

Sinusitis. Antimicrobial agents effective for treatment of acute otitis media also are likely to be effective for acute sinusitis and are recommended.

Image 80.1
Periorbital cellulitis with purulent exudate in an infant. *Streptococcus pneumoniae* was isolated from blood culture. The CSF culture was sterile.

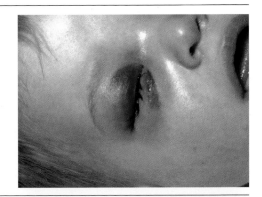

Image 80.2
A 3½-year-old white male with acute *Streptococcus pneumoniae* suppurative otitis media and mastoiditis. Note the protuberance of the right external ear secondary to mastoid swelling.

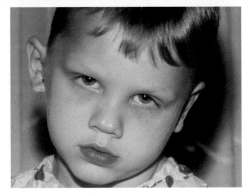

Image 80.3
Streptococcus pneumoniae sepsis with purpura fulminans in a child who had undergone splenectomy for refractory idiopathic thrombocytopenic purpura..

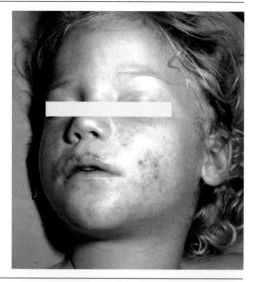

Image 80.4
Segmental (nodular) pneumonia due to *Streptococcus pneumoniae*.

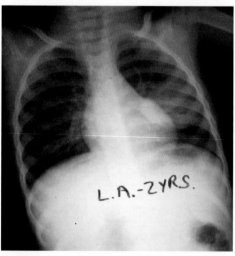

Image 80.5
Pneumonia, with right subpleural empyema, due to *Streptococcus pneumoniae* in a child with sickle cell disease.

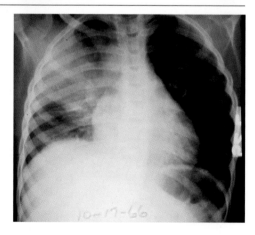

Image 80.6

Streptococcus pneumoniae in pleural exudate (Gram stain).

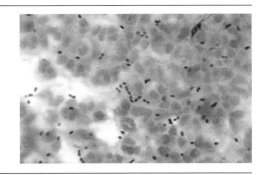

Image 80.7

Pericarditis due to *Streptococcus pneumoniae* treated with penicillin and pericardiostomy tube drainage, which resulted in recovery.

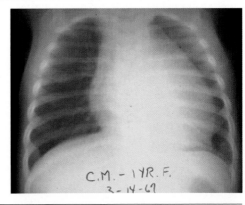

Image 80.8

The purulent exudate on this brain was caused by meningeal infection with *Streptococcus pneumoniae*.

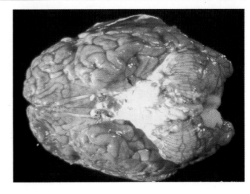

81

Pneumocystis jiroveci Infections

Clinical Manifestations

Infants and children develop a characteristic syndrome of subacute diffuse pneumonitis with dyspnea, tachypnea, oxygen desaturation, nonproductive cough, and fever. However, the intensity of these signs and symptoms can vary, and in some immunocompromised children and adults, onset can be acute and fulminant. The chest radiograph often shows bilateral diffuse interstitial or alveolar disease; rarely, lobar, miliary, and nodular lesions or even no lesions are seen. The mortality rate in immunocompromised patients ranges from 5% to 40% if treated and approaches 100% if untreated.

Etiology

Nomenclature for *Pneumocystis* species is in evolution. *Pneumocystis jiroveci* has been proposed, denoting the fact that *Pneumocystis carinii* only infects rats. At present, *P carinii* or *P carinii f sp hominis* continue to be used. *P jiroveci* is classified as a fungus on the basis of DNA sequence analysis. However, *P jiroveci* retains several morphologic and biologic similarities to protozoa, including susceptibility to a number of antiprotozoal agents but resistance to most antifungal agents.

Epidemiology

P jiroveci is ubiquitous in mammals worldwide, particularly rodents, and has a tropism for growth on respiratory tract surfaces. *P jiroveci* isolates recovered from mice, rats, and ferrets are diverse genetically from each other and from human *P jiroveci*; isolates from one animal species do not cross-infect other animal species. Asymptomatic infection occurs early in life, with more than 85% of healthy children acquiring antibody by 20 months of age. *P jiroveci* often is found postmortem in lungs of infants with a diagnosis of sudden infant death syndrome, but a causal relationship is uncertain. In resource-limited countries and in times of famine, *P jiroveci* pneumonia (PCP) has occurred in epidemics, primarily affecting malnourished infants and children.

Epidemics also have occurred in preterm infants. In industrialized countries, PCP occurs almost entirely in immunocompromised people with deficient cell-mediated immunity, particularly people with HIV infection, recipients of immunosuppressive therapy after organ transplantation or treatment for malignant neoplasm, and children with congenital immunodeficiency syndromes. Although decreasing in frequency because of effective prophylaxis and antiretroviral therapy, PCP remains one of the most common serious opportunistic infections in infants and children with perinatally acquired HIV infection. Although onset of disease can occur at any age, including rare instances during the first month of life, PCP most commonly occurs in HIV-infected children in the first year of life. The mode of transmission is unknown. Animal studies have demonstrated animal-to-animal transmission by the airborne route, suggesting the possibility that person-to-person transmission may occur in humans. Primary infection probably accounts for disease during infancy. Studies of patients with AIDS with more than one episode of PCP suggest reinfection rather than relapse. In patients with cancer, the disease can occur during remission or relapse. The period of communicability is unknown.

Incubation Period

Unknown.

Diagnostic Tests

A definitive diagnosis of PCP is made by demonstration of organisms in lung tissue or respiratory tract secretion specimens. The most sensitive and specific diagnostic procedures are open lung biopsy and, in older children, transbronchial biopsy. However, bronchoscopy with bronchoalveolar lavage, induction of sputum in older children and adolescents, and intubation with deep endotracheal aspiration are less invasive, can be diagnostic, and are sensitive in patients with HIV infection who have an increased number of organisms. Methenamine silver, toluidine blue O, calcofluor white, and fluorescein-conjugated monoclonal antibody are the most useful stains for identifying the thick-walled cysts of *P jiroveci*. Extracystic trophozoite forms are identified with Giemsa stain, modified Wright-Giemsa stain, and fluorescein-conjugated monoclonal antibody stain. PCR assays for detecting *P jiroveci* infection are experimental. Serologic tests are not useful.

Treatment

The drug of choice is intravenous trimethoprim-sulfamethoxazole. Oral therapy should be reserved for patients with mild disease who do not have malabsorption or diarrhea or for patients with a favorable clinical response to initial intravenous therapy. The rate of adverse reactions (rash, neutropenia, anemia, renal dysfunction, nausea, vomiting, and diarrhea) to trimethoprim-sulfamethoxazole is higher in HIV-infected children than in other patients. If the adverse reaction is not severe, continuation of therapy is recommended. Half of patients with adverse reactions subsequently have been treated successfully with trimethoprim-sulfamethoxazole.

Intravenously administered pentamidine is an alternative drug for children and adults who cannot tolerate trimethoprim-sulfamethoxazole or who have severe disease and have not responded to trimethoprim-sulfamethoxazole after 5 to 7 days of therapy. The therapeutic efficacy of parenteral pentamidine in adults with PCP is similar to that of trimethoprim-sulfamethoxazole. Pentamidine is associated with a high incidence of adverse reactions, including pancreatitis, renal dysfunction, hypoglycemia, hyperglycemia, hypotension, fever, and neutropenia. Pentamidine should not be administered concomitantly with didanosine because both drugs cause pancreatitis.

Atovaquone is approved for the oral treatment of mild to moderate PCP in adults who are intolerant of trimethoprim-sulfamethoxazole. Experience with the use of atovaquone in children is limited. Other potentially useful drugs in adults include clindamycin with primaquine, dapsone with trimethoprim, and trimetrexate with leucovorin. Experience with the use of these combinations in children is limited.

Corticosteroids seem to be beneficial in treatment of HIV-infected adults with moderate to severe PCP (as defined by an arterial oxygen pressure [PaO_2] of less than 70 mm Hg in room air or an arterial-alveolar gradient of more than 35 mm Hg). For adolescents older than 13 years and adults, oral prednisone in tapering doses through day 21 is recommended. Although no controlled studies of the use of corticosteroids in young children have been performed, most experts would include corticosteroids as part of therapy for children with moderate to severe PCP disease. The optimal dose and duration of corticosteroid therapy for children have not been determined.

Chemoprophylaxis. Prophylaxis against a first episode of PCP is indicated for many patients with significant immunocompromise (see Human Immunodeficiency Virus Infection, p 116) and people with primary or acquired immunodeficiency.

The recommended drug regimen for PCP prophylaxis for all immunocompromised patients is trimethoprim-sulfamethoxazole administered for 3 consecutive days each week. For patients who cannot tolerate the drug, aerosolized pentamidine administered by the Respirgard II nebulizer for people 5 years of age or older is an alternative. Daily oral dapsone is another alternative drug for prophylaxis in children, especially children younger than 5 years. Other drugs with potential for prophylaxis include pyrimethamine plus dapsone plus leucovorin, pyrimethamine-sulfadoxine, and oral atovaquone. Experience with these drugs in adults and children is limited.

Image 81.1

Cysts of *Pneumocystis jiroveci* in smear from bronchoalveolar lavage (Gomori methenamine-silver stain).

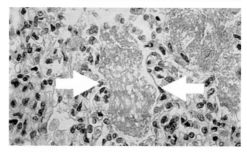

Image 81.2

Foamy intra-alveolar exudate in lung biopsy specimen from a patient with *Pneumocystis jiroveci* pneumonia (hematoxylin-eosin stain).

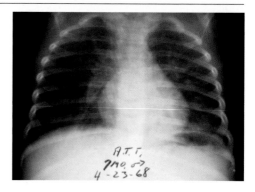

Image 81.3

Pneumocystis jiroveci pneumonia with hyperaeration in an infant with congenital agammaglobulinemia.

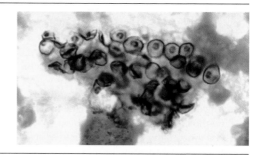

82

Poliovirus Infections

Clinical Manifestations

Approximately 95% of poliovirus infections are asymptomatic. Nonspecific illness with low-grade fever and sore throat (minor illness) occurs in 4% to 8% of people who become infected. Aseptic meningitis, sometimes with paresthesias, occurs in 1% to 5% of patients a few days after the minor illness has resolved. Rapid onset of asymmetric acute flaccid paralysis with areflexia of the involved limb occurs in 0.1% to 2% of infections, and residual paralytic disease involving the motor neurons (paralytic poliomyelitis) occurs in approximately two thirds of people with acute motor neuron disease. Cranial nerve involvement and paralysis of respiratory tract muscles can occur. Findings in CSF are characteristic of viral meningitis with mild pleocytosis and lymphocytic predominance.

Adults who contracted paralytic poliomyelitis during childhood can develop the postpolio syndrome 30 to 40 years later. Postpolio syndrome is characterized by slow and often significant onset of muscle pain and exacerbation of weakness.

Etiology

Polioviruses are enteroviruses and consist of serotypes 1, 2, and 3.

Epidemiology

Poliovirus infections occur only in humans. Spread is by the fecal-oral and respiratory routes. Infection is more common in infants and young children and occurs at an earlier age among children living in poor hygienic conditions. The risk of paralytic disease after infection increases with age. In temperate climates, poliovirus infections are most common during summer and autumn; in the tropics, the seasonal pattern is less pronounced.

The last reported case of poliomyelitis attributable to indigenously acquired, wild-type poliovirus in the United States occurred in 1979 and was caused by a wild type 1 poliovirus. In that outbreak, 10 paralytic cases and 4 other poliovirus infections occurred among unimmunized people. The only identified imported case of paralytic poliomyelitis since 1986 occurred in 1993 in a child transported to the United States for medical care. Since 1979, all other cases have been vaccine-associated paralytic poliomyelitis (VAPP) occurring in vaccine recipients or their contacts and attributable to oral poliovirus (OPV) vaccine. An average of 8 cases of VAPP were reported annually in the United States from 1980 to 1996. Fewer VAPP cases were reported annually between 1997 and 1999 after a shift in US immunization policy to a sequential inactivated poliovirus (IPV)-OPV immunization schedule. Implementation of an all-IPV vaccine schedule in 2000 ended the occurrence of new VAPP cases, thus eliminating the last type of paralytic poliomyelitis in the United States. Circulation of indigenous wild-type poliovirus strains ceased in the United States several decades ago, and the risk of contact with imported wild-type polioviruses is decreasing rapidly, parallel with the success of the global eradication program of the WHO and WHO partners. In 2005 the first identified vaccine-derived poliovirus in the United States and the first transmission in a community since OPV immunizations were discontinued in 2000 was reported. This occurrence raises concerns regarding transmission among people in communities with low levels of immunization and risk of a polio outbreak occurring in the United States.

Communicability of poliovirus is greatest shortly before and after onset of clinical illness, when the virus is present in the throat and excreted in high concentration in feces. The virus persists in the throat for approximately 1 week after onset of illness and is excreted in feces for several weeks. Patients potentially are contagious for as long as fecal excretion persists. In recipients of OPV vaccine, the virus persists in the throat for 1 to 2 weeks and is excreted in feces for several weeks, although in rare cases, excretion for more than 2 months can occur. Immunodeficient patients have excreted virus for periods of more than 10 years.

Incubation Period

3 to 6 days; the onset of paralysis, 7 to 21 days.

Diagnostic Tests

Poliovirus can be recovered from the pharynx, feces, urine and, rarely, CSF by isolation in cell culture. Two or more stool and throat swab specimens for enterovirus isolation should be obtained at least 24 hours apart from patients with suspected paralytic poliomyelitis as early in the course of illness as possible, ideally within 14 days of onset of symptoms. Fecal material is most likely to yield virus. Interpretation of acute and convalescent serologic test results can be difficult.

Image 82.1
An aerial view of a crowd surrounding a city auditorium in San Antonio, TX, awaiting polio immunization, 1962.

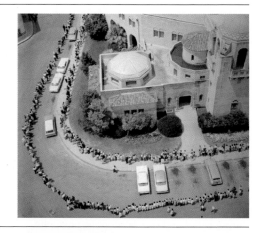

Image 82.2
The physician is shown here examining a tank respirator, also known as an iron lung, during a polio epidemic. The iron lung encased the thoracic cavity externally in an air-tight chamber. The chamber was used to create a negative pressure around the thoracic cavity, thereby causing air to rush into the lungs to equalize intrapulmonary pressure.

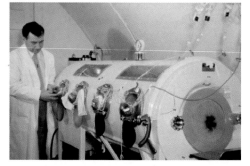

Image 82.3

This child is displaying a deformity of her right lower extremity caused by the poliovirus, an enterovirus member. After initial oropharyngeal inoculation, and multiplication, the virus enters the bloodstream, thereby, finding its way to the CNS and infecting the motor neurons of the anterior horn of the spinal cord and within the brain itself.

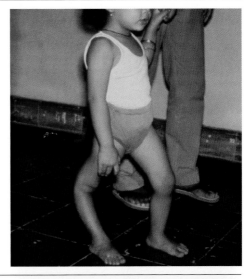

Image 82.4

A young girl with bulbar polio demonstrates the tripod sign when she attempts to sit upright.

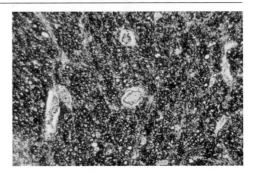

Image 82.5

A photomicrograph of the cervical spinal cord in the region of the anterior horn revealing polio type 3 degenerative changes. The poliovirus has an affinity for the anterior horn motor neurons of the cervical and lumbar regions of the spinal cord. Death of these cells causes muscle weakness of those muscles once innervated by the now dead neurons.

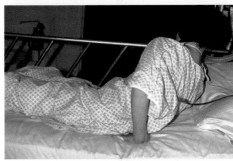

83

Rabies

Clinical Manifestations

Infection with rabies virus characteristically produces an acute illness with rapidly progressive CNS manifestations, including anxiety, dysphagia, and seizures. Some patients can have paralysis. Illness almost invariably progresses to death. The differential diagnosis of acute encephalitic illnesses of unknown cause with atypical focal neurologic signs or with paralysis should include rabies.

Etiology

Rabies virus is an RNA virus classified in the Rhabdoviridae family.

Epidemiology

Understanding the epidemiology of rabies has been aided by strain identification using monoclonal antibodies and nucleotide sequencing. In the United States, the number of cases of human rabies has decreased steadily since the 1950s, reflecting widespread rabies immunization of dogs and the availability of effective immunoprophylaxis after exposure to a rabid animal. Between 1990 and 2004, 34 (72%) of the 47 human rabies deaths in the United States have been associated with bat-variant rabies virus. Since 2000, 14 of 15 cases of indigenously acquired human rabies were associated with bat variants, and only 3 of these 15 human cases had known bat bites. Despite the large focus of rabies in raccoons in the eastern United States, only one human death has been attributed to the raccoon rabies virus variant. Rarely, airborne transmission has been reported in the laboratory and in some caves inhabited by millions of bats. Transmission also has occurred by transplantation of organs, corneas, and other tissues from patients dying of undiagnosed rabies. Person-to-person transmission by bite has not been documented in the United States, although the virus has been isolated from saliva of infected patients.

Wildlife rabies exists throughout the United States except in Hawaii, which remains rabies-free. Wild animals, including raccoons, skunks, foxes, coyotes, bats, and other species, are the most important potential source of infection for humans and domestic animals. Rabies in small rodents (squirrels, hamsters, guinea pigs, gerbils, chipmunks, rats, and mice) and lagomorphs (rabbits and hares) is rare, but rabies can occur in woodchucks or other large rodents in areas where raccoon rabies is common. The virus is present in saliva and is transmitted by bites or, rarely, by contamination of mucosa or skin lesions by saliva or other potentially infectious material (eg, neural tissue). Worldwide, most rabies cases in humans result from dog bites in areas where canine rabies is enzootic. Most rabid dogs, cats, and ferrets can shed virus for a few days before there are obvious signs of illness. No case of human rabies in the United States has been attributed to a dog, cat, or ferret that has remained healthy throughout the standard 10-day period of confinement.

Incubation Period

4 to 6 weeks in humans (range, 5 days to up to 6 years).

Diagnostic Tests

Infection in animals can be diagnosed by demonstration of virus-specific fluorescent antigen in brain tissue. Suspected rabid animals should be euthanized in a manner that preserves brain tissue for appropriate examination. Virus can be isolated from saliva, brain, and other tissues in suckling mice or in tissue culture and can be detected by identification of viral antigens or nucleotides in affected tissues. The diagnosis can be made postmortem by either immunofluorescent or immunohistochemical examination of the brain. Antemortem diagnosis can be made by fluorescent microscopy of skin biopsy specimens from the nape of the neck, by isolation of the virus from saliva, by detection of antibody in the CSF or serum in unimmunized people, and by detection of viral antigens and nucleic acid in infected tissues. Laboratory personnel should be consulted before submission of specimens so that appropriate collection and transport of materials can be arranged.

Treatment

Once symptoms have developed, neither vaccine nor rabies immune globulin improves the prognosis. There is no specific treatment.

Very few patients with human rabies have survived, even with intensive supportive care.

Image 83.1

Raccoons can be vectors of the rabies virus, transmitting the virus to humans and other animals. Rabies virus belongs to the order *Mononegavirales*. Raccoons continue to be the most frequently reported rabid wildlife species and involved 37.7% of all animal-transmitted cases during 2000 in the United States.

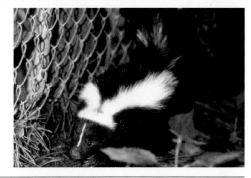

Image 83.2

Approximately a third of reported animal rabies in the United States is attributed to the wild skunk population. Wild animals accounted for 93% of reported animal cases of rabies in the year 2000. Skunks were responsible for 30.1% of this number.

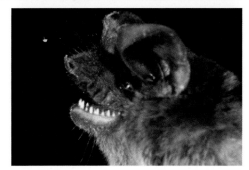

Image 83.3

This bat, *Artibeus jamaicensis,* is also known as the Jamaican fruit bat. Most of the recent human rabies cases in the United States have been caused by rabies virus that was transmitted through a bat vector.

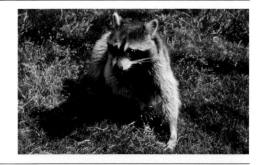

Image 83.4
Close-up of a dog's face during late-stage "dumb" paralytic rabies. Animals with "dumb" rabies appear depressed, lethargic, and unco-ordinated. Gradually they become completely paralyzed. When their throat and jaw muscles are paralyzed, the animals will drool and have difficulty swallowing.

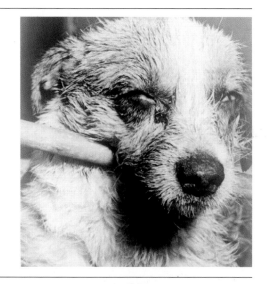

Image 83.5
Photomicrograph of brain tissue from a rabies encephalitis patient (hematoxylin-eosin stain) displaying the pathognomonic finding of Negri bodies within the neuronal cytoplasm.

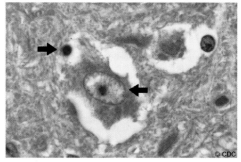

84

Rat-Bite Fever

Clinical Manifestations

Rat-bite fever is caused by *Streptobacillus moniliformis* or *Spirillum minus*. *S moniliformis* infection (streptobacillary fever or Haverhill fever) is characterized by fever, rash, and arthritis. There is an abrupt onset of fever, chills, muscle pain, vomiting, headache and, occasionally, adenopathy. A maculopapular or petechial rash develops, predominantly on the extremities, typically within a few days of fever onset. The bite site usually heals promptly and exhibits no or minimal inflammation. Nonsuppurative migratory polyarthritis or arthralgia follows in approximately 50% of patients. Untreated infection usually has a relapsing course for a mean of 3 weeks. Ulceration at the initial bite wound and regional lymphadenopathy do not occur. Complications include soft tissue and solid-organ abscesses, pneumonia, endocarditis, myocarditis, and meningitis. The case-fatality rate is 7% to 10% in untreated patients. With *S minus* infection, a period of initial apparent healing at the site of the bite usually is followed by fever and ulceration at the site, regional lymphangitis and lymphadenopathy, and a distinctive rash of red or purple plaques. Arthritis is rare. Infection with *S minus* is rare in the United States.

Etiology

The causes of rat-bite fever are *S moniliformis,* a microaerophilic, gram-negative, pleomorphic bacillus, and *S minus,* a small, gram-negative, spiral organism with bipolar flagellar tufts.

Epidemiology

Rat-bite fever is a zoonotic illness. The natural habitat of *S moniliformis* and *S minus* is the upper respiratory tract of rodents. *S moniliformis* is transmitted by bites or scratches from or handling of infected rats; other rodents (eg, mice, gerbils) also can act as reservoirs. Haverhill fever refers to infection after ingestion of milk, water, or food contaminated with *S moniliformis*. *S minus* is transmitted by bites of rats and mice. *S moniliformis* infection accounts for most cases of rat-bite fever in the United States; *S minus* infections occur primarily in Asia.

Incubation Period

S moniliformis is 3 to 10 days (up to 3 weeks); *S minus,* 7 to 21 days.

Diagnostic Tests

S moniliformis is a fastidious, slow-growing organism isolated from specimens of blood, synovial fluid, aspirates from abscesses, or material from the bite lesion by inoculation into bacteriologic media enriched with blood, serum, or ascitic fluid. Cultures should be held up to 3 weeks if *S moniliformis* is suspected. *S minus* has not been recovered on artificial media but can be visualized by dark-field microscopy in wet mounts of blood, exudate of a lesion, and lymph nodes. *S minus* can be recovered from blood, lymph nodes, or local lesions by intraperitoneal inoculation of mice or guinea pigs.

Treatment

Penicillin G procaine intramuscularly or penicillin G intravenously is the drug of choice for rat-bite fever caused by either agent. Doxycycline or streptomycin can be substituted when a patient has a severe hypersensitivity to penicillin. Doxycycline should not be given to children younger than 8 years unless the benefits of therapy are greater than the risks of dental staining. Patients with endocarditis should receive intravenous high-dose penicillin G for at least 4 weeks; streptomycin for initial therapy may be useful.

Image 84.1
Rat bite wounds on the finger of a 5-year-old 12 hours after the bite. Because of fever, chills, headache, and rash 5 days later, blood cultures were obtained and grew *Streptobacillus moniliformis*.

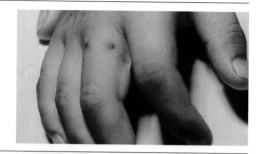

Image 84.2
Five days after being bitten by a rat, this child developed fever, chills, and headache followed 5 days later by a papulovesicular rash on the hands and feet. *Streptobacillus moniliformis* was isolated from blood cultures and he responded to intravenous penicillin therapy without complication.

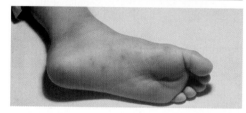

Image 84.3
Close-up view of the rash of an infant who was bitten on the right cheek by a rat. Sodoku, or rat-bite fever caused by *Spirillum minus*, rarely occurs in the United States.

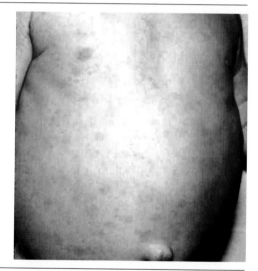

Image 84.4
The rash of rat-bite fever *(Streptobacillus moniliformis)* in an infant bitten by a rat on the right side of the face while sleeping.

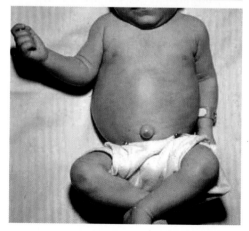

85
Respiratory Syncytial Virus

Clinical Manifestations

RSV causes acute respiratory tract illness in patients of all ages. In infants and young children, RSV is the most important cause of bronchiolitis and pneumonia. During the first few weeks of life, particularly among preterm infants, infection with RSV can produce minimal respiratory tract signs. Lethargy, irritability, and poor feeding, sometimes accompanied by apneic episodes, can be the presenting manifestations in infants. Most previously healthy infants infected with RSV do not require hospitalization, and many who are hospitalized improve with supportive care and are discharged in fewer than 5 days. Characteristics that increase the risk of severe or fatal RSV infection are preterm birth; cyanotic or complicated congenital heart disease, especially conditions causing pulmonary hypertension; underlying pulmonary disease, especially chronic lung disease of prematurity; and immunodeficiency disease or therapy causing immunosuppression at any age. After RSV bronchiolitis, many children will have episodes of recurrent wheezing, which usually diminish in subsequent years. Some children can develop wheezing at older ages or long-term abnormalities in pulmonary function. This association may reflect an underlying predisposition to reactive airway disease rather than a direct consequence of RSV infection.

Almost all children are infected at least once by 2 years of age, and reinfection throughout life is common. RSV infection in older children and adults usually manifests as upper respiratory tract illness, but more serious disease involving the lower respiratory tract also can develop in immunocompromised patients or in the elderly. Exacerbation of acute asthmatic bronchitis or other chronic lung conditions can occur.

Etiology

RSV is an enveloped RNA paramyxovirus that lacks neuraminidase and hemagglutinin surface glycoproteins. Two major strains (groups A and B) have been identified and often circulate concurrently.

Epidemiology

Humans are the only source of infection. Transmission usually is by direct or close contact with contaminated secretions, which can involve droplets or fomites. RSV can persist on environmental surfaces for many hours and for a half hour or more on hands. Infection among hospital personnel and others can occur by self-inoculation with contaminated secretions. Enforcement of infection control policies is important to decrease the risk of health care–related transmission of RSV. Health care–related spread of RSV to organ transplant recipients or patients with cardiopulmonary abnormalities or immunocompromised conditions has been associated with severe and fatal disease in children and adults.

RSV usually occurs in annual epidemics during winter and early spring in temperate climates. Spread among household and child care contacts, including adults, is common. The period of viral shedding usually is 3 to 8 days, but shedding can be longer, especially in young infants and in immunosuppressed individuals, in whom shedding may continue for as long as 3 to 4 weeks.

Incubation Period

2 to 8 days.

Diagnostic Tests

Rapid diagnostic assays, including immunofluorescent and enzyme immunoassay techniques for detection of viral antigen in nasopharyngeal specimens, are available commercially and generally are reliable. The sensitivity of these assays in comparison with culture varies between 53% and 96%, with most in the 80% to 90% range. As with all antigen detection assays, false-positive test results are more likely to occur at the beginning or end of the RSV season when the incidence of disease is low. Therefore, antigen detection assays should not be the solitary basis on which the beginning and end of RSV season is determined.

Viral isolation from nasopharyngeal secretions in cell cultures requires 3 to 5 days, but results and sensitivity vary among laboratories because methods of isolation are exacting and RSV is a labile virus.

Treatment

Primary treatment is supportive and should include hydration, careful clinical assessment of respiratory status, including measurement of oxygen saturation, use of supplemental oxygen, suction of the upper airway and, if necessary, intubation and mechanical ventilation. Ribavirin has in vitro antiviral activity against RSV, but ribavirin aerosol treatment for RSV infection is not recommended routinely. The high cost, aerosol route of administration, concern about potential toxic effects among exposed health care professionals, and conflicting results of efficacy trials have led to controversy about the use of this drug.

Beta-adrenergic Agents. Beta-adrenergic agents are not recommended for routine care of first-time wheezing associated with RSV bronchiolitis.

Corticosteroids. In hospitalized infants with RSV bronchiolitis, corticosteroids are not effective and are not indicated.

Antimicrobial Agents. Antimicrobial agents rarely are indicated because bacterial lung infection and bacteremia are uncommon in infants hospitalized with RSV bronchiolitis or pneumonia. Otitis media occurs in infants with RSV bronchiolitis, but oral antibiotic agents can be used if therapy is necessary.

Image 85.1
Electron micrograph of an RSV. The virion is variable in shape and size (average diameter between 120–300 nm). RSV is the most common cause of bronchiolitis and pneumonia among infants and children younger than 1 year.

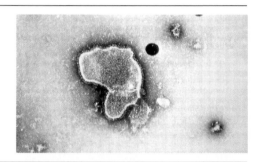

Image 85.2
RSV bronchiolitis and pneumonia. Note the bilateral infiltrates and striking hyperaeration.

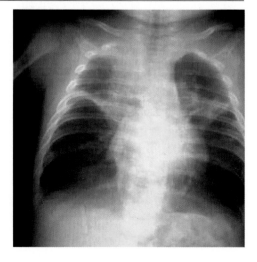

86

Rickettsialpox

Clinical Manifestations

Rickettsialpox is characterized by generalized erythematous papulovesicular eruptions on the trunk, face, extremities (including palms and soles), and mucous membranes after the appearance of an eschar at the site of the bite of a mouse mite. Regional lymph nodes in the area of the primary eschar typically become enlarged. Systemic disease lasts approximately 1 week; manifestations can include fever, chills, headache, drenching sweats, vomiting, myalgias, anorexia, and photophobia. The disease can be moderately severe, is self-limited, and rarely is associated with complications.

Etiology

Rickettsialpox is caused by *Rickettsia akari,* which is classified with the spotted fever group rickettsiae and related antigenically to *Rickettsia rickettsii.*

Epidemiology

The natural host for *R akari* in the United States is *Mus musculus,* the common house mouse. The disease is transmitted by the mouse mite *(Liponyssoides sanguineus).* Disease risk is heightened in areas infested with mice. The disease can be found wherever the hosts, pathogens, and humans coexist but is found mostly in large urban settings and has been recognized in the northeastern United States, especially in New York City, but also in Ohio, North Carolina, Utah, Croatia, Ukraine, Turkey, Russia, Korea, and South Africa. All age groups can be affected. No seasonal pattern of disease occurs. The disease is not com-

municable and is reported rarely in the United States; however, it is likely that rickettsialpox is underdiagnosed at present.

Incubation Period

9 to 14 days.

Diagnostic Tests

R akari can be isolated from blood during the acute stage of disease, but culture is not attempted routinely and is available only in specialized laboratories. Because antibodies to *R akari* have extensive cross-reactivity with antibodies against *R rickettsii,* an indirect immunofluorescent antibody assay for *R rickettsii* (the cause of Rocky Mountain spotted fever) may demonstrate a 4-fold change in antibody titers between acute and convalescent serum specimens taken 3 to 4 weeks apart. Absorption of serum specimens before indirect immunofluorescent antibody assay can distinguish between antibody responses to *R rickettsii* and *R akari.* Direct fluorescent antibody or immunohistochemical testing of paraffin-embedded eschars and histopathologic examination of papulovesicles for distinctive features are useful diagnostic techniques.

Treatment

Doxycycline will shorten the course of disease; symptoms resolve within 48 hours after initiation of therapy. Despite concerns regarding dental staining after use of tetracyclines in children younger than 8 years, doxycycline is the drug of choice for this potentially severe disease. Relapse is rare. Chloramphenicol and a fluoroquinolone are alternative drugs.

Image 86.1
Eschar on posterior right calf of patient with rickettsialpox.

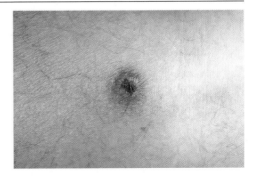

Image 86.2

Multiple papulovesicular lesions involving the upper trunk on a patient with rickettsialpox.

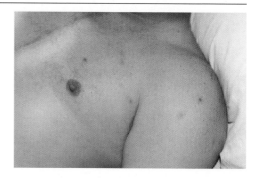

87

Rocky Mountain Spotted Fever

Clinical Manifestations

Rocky Mountain spotted fever (RMSF) is a systemic, small-vessel vasculitis with a characteristic rash that usually occurs before the sixth day of illness. Fever, myalgia, severe headache, nausea, vomiting, and anorexia are major clinical features. Abdominal pain and diarrhea often are present and can obscure the diagnosis. The rash initially is erythematous and macular and later can become maculopapular and, often, petechial. Rash usually appears first on the wrists and ankles, often spreading within hours proximally to the trunk. The palms and soles typically are involved. Although early development of a rash is a useful diagnostic sign, rash fails to develop in up to 20% of cases. Thrombocytopenia of varying severity and hyponatremia develop in many cases. The white blood cell count typically is normal, but leukopenia and anemia can occur. The illness can last as long as 3 weeks and can be severe, with prominent CNS, cardiac, pulmonary, gastrointestinal tract, and renal involvement; disseminated intravascular coagulation; and shock leading to death. Significant long-term sequelae are common in patients with severe RMSF, including neurologic (paraparesis; hearing loss; peripheral neuropathy; bladder and bowel incontinence; and cerebellar, vestibular, and motor dysfunction) and non-neurologic effects (disability from limb amputation).

Etiology

Rickettsia rickettsii is an obligate intracellular pathogen and a member of the spotted fever group of rickettsiae. The primary targets of infection in mammalian hosts are endothelial cells lining the small vessels of all major tissues and organs.

Epidemiology

The disease is transmitted to humans by the bite of an *Ixodes* species tick. Many small wild animals and dogs have antibodies to *R rickettsii,* but their role as natural reservoirs is not clear. Ticks are both reservoirs and vectors of *R rickettsii.* In ticks, the agent is trans-mitted transovarially and between stages. People with occupational or recreational exposure to the tick vector (eg, pet owners, animal handlers, and people who spend time outdoors) are at increased risk of acquiring the organism. People of all ages can be infected, but national surveillance indicates that most cases occur in people younger than 15 years. April through September are the months of highest incidence in the United States. Laboratory-acquired infection has resulted from accidental inoculation and aerosol contamination. Transmission has occurred on rare occasions by blood transfusion. Mortality is highest in males, people older than 50 years, and people with no recognized tick bite or attachment. Lack of confirmed recent tick bite does not exclude the diagnosis. Delay in disease recognition and initiation of antirickettsial therapy increase the risk of death. Factors contributing to delayed diagnosis include absence of rash, initial presentation before the fourth day of illness, and onset of illness during months other than May through August.

The disease is widespread in the United States. Most cases are reported in the south Atlantic, southeastern, and south central states. The principal recognized vectors of *R rickettsii* are *Dermacentor variabilis* (the American dog tick) in the eastern and central United States and *Dermacentor andersoni* (the Rocky Mountain wood tick) in western United States. Another common tick throughout the world that feeds on dogs, *Rhipicephalus sanguineus* (the brown dog tick), has been implicated as a vector of *R rickettsii* in Arizona. Transmission parallels the tick season in a given geographic area. RMSF also occurs in Canada, Mexico, and Central and South America.

Incubation Period

Approximately 1 week (range, 2–14 days).

Diagnostic Tests

The diagnosis can be established by one of the multiple rickettsial group-specific serologic tests. A 4-fold or greater change in titer between acute and convalescent serum specimens obtained 2 to 3 weeks apart is diagnostic when determined by indirect immunofluorescent antibody (IFA) assay, enzyme immuno-assay, complement fixation, latex agglutination, indirect hemagglutination, or microagglutination tests. The IFA assay is the most widely available confirmatory test. Antibodies generally are detected by IFA assay 7 to 10 days after onset of illness. A probable diagnosis can be established by a single serum titer of 1:64 or greater by IFA assay. The nonspecific and insensitive Weil-Felix serologic test (*Proteus vulgaris* OX-19 and OX-2 agglutinins) is not recommended.

Culture of *R rickettsii* should be conducted only by laboratories with adequate biohazard containment equipment. *R rickettsii* can be identified by immunohistochemical staining or PCR of tissue specimens (biopsy or autopsy). Ideally, a specimen from the site of the rash should be obtained before antimicrobial therapy is initiated or soon thereafter because sensitivity diminishes quickly afterward. Isolation or PCR assays for detection of *R rickettsii*

in blood and biopsy specimens during the acute phase of illness confirm the diagnosis.

Treatment

Doxycycline is the drug of choice; chloramphenicol or a fluoroquinolone are alternative drugs. Although tetracyclines generally are not given to children younger than 8 years because of the risk of dental staining, most experts consider doxycycline to be the drug of choice for children of any age. Reasons for this preference include the following: (1) tetracycline staining of teeth is related to the total dose; (2) doxycycline is less likely than other tetracyclines to stain developing teeth; (3) doxycycline is effective against ehrlichiosis, which may mimic RMSF, but chloramphenicol may not be (see *Ehrlichia* and *Anaplasma* Infections, p 63); and (4) use of chloramphenicol is problematic because of serious adverse effects, the need to monitor serum concentrations, and lack of an oral preparation in the United States.

Image 87.1
This is a female Lone star tick, *Amblyomma americanum,* that is found in the southeastern and mid-Atlantic United States. This tick is a vector of several zoonotic diseases including human monocytic ehrlichiosis and Rocky Mountain spotted fever.

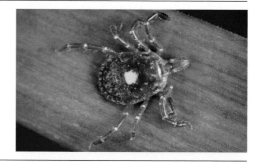

Image 87.2
Rocky Mountain spotted fever in an 8-year-old male—sixth day of rash without treatment.

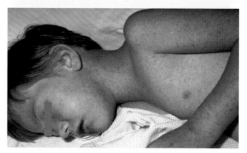

Image 87.3

Rocky Mountain spotted fever—sixth day of rash without treatment.

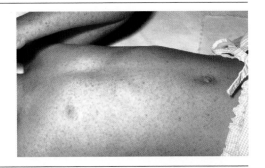

Image 87.4

Rocky Mountain spotted fever—sixth day of rash without treatment.

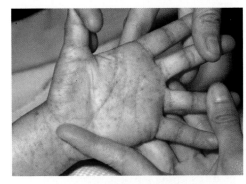

Image 87.5

A 2-year-old boy with obtundation and disorientation from Rocky Mountain spotted fever showing petechial rash and edema of the upper extremity. The rickettsiae multiply in the endothelial lining of small blood vessels and produce a widespread vasculitis.

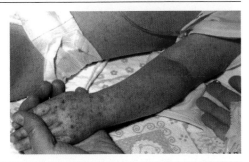

Image 87.6

A 2-year-old boy with Rocky Mountain spotted fever showing petechiae and edema of the foot typical of the vasculitis in this infection.

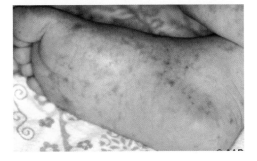

Image 87.7

A 33-year-old man with Rocky Mountain spotted fever (foot), day 11 of the illness. Note the edema in addition to the petechiae and purpura, which can mimic meningococcemia.

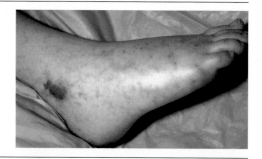

Image 87.8

A 2-year-old boy admitted with the typical rash of Rocky Mountain spotted fever and respiratory distress caused by rickettsial pneumonia.

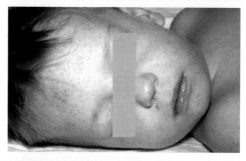

Image 87.9

A child's right hand and wrist displaying the spotted rash and edema of Rocky Mountain spotted fever.

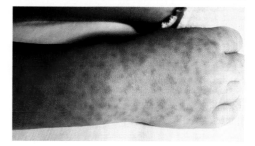

88

Rotavirus Infections

Clinical Manifestations

Infection causes nonbloody diarrhea, often preceded or accompanied by vomiting and fever. Symptoms generally persist for 3 to 8 days. In severe cases, dehydration, electrolyte abnormalities, and acidosis can occur. Almost all children are infected by 5 years of age; those younger than 1 year are most likely to experience dehydration. In immunocompromised children, including children with HIV, persistent infection and diarrhea can develop.

Etiology

Rotaviruses are segmented, double-stranded RNA viruses belonging to the family Reoviridae, with at least 7 distinct antigenic groups (A–G). Group A viruses are the major causes of rotavirus diarrhea worldwide. Serotyping is based on the VP7 glycoprotein (G) and VP4 protease-cleaved hemagglutinin (P); G types 1 through 4 and 9 and P types 1A and 1B are most common.

Epidemiology

Most human infections result from direct or indirect contact with infected people. Rotavirus is present in high titer in stools of infected patients with diarrhea, which is the only body specimen consistently positive for the virus. Rotavirus can be detected in stool before onset of diarrhea and may persist for as long as 21 days after the onset of symptoms in immunocompetent hosts. Transmission is presumed to be by the fecal-oral route. Rotavirus can be found on toys and hard surfaces in child care centers, indicating that fomites may serve as a mode of transmission. Spread within families and institutions is common. Rotavirus is the most common cause of health care–acquired diarrhea in children and is an important cause of acute gastroenteritis in children attending child care. Rarely, common-source outbreaks from contaminated water or food have been reported.

Human rotavirus infections are ubiquitous. Rotavirus gastroenteritis is the most common cause of severe diarrhea in children younger than 5 years. Severe rotavirus infections occur most commonly in infants and children between 4 and 24 months of age. Rotavirus-related hospitalizations can account for as many as 5% of all hospitalizations of children. Approximately 20% of adult household contacts of infected infants will develop symptomatic infection. Breastfeeding is associated with milder disease.

In temperate climates, disease is most prevalent during the cooler months. In North America, the annual epidemic usually starts during the autumn in Mexico and the southwestern United States and moves sequentially to reach the northeastern United States and Canada by spring. The seasonal pattern of disease is less pronounced in tropical climates, but rotavirus infection is more common during the cooler, drier months.

Incubation Period

2 to 4 days.

Diagnostic Tests

It is not possible to diagnose rotavirus infection by clinical presentation or nonspecific laboratory tests. Enzyme immunoassay and latex agglutination assays for group A rotavirus antigen detection in stool are available commercially. Both assays have high specificity, but false-positive results and nonspecific reactions can occur in neonates and in people with underlying intestinal disease. Nonspecific reactions can be distinguished from true positive reactions by performance of confirmatory assays. Virus also can be identified in stool by electron microscopy and by specific nucleic acid amplification techniques.

Treatment

No specific antiviral therapy is available. Oral or parenteral fluids and electrolytes are given to prevent and correct dehydration.

Image 88.1

Transmission electron micrograph of intact rotavirus particles with their distinctive rim of radiating capsomeres.

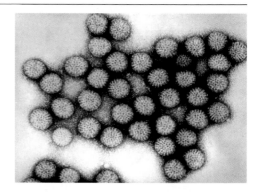

89

Rubella

Clinical Manifestations

Postnatal Rubella. Many cases of rubella are subclinical. Clinical disease usually is mild and characterized by a generalized erythematous maculopapular rash, lymphadenopathy, and slight fever. The rash starts on the face, becomes generalized in 24 hours, and lasts a median of 3 days. Lymphadenopathy, which may precede rash, often involves posterior auricular or suboccipital lymph nodes, can be generalized, and lasts between 5 and 8 days. Conjunctivitis and palatal enanthem have been noted. Transient polyarthralgia and polyarthritis rarely occur in children but are common in adolescents and adults, especially females. Encephalitis (1:5000 cases) and thrombocytopenia (1:3000 cases) are rare complications. Maternal rubella during pregnancy can result in miscarriage, fetal death, or a constellation of congenital anomalies (congenital rubella syndrome).

Congenital Rubella Syndrome (CRS). The most commonly described anomalies associated with CRS are ophthalmologic (cataracts, pigmentary retinopathy, microphthalmos, and congenital glaucoma), cardiac (patent ductus arteriosus, peripheral pulmonary artery stenosis), auditory (sensorineural hearing impairment), and neurologic (behavioral disorders, meningoencephalitis, and mental retardation). Neonatal manifestations of congenital rubella syndrome include growth retardation, interstitial pneumonitis, radiolucent bone disease, hepatosplenomegaly, thrombocytopenia, and dermal erythropoiesis (so-called blueberry muffin lesions). Mild forms of the disease can be associated with few or no obvious clinical manifestations at birth. The occurrence of congenital defects is up to 85% if infection associated with maternal rash occurs during the first 12 weeks of gestation, 54% during the first 13 to 16 weeks of gestation, and 25% during the end of the second trimester.

Etiology

Rubella virus is an enveloped, positive-stranded RNA virus classified as a Rubivirus in the Togaviridae family.

Epidemiology

Humans are the only source of infection. Postnatal rubella is transmitted primarily through direct or respiratory droplet contact from nasopharyngeal secretions. The peak incidence of infection is during late winter and early spring. Approximately 25% to 50% of infections are asymptomatic. Immunity from wild-type or vaccine virus usually is prolonged, but reinfection on rare occasions has been demonstrated and rarely has resulted in congenital rubella. The period of maximal communicability extends from a few days before to 7 days after onset of rash. A small number of infants with congenital rubella continue to shed virus in nasopharyngeal secretions and urine for 1 year or more and can transmit infection to susceptible contacts. Rubella virus has been recovered in high titer from lens aspirates in children with congenital cataracts for up to several years.

Before widespread use of rubella vaccine, rubella was an epidemic disease, occurring in 6- to 9-year cycles, with most cases occurring in children. The incidence of rubella in the United States has decreased by approximately 99% from the prevaccine era. Currently, rubella has been eradicated in the United States. In the vaccine era, most cases in the 1970s and 1980s occurred in young, unimmunized adults in outbreaks on college campuses and in occupational settings. More recent outbreaks have occurred in foreign-born or unimmunized individuals. Although the number of susceptible people has decreased since introduction and widespread use of rubella vaccine, recent serologic surveys indicate that approximately 10% of the US-born population older than 5 years is susceptible to rubella. The percentage of susceptible people who are foreign born or from areas with poor vaccine coverage is higher. The risk of CRS is highest in infants of women born outside the United States.

Incubation Period

14 to 23 days (usually 16–18 days).

Diagnostic Tests

Detection of rubella-specific IgM antibody usually indicates recent postnatal infection or congenital infection in a newborn infant, but both false-negative and false-positive results occur. Congenital infection also can be confirmed by stable or increasing serum concentrations of rubella-specific IgG over several months. Rubella virus can be isolated most consistently from throat or nasal specimens by inoculation of appropriate cell culture. Laboratory personnel should be notified that rubella is suspected because additional testing is required to detect the virus. Blood, urine, CSF, and throat swab specimens also can yield virus, particularly in congenitally infected infants. Diagnosis of congenital rubella infection in children older than 1 year is difficult. Molecular typing of viral isolates can be useful in defining a source in outbreak scenarios. For diagnosis of postnatally acquired rubella, a 4-fold or greater increase in antibody titer or seroconversion between acute and convalescent serum titers indicates infection. Every effort should be made to establish a laboratory diagnosis when rubella infection is suspected in pregnant women or newborn infants. Enzyme immunoassay tests, latex agglutination, and immunofluorescent assay are sensitive methods to determine rubella immunity.

Treatment

Supportive.

Image 89.1

Rubella rash (face) in a previously unimmunized female. Adenovirus and enterovirus infections can cause exanthems that mimic rubella. Serologic testing is important if the patient is pregnant.

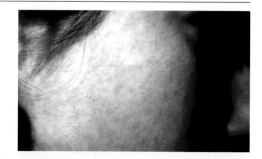

Image 89.2

This patient presented with a generalized rash on the abdomen caused by German measles (rubella). The rash usually lasts about 3 days and may be accompanied by a low-grade fever.

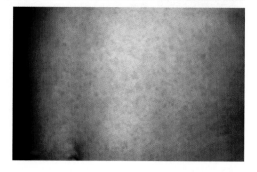

Image 89.3
Postauricular lymphadenopathy in the
17-year-old in Image 89.2 with rubella.

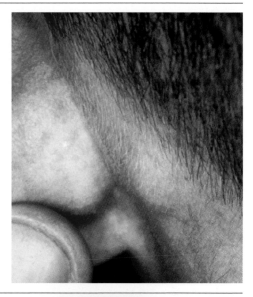

Image 89.4
Male infant with congenital rubella
and microcephaly.

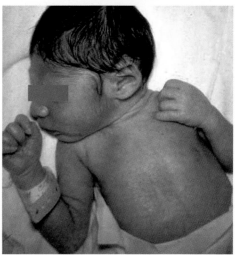

Image 89.5
Newborn with congenital rubella (blueberry
muffin) facial rash.

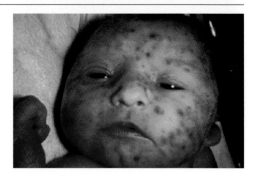

Image 89.6

This photograph shows the cataracts in an infant with congenital rubella syndrome. Rubella is a viral disease that can affect susceptible persons of any age. Although generally a mild illness, if contracted in early pregnancy, rubella can cause a high rate of fetal wastage or birth defects.

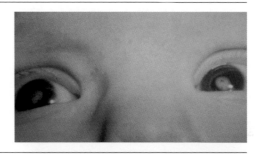

Image 89.7

Radiograph of the lower extremity showing metaphyseal radiolucent changes (celery stalk), which are found in 10% to 20% of infants with congenital rubella.

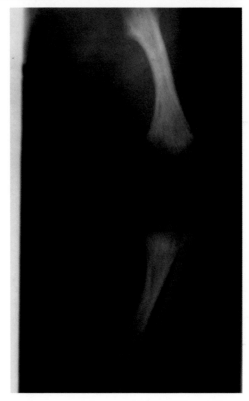

90

Salmonella Infections

Clinical Manifestations

Nontyphoidal *Salmonella* organisms cause asymptomatic carriage, gastroenteritis, bacteremia, and focal infections (such as meningitis and osteomyelitis). These disease categories are not mutually exclusive but represent a spectrum of illness. The most common illness associated with nontyphoidal *Salmonella* infection is gastroenteritis, in which diarrhea, abdominal cramps, and fever are common manifestations. The site of infection usually is the small intestine, but colitis can occur. Sustained or intermittent bacteremia can occur, and focal infections are recognized in as many as 10% of patients with *Salmonella* bacteremia.

Salmonella serotype Typhi and several other *Salmonella* serotypes can cause a protracted bacteremic illness often referred to as enteric or typhoid fever. The onset of illness typically is gradual, with manifestations such as fever, constitutional symptoms (eg, headache, malaise, anorexia, and lethargy), abdominal pain and tenderness, hepatomegaly, splenomegaly, rose spots, and change in mental status. Enteric fever can manifest as a mild, nondescript febrile illness in young children, in whom sustained or intermittent bacteremia can occur. Constipation can be an early feature. Diarrhea commonly occurs in children.

Etiology

Salmonella organisms are gram-negative bacilli that belong to the Enterobacteriaceae family. Currently, there are more than 2460 *Salmonella* serotypes; most serotypes causing human disease are divided among O-antigen groups A through E. *Salmonella* serotype Typhi is classified in serogroup D. In 2004 the most commonly reported human isolates in the United States were *Salmonella* serotype Typhimurium (serogroup B), *Salmonella* serotype Enteritidis (D), and *Salmonella* serotype Newport (C2); these 3 serotypes accounted for nearly half of all *Salmonella* infections. The *Salmonella* nomenclature is shown in Table 90.1.

Epidemiology

The principal reservoirs for nontyphoidal *Salmonella* organisms include poultry, livestock, reptiles, and pets. The major vehicle of transmission is food of animal origin, such as poultry, beef, eggs, and dairy products. Other food vehicles (eg, fruits, vegetables, and bakery products) have been implicated in outbreaks, in which the food was contaminated by contact with an infected animal product or human. Other modes of transmission include ingestion of contaminated water; contact with infected reptiles or amphibians (eg, pet turtles, iguanas, lizards, snakes, frogs, toads, newts, salamanders) and possibly rodents; and exposure to contaminated medications, dyes, and medical instruments.

Table 90.1
Nomenclature for Salmonella Organisms[1]

Complete Name	CDC Designation	Commonly Used Name
S enterica[2] subsp *enterica* serotype Typhi	*S* ser Typhi	*S typhi*
S enterica subsp *enterica* serotype Typhimurium	*S* ser Typhimurium	*S typhimurium*
S enterica subsp *enterica* serotype Newport	*S* ser Newport	*S newport*
S enterica subsp enterica serotype *Choleraesuis*	*S* ser Choleraesuis	*S choleraesuis*
S enterica subsp *arizona* serotype 18:z_4,z_{23}:-	*S* ser 18:z_4,z_{23}:-	*Arizona hinshawii*
S enterica subsp *houtenae* serotype Marina	*S* ser IV48:g,z51:-	*S marina*

[1] CDC indicates Centers for Disease Control and Prevention.
[2] Some also use *choleraesuis* and *enteritidis* as species names.

Unlike nontyphoidal *Salmonella* serotypes, S serotype Typhi is found only in humans, and infection implies direct contact with an infected person or with an item contaminated by a carrier. Although uncommon in the United States (approximately 400 cases per year), typhoid fever is endemic in many countries. Consequently, typhoid fever infections in the United States usually are acquired during international travel.

Age-specific attack rates for *Salmonella* infection are highest in people 1 to 4 years of age. Rates of invasive infections and mortality are higher in infants, elderly people, and people with immunosuppressive conditions, hemoglobinopathies (including sickle cell disease), malignant neoplasms, and HIV infection. Most reported cases are sporadic, but widespread outbreaks, including nosocomial, institutional, and nursery outbreaks, have been reported. Every year *Salmonella* organisms are one of the most common causes of laboratory-confirmed cases of enteric disease reported by the Foodborne Diseases Active Surveillance Network.

The risk of transmission exists for the duration of fecal excretion of organisms. Twelve weeks after infection, 45% of children younger than 5 years excrete *Salmonella* organisms, compared with 5% of older children and adults; antimicrobial therapy can prolong excretion. Approximately 1% of patients continue to excrete *Salmonella* organisms for more than 1 year (chronic carriers).

Incubation Period

Gastroenteritis, usually 12 to 36 hours (range, 6–72 hours); enteric fever, usually 7 to 14 days (range, 3–60 days).

Diagnostic Tests

Isolation of *Salmonella* organisms from cultures of stool, blood, urine, and material from foci of infection is diagnostic. Gastroenteritis is diagnosed by stool culture. Rapid tests using enzyme immunoassay, latex agglutination, DNA probes, and monoclonal antibodies have been developed and are in use in some labora-

tories. Serologic tests for *Salmonella* agglutinins (febrile agglutinins [the Widal test]) are not recommended.

Treatment

Antimicrobial therapy usually is not indicated for patients with either asymptomatic infection or uncomplicated (noninvasive) gastroenteritis caused by nontyphoidal *Salmonella* species because therapy does not shorten the duration of disease and can prolong the duration of fecal excretion. Although of unproven benefit, antimicrobial therapy is recommended for gastroenteritis caused by *Salmonella* species in people at increased risk of invasive disease, including infants younger than 3 months and people with chronic gastrointestinal tract disease, malignant neoplasms, hemoglobinopathies, HIV infection, or other immunosuppressive illnesses or therapies.

If antimicrobial therapy is initiated in people with gastroenteritis, ampicillin, amoxicillin, or trimethoprim-sulfamethoxazole is recommended for susceptible strains. Resistance to these antimicrobial agents is becoming more frequent, especially in resource-limited countries. In areas where ampicillin and trimethoprim-sulfamethoxazole resistance is frequent, ceftriaxone, cefotaxime, or fluoroquinolones usually are effective. However, fluoroquinolones are not approved for this indication in people younger than 18 years and are not recommended unless the benefits of therapy outweigh the potential risks with use of the drug.

For people with localized invasive disease (eg, osteomyelitis, abscess, meningitis, or bacteremia in people infected with HIV), empiric therapy with an expanded-spectrum cephalosporin (cefotaxime or ceftriaxone) is recommended. Once antimicrobial susceptibility test results are available, ampicillin, ceftriaxone, or cefotaxime for susceptible strains is recommended.

For invasive, nonfocal infections, such as bacteremia or enteric fever, caused by nontyphoidal *Salmonella* or S serotype Typhi, drugs of choice, route of administration, and duration of therapy are based on susceptibility of the organism, site of infection, host, and clinical response. Relapse of enteric fever occurs in up to 15% of patients and requires re-treatment.

Chronic (≥1 year) S serotype Typhi carriage, unusual in children, may be eradicated by high-dose parenteral ampicillin or high-dose oral amoxicillin combined with probenecid. Ciprofloxacin is the drug of choice for elimination of organisms from adult carriers

of S serotype Typhi. Cholecystectomy may be indicated in some adults in whom gallstones contribute to chronic carrier states.

Corticosteroids may be beneficial in patients with severe enteric fever, which is characterized by delirium, obtundation, stupor, coma, or shock. These drugs should be reserved for critically ill patients in whom relief of the manifestations of toxemia may be lifesaving.

Image 90.1
Young African American child with sickle cell disease and *Salmonella* sepsis with dactylitis.

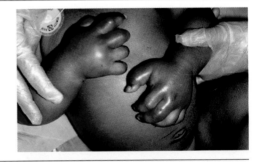

Image 90.2
Young child with sickle cell dactylitis of the foot and *Salmonella* sepsis. This is the same patient as in Image 90.1.

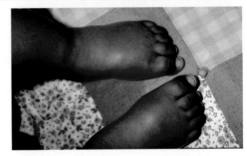

Image 90.3
Typhoid fever cholecystitis with an ulceration and perforation of the gallbladder into the jejunum. *Salmonella typhi,* the bacterium responsible for typhoid fever, has a preference for the gallbladder, and if present will colonize the surface of gallstones, which is how people become long-term carriers of the infection.

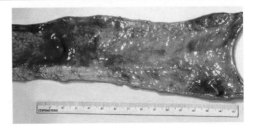

Image 90.4
Osteomyelitis (chronic) due to *Salmonella* infection of proximal femur.

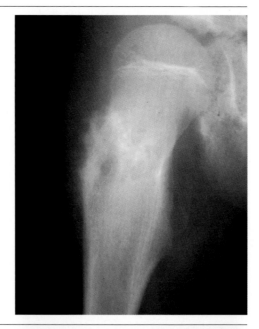

Image 90.5
A CT scan showing a large brain abscess in the posterior parietal region as a complication of *Salmonella* meningitis in a neonate.

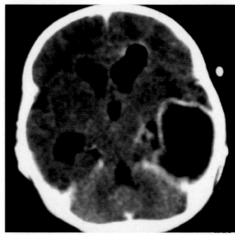

Image 90.6
Histopathologic changes in brain tissue due to *Salmonella* meningitis. *Salmonella* septicemia has been associated with subsequent infection of virtually every organ system, and the nervous system is no exception.

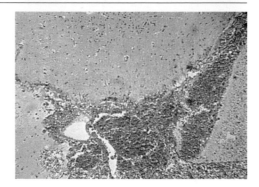

91

Scabies

Clinical Manifestations

Scabies is characterized by an intensely pruritic, erythematous, papular eruption caused by burrowing of adult female mites in upper layers of the epidermis, creating serpiginous burrows. Itching is most intense at night. In older children and adults, the sites of predilection are interdigital folds, flexor aspects of wrists, extensor surfaces of elbows, anterior axillary folds, waistline, thighs, navel, genitalia, areolae, abdomen, intergluteal cleft, and buttocks. In children younger than 2 years, the eruption generally is vesicular and often occurs in areas usually spared in older children and adults, such as the head, neck, palms, and soles. The eruption is caused by a hypersensitivity reaction to the proteins of the parasite.

The characteristic scabietic burrows appear as gray or white, tortuous, thread-like lines. Excoriations are common, and most burrows are obliterated by scratching before a patient is seen by a physician. Occasionally, 2- to 5-mm red-brown nodules are present, particularly on covered parts of the body, such as the genitalia, groin, and axilla. These scabies nodules are a granulomatous response to dead mite antigens and feces; the nodules can persist for weeks and even months after effective treatment. Cutaneous secondary bacterial infection can occur and usually is caused by *Streptococcus pyogenes* or *Staphylococcus aureus.*

Norwegian scabies is an uncommon clinical syndrome characterized by a large number of mites and widespread, crusted, hyperkeratotic lesions. Norwegian scabies usually occurs in debilitated, developmentally disabled, or immunologically compromised people but has occurred in otherwise healthy children after long-term use of topical corticosteroid therapy.

Etiology

The mite, *Sarcoptes scabiei* subsp *hominis,* is the cause of scabies. *Sarcoptes scabiei* subsp *canis,* acquired from dogs (with clinical mange), can cause a self-limited and mild infestation usually involving the area in direct contact with the infested animal that will resolve without specific treatment.

Epidemiology

Humans are the source of infestation. Transmission usually occurs through prolonged, close, personal contact. Because of the large number of mites in exfoliating scales, even minimal contact with a patient with crusted (Norwegian) scabies can result in transmission. Infestation acquired from dogs and other animals is uncommon, and these mites do not replicate in humans. Scabies of human origin can be transmitted as long as the patient remains infested and untreated, including the interval before symptoms develop. Scabies is endemic in many countries and occurs worldwide in cycles thought to be 15 to 30 years long. Scabies affects people from all socioeconomic levels without regard to age, gender, or standards of personal hygiene. Scabies in adults often is acquired sexually.

Incubation Period

Without previous exposure, 4 to 6 weeks; if previously infested, 1 to 4 days .

Diagnostic Tests

Diagnosis is confirmed by identification of the mite or mite eggs or scybala (feces) from scrapings of papules or intact burrows, preferably from the terminal portion where the mite generally is found. Mineral oil, microscope immersion oil, or water applied to skin facilitates collection of scrapings. A broad-blade scalpel is used to scrape the burrow. Scrapings and oil can be placed on a slide under a glass coverslip and examined microscopically under low power. Adult female mites average 330 to 450 μm in length.

Treatment

Infested children and adults should apply lotion or cream containing a scabicide over their entire body below the head. Because scabies can affect the head, scalp, and neck in infants and young children, treatment of the entire head, neck, and body in this age group is required. The drug of choice, particularly for infants, young children, and pregnant or nursing women, is 5% permethrin cream (not approved for children younger than 2 months), a synthetic pyrethroid. Alternative drugs are 10% crotamiton, ivermectin, or 1% lindane cream or lotion. Permethrin should be removed by bathing after 8 to 14 hours. Crotamiton is associated with frequent treatment failures and has not been approved for use in children. Ivermectin in a single dose administered orally is effective for treatment of severe or crusted (Norwegian) scabies and should be considered for patients whose infestation is refractory or who cannot tolerate topical therapy.

Lindane preparations should be reserved for treatment of patients who fail to respond to other preparations. Lindane is contraindicated in patients with crusted scabies, preterm infants, people with known seizure disorders, people with hypersensitivity to the product, young infants, women who are pregnant or breastfeeding, and patients who have extensive dermatitis. Lindane should not be used immediately after a bath or shower.

Because scabietic lesions are the result of a hypersensitivity reaction to the mite, itching may not subside for several weeks despite successful treatment. The use of oral antihistamines and topical corticosteroids can help relieve this itching. Topical or systemic antimicrobial therapy is indicated for secondary bacterial infections of the excoriated lesions.

Image 91.1
Linear papulovesicular burrows often contain female scabies mites when examined in mineral oil, which confirms the diagnosis of scabies.

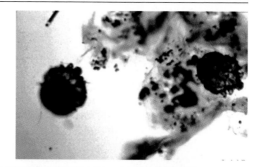

Image 91.2
Scabies rash in an infant.

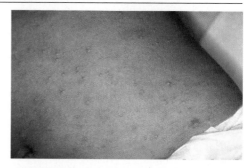

Image 91.3
Scabies of the hands of the mother of the infant in Image 91.2.

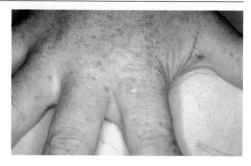

Image 91.4

Papulopustules and a widespread eczematous eruption, which represents a hypersensitivity reaction to a scabies infestation.

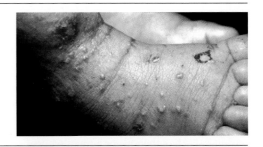

Image 91.5

Older children, adolescents, and adults with scabies exhibit erythematous papules, nodules, or burrows in the interdigital webs as in this patient.

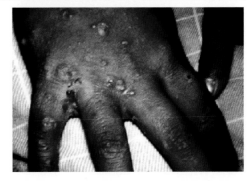

92

Schistosomiasis

Clinical Manifestations

Initial entry of the infecting larvae (cercariae) through skin commonly is accompanied by a transient, pruritic, papular rash (cercarial dermatitis). After penetration, the organism enters the bloodstream and migrates through the lungs. Each of the 3 major human schistosome parasites lives in some part of the venous plexus that drains the intestines or the bladder. Four to 8 weeks after exposure to *Schistosoma mansoni* or *Schistosoma japonicum,* an acute illness that manifests as fever, malaise, cough, rash, abdominal pain, hepatosplenomegaly, diarrhea, nausea, lymphadenopathy, and eosinophilia (Katayama fever), can develop. Heavy infection can result in mucoid bloody diarrhea accompanied by tender hepatomegaly. The severity of symptoms associated with chronic disease is related to the worm burden. People with low to moderate worm burdens may never develop overt clinical illness; people with significant worm burdens can have a range of symptoms caused primarily by inflammation and fibrosis triggered by eggs produced by adult worms. Portal hypertension can develop and cause hepatosplenomegaly, ascites, and esophageal varices and hematemesis. Long-term involvement of the colon produces abdominal pain and bloody diarrhea. In *Schistosoma haematobium* infections, the bladder can become inflamed and fibrotic. Symptoms and signs include dysuria, urgency, terminal microscopic and gross hematuria, secondary urinary tract infections, and nonspecific pelvic pain. An association between *S haematobium* and bladder cancer has been reported. Other organ systems can be involved from embolized eggs, for example, to the lungs, causing pulmonary hypertension; or to the CNS, notably the spinal cord in *S mansoni* or *S haematobium* infections and the brain in *S japonicum* infection.

Swimmer's itch (cercarial dermatitis or schistosome dermatitis) is caused by the larvae of other avian and mammalian schistosome species that penetrate human skin but do not complete the life cycle and do not cause chronic fibrotic disease. Manifestations include mild to moderate pruritus at the penetration site a few hours after exposure, followed in 5 to 14 days by an intermittent pruritic, sometimes papular, eruption. In previously sensitized people, more intense papular eruptions may occur for 7 to 10 days after exposure.

Etiology

The trematodes (flukes) *S mansoni, S japonicum, S haematobium* and, rarely, *Schistosoma mekongi* and *Schistosoma intercalatum* cause disease. All species have similar life cycles. Swimmer's itch is caused by multiple avian and mammalian species of *Schistosoma.*

Epidemiology

Humans are the principal hosts for the major species. Persistence of schistosomiasis depends on the presence of an appropriate snail as an intermediate host. Eggs excreted in stool (*S mansoni, S japonicum, S mekongi,* and *S intercalatum*) or urine (*S haematobium*) into freshwater hatch into motile miracidia, which infect snails. After development in snails, cercariae emerge and penetrate the skin of humans encountered in the water. Children commonly are infected after infancy when they begin to explore the environment. Children also are involved in transmission because of habits of uncontrolled defecation and urination and frequent wading in infected waters. Communicability lasts as long as live eggs are excreted in the urine and feces.

S mansoni occurs throughout tropical Africa, in several Caribbean islands, and in Venezuela, Brazil, Suriname, and the Arabian Peninsula. *S japonicum* is found in China, the Philippines, and Indonesia. *S haematobium* occurs in Africa and the eastern Mediterranean region. *S mekongi* is found in Cambodia, Laos, Japan, the Philippines, and Central Indonesia. *S intercalatum* is found in West and Central Africa. Adult worms of *S mansoni* can live as long as 30 years in the human host. Thus schistosomiasis can be diagnosed in patients many years after they have left an area with endemic infection. Swimmer's itch occurs in all regions of the world after exposure to freshwater, brackish water, or saltwater-containing larvae that do not complete their life cycle in humans. Immunity does not develop after infection; thus reinfection commonly occurs.

Incubation Period

Approximately 4 to 6 weeks for *S japonicum*, 6 to 8 weeks for *S mansoni*, and 10 to 12 weeks for *S haematobium*.

Diagnostic Tests

Infection with *S mansoni* and other species (except *S haematobium*) is determined by microscopic examination of concentrated stool specimens to detect characteristic eggs. In light infections, several specimens may need to be examined before eggs are found, or a biopsy of the rectal mucosa may be necessary. *S haematobium* is diagnosed by examining filtered urine for eggs. Egg excretion often peaks between noon and 3 pm. Biopsy of the bladder mucosa may be necessary. Serologic tests, available through the CDC and some commercial laboratories, are 50% to 99% sensitive for detecting infection attributable to

S mansoni, S haematobium, and *S japonicum,* respectively. Specific serologic tests can be particularly helpful for detecting light infections or before eggs appear in the stool or urine. These tests remain positive for many years and are not useful in differentiating ongoing infection from past infection or reinfection.

Swimmer's itch can be difficult to differentiate from other causes of dermatitis. A skin biopsy may demonstrate larvae, but their absence does not exclude the diagnosis.

Treatment

The drug of choice for schistosomiasis caused by any species is praziquantel; the alternative drug for *S mansoni* is oxamniquine. Praziquantel does not kill developing worms; therapy given during the 4 to 8 weeks of exposure should be repeated 1 to 2 months later. Swimmer's itch is a self-limited disease that requires only symptomatic treatment of the urticarial rash.

Image 92.1
A boy with hepatosplenomegaly due to schistosomiasis (bilharziasis).

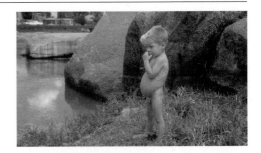

Image 92.2
A, B: Cross-section of different human tissues showing *Schistosoma* species eggs. *Schistosoma* species in liver (A) and bladder (B).

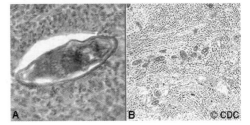

Image 92.3
Histopathology of bladder shows eggs of
Schistosoma haematobium surrounded by
intense infiltrates of eosinophils.

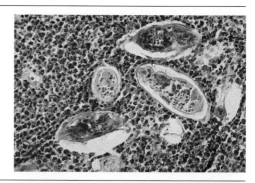

Image 92.4
This micrograph reveals signs of schistosomiasis
infection of the liver, also known as pipestem
cirrhosis (500x). Pipe stem cirrhosis occurs
when schistosomes infect the liver (ie, hepatic
schistosomiasis), which causes scarring to
occur, thereby, entrapping parasites and
their ova in and around the hepatic portal
circulatory vessels.

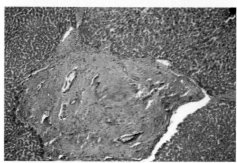

Image 92.5
Swimmer's itch showing symmetric, widespread,
edematous red plaques with central vesicles
and pustules.

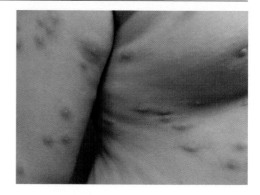

93

Shigella Infections

Clinical Manifestations

Shigella species primarily infect the large intestine, causing clinical manifestations that range from watery or loose stools with minimal or no constitutional symptoms to more severe symptoms, including fever, abdominal cramps or tenderness, tenesmus, and mucoid stools with or without blood. Clinical presentations vary with *Shigella* species; patients with *Shigella sonnei* infection usually exhibit watery diarrhea; people with *Shigella flexneri, Shigella boydii,* and *Shigella dysenteriae* infection typically have bloody diarrhea and severe systemic symptoms. Rare complications include bacteremia, Reiter syndrome (after *S flexneri* infection), hemolytic-uremic syndrome (after *S dysenteriae* type 1 infection), toxic megacolon and intestinal perforation, and toxic encephalopathy (ekiri).

Etiology

Shigella species are aerobic, gram-negative bacilli in the family Enterobacteriaceae. Four species (with >40 serotypes) have been identified. Among *Shigella* isolates reported in the United States in 2003, approximately 88% were *S sonnei,* 11% were *S flexneri,* 1% were *S boydii,* and 0.3% were *S dysenteriae. S dysenteriae* is rare in the United States but is endemic in rural Africa and the Indian subcontinent.

Epidemiology

Humans are the natural host for *Shigella,* although other primates may be infected. The primary mode of transmission is fecal-oral. Children 5 years of age or younger in child care settings, their caregivers, and other people living in crowded conditions are at increased risk of infection. Travel to resource-limited countries with inadequate sanitation can place the traveler at risk of infection. Ingestion of as few as 10 to 200 organisms is sufficient for infection to occur, depending on *Shigella* species. Predominant modes of transmission include person-to-person contact, contact with a contaminated inanimate object, ingestion of contaminated food or water, and sexual

contact. Houseflies also may be vectors through physical transport of infected feces. *S flexneri, S boydii,* and *S dysenteriae* infections are more common in older children and adults, and these infections often are associated with sources outside the United States. Transmission can occur as long as the organism is present in feces. Even without antimicrobial therapy, the carrier state usually ceases within 4 weeks of the onset of illness; chronic carriage (>1 year) is rare.

Incubation Period

1 to 7 days (typically 2–4 days).

Diagnostic Tests

Isolation of *Shigella* from feces or rectal swab specimens containing feces is diagnostic but lacks sensitivity. The presence of fecal leukocytes on a methylene blue–stained stool smear is sensitive for the diagnosis of colitis but is not specific for *Shigella* species. An enzyme immunoassay for Shiga toxin may be useful for detection of *S dysenteriae* type 1 in stool. Although bacteremia is rare, blood should be cultured in severely ill, immunocompromised, or malnourished patients. Other testing modalities, including the fluorescent antibody test, PCR assay, and enzyme-linked DNA probes, are available in research laboratories.

Treatment

Most clinical infections with *S sonnei* are self-limited (48–72 hours) and do not require antimicrobial therapy. However, antimicrobial therapy is effective in shortening the duration of diarrhea and eradicating organisms from feces. Treatment is recommended for patients with severe disease, dysentery, or underlying immunosuppressive conditions; in these patients, empirical therapy should be given while awaiting culture and susceptibility results. In mild disease, the primary indication for treatment is to prevent spread of the organism.

Antimicrobial susceptibility testing of clinical isolates is indicated because susceptibility data can guide appropriate therapy. In the United States, sentinel surveillance data in 2002 indicated that 77% of *Shigella* species were resistant to ampicillin, 37% were resistant to trimethoprim-sulfamethoxazole, and less than 1% were resistant to ceftriaxone and ciprofloxacin.

For cases in which susceptibility is unknown or an ampicillin and trimethoprim-sulfamethoxazole–resistant strain is isolated, parenteral cefotaxime or ceftriaxone, a fluoroquinolone (such as ciprofloxacin), or azithromycin can be given. Oral cephalosporins are not useful for treatment. For susceptible strains, ampicillin and trimethoprim-sulfamethoxazole are effective; amoxicillin is less

effective because of its rapid absorption from the gastrointestinal tract. The oral route of therapy is recommended except for seriously ill patients.

Antidiarrheal compounds that inhibit intestinal peristalsis are contraindicated because they can prolong the clinical and bacteriologic course of disease. Nutritional supplementation, including vitamin A (200 000 IU), can be given to hasten clinical resolution in geographic areas where children are at risk of malnutrition.

Image 93.1
Characteristic bloody mucoid stool of child with shigellosis.

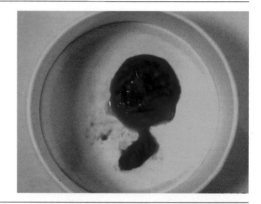

Image 93.2
Fecal leukocytes (shigellosis) (methylene blue stain). The presence of fecal leukocytes suggests a bacterial diarrhea, but is specific for *Shigella* infection.

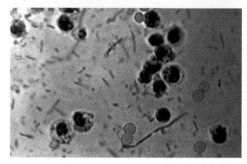

94

Smallpox

(Variola)

In 1979 the WHO declared that smallpox (variola) had been eradicated successfully worldwide. The last naturally occurring case of smallpox occurred in Somalia in 1977, followed by 2 cases attributable to laboratory exposure in 1978. The United States discontinued routine childhood immunization against smallpox in 1972 and routine immunization of health care professionals in 1976. The US military continued to immunize military personnel until 1995. Since 1980, the vaccine has been recommended only for people working with nonvariola orthopoxviruses. Two WHO reference laboratories were authorized to maintain stocks of variola virus. There is concern that the virus and the expertise to use it as a weapon of bioterrorism may have been misappropriated.

Clinical Manifestations

An individual infected with variola major develops a severe prodromal illness characterized by high fever (38.9°C–40.0°C [102°F–104°F]) and constitutional symptoms, including malaise, severe headache, backache, abdominal pain, and prostration, lasting for 2 to 5 days. Abdominal pain and back pain can be mistaken for focal pathology. Infected children can suffer from vomiting and seizures during this prodromal period. Most patients with smallpox tend to be severely ill and bedridden during the febrile prodrome. The prodromal period is followed by enanthemas (lesions on the mucosa of the mouth or pharynx), which may not be noticed by the patient. This stage occurs less than 24 hours before the onset of rash, which usually is the first recognized manifestation of infectiousness. With the onset of enanthemas, the patient becomes infectious and remains so until all skin crust lesions have separated. The exanthem, or rash, typically begins on the face and rapidly progresses to involve the forearms, trunk, and legs in a centrifugal distribution (greatest concentration of lesions on the face and distal extremities). Many patients will have lesions on the palms and soles. With rash onset, fever

decreases but the patient does not defervesce fully. Lesions begin as maculae that progress to papules, then firm vesicles, and then deep-seated, hard pustules described as "pearls of pus," with each stage lasting 1 to 2 days. By the sixth or seventh day of rash, lesions may begin to umbilicate or become confluent. Lesions increase in size for approximately 8 to 10 days, after which they begin to crust. Once all the lesions have separated, 3 to 4 weeks after the onset of rash, the patient no longer is infectious. Infected people sustain significant scarring after separation of the crusts. Because of the relatively slow and steady evolution of rash lesions, all lesions on any one part of the body are in the same stage of development. Variola minor is clinically indistinguishable except that it causes fewer systemic symptoms, less extensive rash, little persistent scarring, and fewer fatalities.

In addition to the typical presentation of smallpox (≥90% of cases), there are 2 uncommon forms of variola major: hemorrhagic (characterized by hemorrhage into skin lesions and disseminated intravascular coagulation) and malignant or flat type (in which the skin lesions do not progress to the pustular stage but remain flat and soft). Each variant occurred in approximately 5% of cases and was associated with a 95% to 100% mortality rate. Hemorrhagic smallpox rash commonly was confused with meningococcemia or hemorrhagic hematologic disease (eg, leukemia). Flat-type (velvety) smallpox occurred more commonly in children. By contrast, variola minor, or alastrim, was associated with fewer lesions, more rapid progression of rash, and a much lower mortality rate (approximately 1%) than variola major or typical smallpox.

Variola major in unimmunized people was associated with case fatality rates of 30% during epidemics of smallpox. The mortality rate was highest in children younger than 1 year and adults older than 30 years. The potential for modern supportive therapy in improving outcome is not known. Death was most likely to occur during the second week of illness and has been attributed to cytopathic effects from viral damage and inflammation. Secondary bacterial infections occurred but were a less significant cause of mortality.

Etiology

Variola is a member of the Poxviridae family (genus *Orthopoxvirus*). These DNA viruses are among the largest and most complex viruses known and differ from most other DNA viruses by multiplying in the cytoplasm. Monkeypox, vaccinia, and cowpox are other members of the genus and can cause zoonotic infection of humans but usually do not spread from person to person. Humans are the only natural reservoir for variola virus (smallpox).

Epidemiology

Smallpox is spread most commonly in droplets from the oropharynx of infected individuals, although rare transmission from aerosol and direct contact with infected lesions, clothing, or bedding has been reported. Patients are not infectious during the incubation period or febrile prodrome but become infectious with the onset of mucosal lesions (enanthemas), which occur within hours of the rash. The first week of rash illness is regarded as the most infectious period, although patients remain infectious until all scabs have separated. Because most patients with smallpox are extremely ill and bedridden, spread generally is limited to household contacts, hospital workers, and other health care professionals.

Incubation Period

7 to 17 days.

Diagnostic Tests

Variola virus can be detected in vesicular or pustular fluid by culture or by PCR assay. Electron microscopy detects orthopoxvirus infection but cannot distinguish between viruses. Variola diagnostic testing is conducted only at the CDC. If a patient is suspected of having smallpox, standard, contact, and airborne precautions should be implemented immediately.

Treatment

There is no known effective antiviral therapy available to treat smallpox. Infected patients should receive supportive care. Cidofovir, licensed for CMV retinitis, has been suggested as having a role in smallpox therapy, but data to support its use in smallpox are not available. The drug is associated with significant renal toxicity.

Image 94.1
Variola minor lesions on the face of a 2-year-old Latin American male.

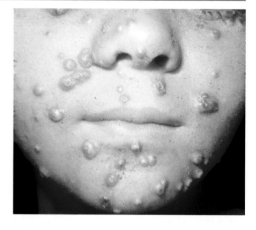

Image 94.2

A 7-year-old male residing in India with smallpox lesions in a typical centripetal distribution.

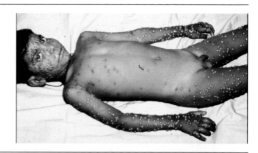

Image 94.3

This photograph reveals the back of a Nigerian child with smallpox. Note the pustules are centripetal in distribution, radiating from their densest area of eruption on the upper back, and outward along the extremities. All the skin lesions are at the same stage of development.

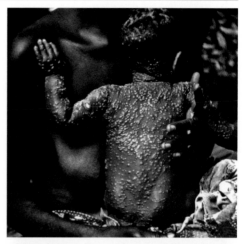

Image 94.4

Generalized vaccinia reaction secondary to smallpox vaccination. No vaccinia Ig treatment was required for resolution. Note the primary vaccination reaction on the left deltoid area.

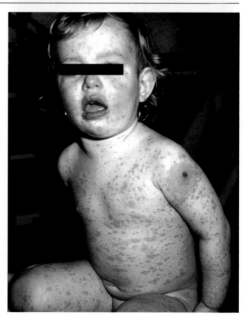

Image 94.5
The right foot of a 6-year-old boy with smallpox. The palms and soles are characteristically involved in smallpox patients.

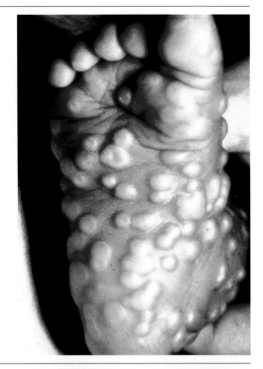

Image 94.6
Early smallpox pustules on the face of an infant. If this infant survives, smallpox lesions, or pustules, will eventually form scabs that will fall off, leaving marks on the skin. The patient is contagious to others until all of the scabs have fallen off.

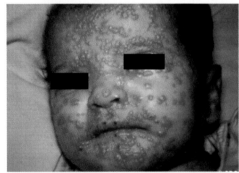

Image 94.7
A woman with generalized eczema developed severe eczema vaccinatum following smallpox vaccination given in error.

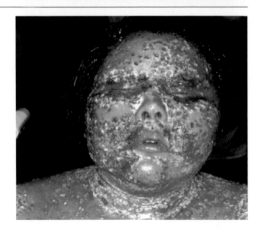

Image 94.8
This young girl in Bangladesh was infected with smallpox in 1973.

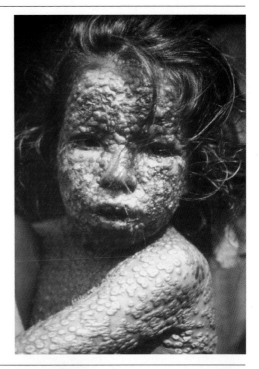

Image 94.9
Freedom from smallpox was declared in Bangladesh in December 1977 when a WHO international commission officially certified that smallpox had been eradicated from that country.

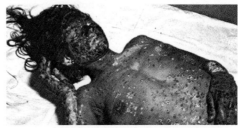

Image 94.10
These are eczema vaccinatum lesions on the skin of a smallpox vaccine recipient. Persons who have ever been diagnosed with eczema or atopic dermatitis should not be vaccinated unless the benefit is considered to outweigh the risk, even if the condition is currently not active, for they are at a high risk of developing eczema vaccinatum, a potentially severe, sometimes fatal complication.

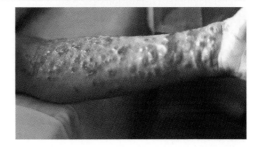

95

Sporotrichosis

Clinical Manifestations

Sporotrichosis manifests most commonly as the lymphocutaneous form. Inoculation occurs at a site of minor trauma, causing a painless papule that enlarges slowly to become a nodular lesion that can develop a violaceous hue or can ulcerate. Secondary lesions follow the same evolution and develop along the lymphatic distribution proximal to the initial lesion. Fixed cutaneous sporotrichosis, common in children, presents as a solitary crusted papule, papuloulcerative, or nodular lesion in which lymphatic spread is not observed. The extremities and face are the most common sites of infection in children. A disseminated cutaneous form is rare, usually occurring in children with immunocompromise.

Extracutaneous sporotrichosis commonly affects bones and joints, particularly those of the hands, elbows, ankles, or knees, but any organ can be affected. Osteoarticular structures are involved after local inoculation or hematogenous spread. Disseminated disease generally occurs after hematogenous spread from primary skin or lung infection. Disseminated sporotrichosis can involve multiple foci (eg, eyes, genitourinary system, or CNS) and occurs predominantly in immunocompromised patients. Pulmonary sporotrichosis clinically resembles tuberculosis and occurs after inhalation or aspiration of aerosolized spores. Pulmonary and disseminated sporotrichosis are uncommon in children.

Etiology

Sporothrix schenckii is a thermally dimorphic fungus that grows as a mold at room temperature and as a yeast at 37°C (98°F) and in host tissues.

Epidemiology

S schenckii is a ubiquitous organism that has worldwide distribution but is most common in tropical and subtropical regions of Central and South America and parts of North America. The fungus is isolated from soil and plants, including hay, straw, thorny plants (especially roses), sphagnum moss, and decaying vegetation. Cutaneous disease occurs from inoculation of debris containing the organism. People engaging in gardening or farming are at risk of infection. Inhalation of spores can lead to pulmonary disease. Rarely, transmission from infected cats has led to cutaneous disease.

Incubation Period

7 to 30 days after cutaneous inoculation.

Diagnostic Tests

Culture of *S schenckii* from a tissue, wound drainage, or sputum specimen is diagnostic of infection. Culture of *S schenckii* from a blood specimen suggests the disseminated form of infection associated with immunodeficiency. Histopathologic examination of tissue may not be helpful because the organism seldom is abundant. Special fungal stains to visualize the oval or cigar-shaped organism are required. A latex agglutination assay for detection of *Sporothrix* antigen in serum or CSF is available commercially.

Treatment

Sporotrichosis usually does not resolve without treatment. Itraconazole is the drug of choice for lymphocutaneous and fixed cutaneous disease in adults. For extracutaneous disease, amphotericin B or itraconazole is the drug of choice. Oral fluconazole is less effective. The time honored treatment for sporotrichosis, a saturated solution of potassium iodide, is much less costly and still is recommended as an alternative treatment. Saturated solution of potassium iodide is given orally until several weeks after all lesions are healed. Itraconazole is the treatment of choice for osteoarticular infection because this form of sporotrichosis rarely is accompanied by systemic illness. Amphotericin B and itraconazole are treatment options for pulmonary infections, depending on severity. Amphotericin B is the drug of choice for disseminated sporotrichosis, including meningeal sporotrichosis, and infection in children with immunodeficiency, including HIV infection. Itraconazole may be required for lifelong maintenance therapy after initial treatment with amphotericin B in children with HIV infection. Pulmonary and disseminated infection respond less well than cutaneous infection, despite prolonged therapy. Surgical debride-ment or excision may be necessary to achieve resolution of cavitary pulmonary disease.

Image 95.1

Sporothrix schenkii, mold phase (48-hour potato dextrose agar, lactophenol cotton blue preparation); small tear-shaped conidia forming rosette-like clusters.

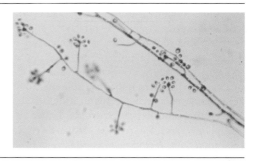

Image 95.2

Cutaneous sporotrichosis of the face in a preschool-aged child.

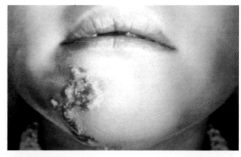

Image 95.3

Sporothrix schenckii was cultured from the biopsy specimen from an abscessed cervical lymph node of this 10-year-old boy. Stained smears of purulent material aspirated from a cervical lymph node were negative.

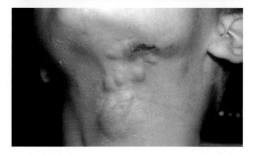

96

Staphylococcal Infections

Clinical Manifestations

Staphylococcus aureus causes a variety of localized and invasive suppurative infections and 3 toxin-mediated syndromes: toxic shock syndrome, scalded skin syndrome, and food poisoning. Localized infections include hordeola, furuncles, carbuncles, impetigo (bullous and nonbullous), paronychia, ecthyma, cellulitis, omphalitis, parotitis, lymphadenitis, and wound infections. *S aureus* also causes foreign body infections, including infections associated with intravascular catheters or grafts, pacemakers, peritoneal catheters, CSF shunts, and prosthetic joints, which can be associated with bacteremia. Bacteremia can be complicated by septicemia; endocarditis; pericarditis; pneumonia; pleural empyema; soft tissue, muscle, or visceral abscesses; arthritis; osteomyelitis; septic thrombophlebitis of large vessels; and other foci of infection. Meningitis is rare. *S aureus* infections can be fulminant and commonly are associated with metastatic foci and abscess formation, often requiring prolonged antimicrobial therapy, drainage, and foreign body removal to achieve cure. Risk factors for severe *S aureus* infections include chronic diseases such as diabetes mellitus and cirrhosis, immunodeficiency, nutritional disorders, surgery, and transplantation.

Staphylococcal scalded skin syndrome (SSSS) is a toxin-mediated disease caused by circulation of exfoliative toxins A and B produced by *S aureus*. The manifestations of SSSS are age related and include Ritter disease (generalized exfoliation) in the neonate, a tender scarlatiniform eruption and localized bullous impetigo in older children, and a combination of these with thick white/brown flaky desquamation of the entire skin, especially on the face and neck, in older infants and toddlers. The hallmark of SSSS is the toxin-mediated cleavage of the stratum granulosum layer of the epidermis (Nikolsky sign). Healing occurs without scarring. Bacteremia is rare, but dehydration and superinfection can occur with extensive exfoliation.

Coagulase-Negative Staphylococci: Most coagulase-negative staphylococci (CoNS)

isolates from patient specimens represent contamination of culture material. Of the isolates that do not represent contamination, most come from infections that are health care–associated, in patients who have obvious disruptions of host defenses caused by surgery, medical device insertion, or immunosuppression. CoNS are the most common cause of late-onset septicemia among preterm infants, especially infants weighing less than 1500 g at birth, and of episodes of health care–associated bacteremia in all age groups. CoNS are responsible for bacteremia in children undergoing treatment for leukemia, lymphoma, or solid tumors as well as in stem cell transplant recipients. Infections often are associated with intravascular catheters, CSF shunts, peritoneal or urinary catheters, vascular grafts or intracardiac patches, prosthetic cardiac valves, pacemaker wires, or prosthetic joints. Mediastinitis after open-heart surgery, endophthalmitis after intraocular trauma, and omphalitis and scalp abscesses in neonates have been described. CoNS also can enter the bloodstream from the respiratory tract of mechanically ventilated preterm infants or from the gastrointestinal tract of infants with necrotizing enterocolitis. Some species of CoNS are associated with urinary tract infection, including *Staphylococcus saprophyticus* in adolescent girls and young adult women, often after sexual intercourse, and *Staphylococcus epidermidis* and *Staphylococcus haemolyticus* in hospitalized patients with urinary tract catheters. In general, CoNS infections have an indolent clinical course in children with intact immune function and even in children who are immunocompromised.

Etiology

Staphylococci are catalase-positive, gram-positive cocci that appear microscopically as grape-like clusters. There are 32 species that are related closely on the basis of DNA base composition, but only 17 species are indigenous to humans. *S aureus* is the only species that produces coagulase. Of the 16 CoNS, *S epidermidis, S haemolyticus, S saprophyticus, Staphylococcus schleiferi,* and *Staphylococcus lugdunensis* most often are associated with human infections. Staphylococci are ubiquitous and can survive extreme conditions of drying, heat, and low-oxygen and high-salt environments. *S aureus* has many surface proteins, including the microbial surface components recognizing adhesive matrix molecule (MSCRAMM) receptors that allow the organism to bind to tissues and foreign bodies coated with fibronectin, fibrinogen, and collagen. This permits a low inoculum of organisms to adhere to sutures, catheters, prosthetic valves, and other devices. Many CoNS produce an exopolysaccharide slime biofilm that makes these organisms, as they bind to medical devices (eg, catheters), relatively inaccessible to host defenses and to antimicrobial agents.

Epidemiology

S aureus. *S aureus,* which is second only to CoNS as a cause of health care–associated bacteremia, is equal to *Pseudomonas aeruginosa* as the most common cause of health care–associated pneumonia in adults and is responsible for most health care–associated surgical site infections. *S aureus* colonizes the skin and mucous membranes of 30% to 50% of healthy adults and children. The anterior nares, throat (infants and young children), axilla, perineum, vagina, or rectum are the usual sites of colonization. The anterior nares are colonized most densely, and colonization can persist for years in 10% to 20% of affected people. From 25% to 50% of nasal carriers transiently carry the organism on their hands and other skin areas. Rates of carriage of more than 50% occur in children with desquamating skin disorders or burns and in people with frequent needle use (eg, diabetes mellitus, hemodialysis, recreational drug use, allergy shots).

Transmission of S aureus *in Hospitals.*
S aureus is transmitted most often by direct contact. Health care professionals and family members who have colonization of *S aureus* in the nares or on the skin can serve as an important reservoir for transmission of *S aureus* to patients. Health care professionals also can acquire transient hand colonization while caring for one patient and then transmit the organism to another patient. The role of clothing, gowns, environmental surfaces, and other fomites in transmission of *S aureus* is unclear.

Transmission by large droplets can occur when patients have draining wounds, burns, or areas of dermatitis that are colonized or infected. Changing dressings or linens can cause these organisms to become droplet nuclei, leading to airborne transmission. Dissemination of *S aureus* from people, including infants, with nasal carriage is related to density of colonization, and increased dissemination occurs during viral upper respiratory tract infections. Additional risk factors for health care–associated acquisition of *S aureus* include illness requiring care in high-risk locations, such as neonatal or pediatric intensive care or burn units; surgical procedures; prolonged hospitalization; local epidemic of *S aureus* infection; and the presence of indwelling vascular catheters or prosthetic devices. Previous antimicrobial therapy increases the risk of acquiring an antimicrobial-resistant strain.

S aureus *Colonization and Disease.* Nasal and skin carriage are the primary reservoirs for *S aureus.* Adults who carry *S aureus* in the nose preoperatively are more likely to develop surgical site infections after general, cardiac, orthopedic, or solid organ transplant surgery than patients who are not carriers. Heavy cutaneous colonization at the insertion site is the single most important predictor of intravenous catheter-related infections for short-term percutaneously inserted catheters. For patients with *S aureus* skin colonization receiving hemodialysis, the incidence of vascular access-related bacteremia is 6-fold higher than for patients without skin colonization. After head trauma, adults who are nasal carriers of *S aureus* are more likely to develop *S aureus* pneumonia than are noncolonized patients.

Health Care–Associated Methicillin-Resistant S aureus. Methicillin-resistant *S aureus* (MRSA) accounts for 50% of health care–associated *S aureus* infections in large hospitals with 500 or more beds. Health care–associated MRSA strains are resistant to all beta-lactamase resistant (BLR) beta-lactam and cephalosporin antimicrobial agents as well as to antimicrobial agents of several other classes (multidrug resistance).

Risk factors for nasal carriage of health care–associated MRSA include hospitalization within the previous year, recent (within the previous 60 days) antimicrobial use, prolonged hospital stay, frequent contact with a health care environment, presence of an intravascular catheter or tracheal tube, increased number of surgical procedures, or frequent contact with an individual with one or more of the preceding risk factors. A discharged patient known to have had colonization with MRSA should be assumed to have continued colonization when rehospitalized because carriage can persist for years.

Epidemic Strains of MRSA. Most health care–associated MRSA infections result from the patient's own organism or from endemic strains transmitted to the patient by hands of health care professionals. On occasion, a strain of MRSA will be introduced into a community or a health care facility environment where the organism spreads rapidly despite measures that contain the spread of nonepidemic strains. Identification of these epidemic MRSA strains using pulsed-field gel electrophoresis is important because containment of epidemic MRSA strains requires strict adherence to and enhancement of infection control policies.

MRSA and methicillin-resistant CoNS are responsible for a large portion of health care–associated infections. These strains particularly are difficult to treat because they usually are multidrug resistant and predictably susceptible only to vancomycin.

Community-Associated MRSA. Unique clones of MRSA increasingly are responsible for community-associated infections in healthy children and adults without typical risk factors for health care–associated MRSA infections. The most frequent manifestation of these community-associated MRSA infections is skin and soft tissue infection, but invasive disease and pneumonia also occur. The antimicrobial susceptibility patterns of these strains differ from those of health care–associated strains. Although they are resistant to all beta-lactam antimicrobial agents, they typically are susceptible to multiple antimicrobial agents, including trimethoprim-sulfamethoxazole, gentamicin, and doxycycline. These community-associated MRSA strains have been isolated from people without risk factors from most cities in the United States and elsewhere and from child care centers.

Vancomycin-Intermediately Susceptible S aureus. Strains of MRSA with intermediate susceptibility to vancomycin (minimum inhibitory concentration [MIC] ≥4 µg/mL and ≤16 µg/mL) were isolated from 48 adults in the United States from 1996 to 2001. Each person had received multiple courses of vancomycin for an MRSA infection. Strains of MRSA can be heterogeneous for vancomycin resistance. Extensive vancomycin use allows the vancomycin-intermediately susceptible S aureus (VISA) strains to grow. Rapid and aggressive control measures have focused on containing VISA strains to prevent spread. Recommended measures from the CDC have included rapid diagnostic tests to detect VISA, confirmatory testing of isolated strains, measures to restrict vancomycin use, and strict infection control measures for the infected patient and the institution. Although rare, outbreaks of MRSA with decreased susceptibility to vancomycin and heteroresistance have been reported in France, Spain, and Japan. Communicability persists as long as lesions or the carrier state are present.

Vancomycin-Resistant S aureus. In 2002, 2 isolates of vancomycin-resistant S aureus (VRSA; MIC ≥32 µg/mL) were identified in adults from 2 different states. Since then, an additional isolate from an adult in a third state has been reported. A concern is that automated antimicrobial susceptibility testing methods commonly used in the United States were unable to detect vancomycin resistance in these isolates. The guidelines for detecting these organisms and preventing spread are similar to those recommended for VISA.

Coagulase-Negative Staphylococci. Coagulase-negative staphylococci are common inhabitants of the skin and mucous membranes. Virtually all infants have colonization at multiple sites by 2 to 4 days of age. The most frequently isolated CoNS is S epidermidis. The frequency of nosocomial CoNS infections has increased steadily during the past

3 decades. Infants and children in intensive care units, including neonatal intensive care units, have the highest incidence of CoNS bloodstream infections. CoNS colonizing the skin can be introduced at the time of medical device placement, through mucous membrane or skin breaks, or during catheter manipulation. Less often, health care professionals with environmental CoNS colonization on the hands transmit the organism. The roles of the environment or fomites in CoNS transmission are not known.

Methicillin-Resistant CoNS. Methicillin-resistant CoNS account for most health care–associated CoNS infections. Methicillin-resistant strains are resistant to all beta-lactam drugs, including cephalosporins, and usually several other drug classes. As for MRSA, once these strains become endemic in a hospital, eradication is difficult, even when strict infection control techniques are followed.

Incubation Period

Variable.

Diagnostic Tests

Gram-stained smears of material from skin lesions or pyogenic foci can provide presumptive evidence of infection. Isolation of organisms from culture of otherwise sterile body fluid is definitive. *S aureus* almost never is a contaminant when isolated from a blood culture. CoNS isolated from a blood culture commonly are dismissed as "contaminants." In a premature neonate, an immunocompromised person, or a patient with a prosthetic device, repeated isolation of the same phenotypic strain of CoNS (on the basis of antimicrobial susceptibility testing) from blood cultures or another normally sterile body fluid suggests true infection, and genotyping more strongly supports the diagnosis. For catheter-related bacteremia, quantitative cultures from the catheter will have 5 to 10 times more organisms than cultures from a peripheral blood vessel. Criteria that suggest CoNS are pathogens rather than contaminants include the following: (1) 2 or more positive blood cultures from different sites; (2) a positive culture from blood and another usually sterile site (eg, CSF, joint,

abscess) with identical or nearly identical antimicrobial susceptibility patterns for all isolates; (3) growth in continuously monitored blood culture system within 15 hours of incubation; (4) clinical findings of infection in the patient; (5) an intravascular catheter that has been in place for 3 days or more; and (6) similar or identical genotypes among all isolates.

Quantitative antimicrobial susceptibility testing should be performed for all staphylococci, including CoNS, isolated from normally sterile sites. An increasing proportion of community-associated *S aureus* strains are methicillin resistant, and more than 90% of health care–associated *S aureus* as well as CoNS strains are methicillin and multidrug resistant. Because of the high rates of community-associated MRSA infections, clindamycin has become one of the often-used drugs for treatment of presumed *S aureus* infections. Routine antimicrobial susceptibility testing of *S aureus* strains previously has not included a method to detect strains susceptible to clindamycin that rapidly become clindamycin-resistant when exposed to this agent. This clindamycin-inducible resistance can be detected by the D zone test. This test was recommended in 2004 for routine use by microbiology laboratories when an MRSA isolate is determined to be erythromycin-resistant and clindamycin susceptible by routine methods. Patients with MRSA isolates that demonstrate clindamycin-inducible resistance should not receive clindamycin. All *S aureus* strains with an MIC to vancomycin of 4 µg/mL or higher should be confirmed and further characterized. Early detection of VISA is critical to trigger aggressive infection control measures.

S aureus and CoNS strain genotyping has become a necessary adjunct for determining whether several isolates from one patient or from different patients are the same. Typing may facilitate identification of the source, extent, and mechanism of transmission of an outbreak. Multilocus enzyme electrophoresis is another phenotypic tool for use, but pulsed-field gel electrophoresis typing by genotype has proven to be more discriminatory for identifying related isolates.

Treatment

Serious methicillin-susceptible S aureus (MSSA) infections require intravenous therapy with a BLR beta-lactam antimicrobial agent, such as nafcillin or oxacillin, because most S aureus strains produce beta-lactamase enzymes and are resistant to penicillin and ampicillin (Table 96.1). First- or second-generation cephalosporins (eg, cefazolin or cefuroxime) and vancomycin are effective but less so than nafcillin or oxacillin for some sites of infection (eg, endocarditis, meningitis). Furthermore, nafcillin or oxacillin rather than vancomycin (or clindamycin if the S aureus strain is susceptible to this agent) is recommended for treatment of serious MSSA infections to minimize the emergence of vancomycin- or clindamycin-resistant strains. The addition of gentamicin or rifampin to the regimen should be considered for MSSA or MRSA infections, such as endocarditis, persistent bacteremia, meningitis, or ventriculitis, and in consultation with an infectious diseases specialist. A patient who is allergic to penicillin can be treated with a first- or second-generation cephalosporin, if the patient is not also allergic to cephalosporins, or with vancomycin or clindamycin if endocarditis or CNS infection is not a consideration and the S aureus strain is susceptible.

Intravenous vancomycin is recommended for treatment of serious infections attributable to staphylococcal strains resistant to BLR beta-lactam antimicrobial agents (eg, MRSA and all CoNS). For empiric therapy of life-threatening community-acquired as well as hospital-acquired S aureus infections, initial therapy should include vancomycin and a BLR beta-lactam antimicrobial agent (eg, nafcillin or oxacillin). For hospital-acquired CoNS infections, vancomycin is the drug of choice. Subsequent therapy should be determined by antimicrobial susceptibility results.

VISA rarely has been isolated. For seriously ill patients with a history of recurrent MRSA infections or for patients failing vancomycin therapy for whom VISA strains are a consideration, initial therapy could include vancomycin, linezolid, or trimethoprim-sulfamethoxazole, with or without gentamicin.

If antimicrobial susceptibility results document multidrug resistance, alternative agents, such as quinupristin-dalfopristin or daptomycin, could be considered, but neither agent is approved for use in children younger than 18 years.

Duration of therapy for serious MSSA or MRSA infections depends on the site and severity of infection. After initial parenteral therapy, and clinical improvement is noted, completion of the recommended antimicrobial course with an oral drug can be considered in older children if adherence can be ensured and endocarditis or CNS infection is not a consideration. For endocarditis and CNS infection, parenteral therapy is recommended for the entire treatment. Drainage of abscesses and removal of foreign bodies is desirable and almost always required for treatment to be effective.

SSSS in infants should be treated with a parenteral BLR beta-lactam antimicrobial agent or, if MRSA is a consideration, vancomycin. In older children, depending on severity, oral agents can be considered. Skin and soft tissue infections, such as impetigo or cellulitis attributable to S aureus, usually can be treated with oral penicillinase-resistant beta-lactam drugs, such as cloxacillin, dicloxacillin, or a first- or second-generation cephalosporin unless the prevalence of community-associated MRSA in the region is substantial. In the latter circumstance or for the penicillin-allergic patient, trimethoprim-sulfamethoxazole, doxycycline (if 8 years of age or older) or clindamycin (if the strain is susceptible) can be used. For very localized superficial skin lesions, topical antimicrobial therapy with mupirocin or bacitracin and local hygienic measures may be sufficient.

The duration of therapy for central venous catheter infections is controversial and depends on consideration of a number of factors, including the organism (S aureus vs CoNS), the type and location of the catheter, the site of infection (exit site vs tunnel vs bacteremia), the feasibility of using an alternative vessel at a later date, and the presence or absence of a catheter-related thrombus. Infections are more difficult to treat when associated with a thrombus, thrombophlebitis, or intra-atrial thrombus. If blood cultures remain positive for staphylococci for more than 3 to 5 days or if the clinical illness fails to improve, the catheter should be removed, parenteral therapy should be continued, and the patient should be evaluated for metastatic foci of infection. Vegetations or a thrombus in the heart or great vessels always should be considered when an intravascular catheter becomes infected. Transesophageal echocardiography, if feasible, is the most sensitive technique for identifying vegetations. Metastatic spread should be evaluated in patients with *S aureus* bacteremia.

Table 96.1

Parenteral Antimicrobial Agent(s) for Treatment of Bacteremia and Other Serious *Staphylococcus aureus* Infections[1]

Susceptibility	Antimicrobial Agents	Comments
I. Initial empiric therapy (organism of unknown susceptibility)		
Drugs of choice	Vancomycin + nafcillin or oxacillin ± gentamicin	For life-threatening infections (ie, septicemia, endocarditis, CNS infection); linezolid could be substituted if the patient has received several recent courses of vancomycin
	Nafcillin or oxacillin[2]	For non–life-threatening infection without signs of sepsis (eg, skin infection, cellulitis, osteomyelitis, pyarthrosis) when rates of MRSA colonization and infection in the community are very low
	Clindamycin	For non–life-threatening infection without signs of sepsis when rates of MRSA colonization and infection in the community are substantial and prevalence of clindamycin resistance is low
	Vancomycin	For non–life-threatening, hospital-acquired infections
II. Methicillin-susceptible *S aureus*, penicillin-resistant		
Drugs of choice	Nafcillin or oxacillin[2,3]	
Alternatives	Cefazolin[2]	
	Clindamycin (if strain susceptible)	
	Vancomycin	Only for penicillin- and cephalosporin-allergic patients
	Ampicillin + sulbactam	

continued

Table 96.1, continued

Parenteral Antimicrobial Agent(s) for Treatment of Bacteremia and Other Serious *Staphylococcus aureus* Infections[1]

Susceptibility	Antimicrobial Agents	Comments
III. MRSA (oxacillin MIC, ≥4 µg/mL)		
A. Health care–associated (multidrug-resistant)		
Drugs of choice	Vancomycin ± gentamicin or ± rifampin[3]	
Alternatives susceptibility testing results available before alternative drugs are used	Trimethoprim-sulfamethoxazole	
	Linezolid[4]	
	Quinupristin-dalfopristin[4]	
	Fluoroquinolones	Not recommended for people younger than 18 years or as monotherapy
B. Community (not multidrug-resistant)		
Drugs of choice	Vancomycin ± gentamicin (or ± rifampin[3])	For life-threatening infections
	Clindamycin (if strain susceptible)	For pneumonia, septic arthritis, osteomyelitis, skin or soft tissue infections
	Trimethoprim-sulfamethoxazole	For skin or soft tissue infections
Alternative	Vancomycin[3]	
IV. Vancomycin-intermediately susceptible *S aureus* (MIC, >4 µg/mL and ≤16 µg/mL)[3]		
Drugs of choice	Optimal therapy is not known	Dependent on in vitro susceptibility test results
	Linezolid[4]	
	Daptomycin[5]	
	Quinupristin-dalfopristin[4]	
Alternatives	Vancomycin + linezolid ± gentamicin	
	Vancomycin + trimethoprim-sulfamethoxazole[3]	

[1] CNS indicates central nervous system; MRSA, methicillin-resistant *S aureus;* MIC, minimum inhibitory concentration.

[2] Penicillin- and cephalosporin-allergic patients should receive vancomycin as initial therapy for serious infections.

[3] One of the adjunctive agents, gentamicin or rifampin, should be added to the therapeutic regimen for life-threatening infections such as endocarditis or CNS infection or infections with a vancomycin-intermediate *S aureus* strain. Consultation with an infectious diseases specialist should be considered to determine which agent to use and duration of use.

[4] Linezolid and quinupristin-dalfopristin are 2 agents with activity in vitro and efficacy in adults with multidrug-resistant, gram-positive organisms, including *S aureus*. Because experience with these agents in children is limited, consultation with an infectious diseases specialist should be considered before use.

[5] Daptomycin is active in vitro against multidrug-resistant, gram-positive organisms, including *S aureus,* but has not been used in children. Daptomycin is approved by the US Food and Drug Administration only for the treatment of complicated skin and skin structure infections in patients 18 years of age and older.

Image 96.1
Pyoderma caused by *Staphylococcus aureus*.

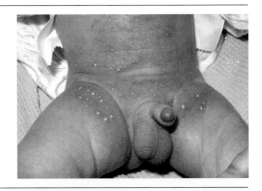

Image 96.2
Bullous impetigo lesions about the eyes, nose, and mouth in a 6-year-old black male. Also note the secondary anterior cervical lymphadenopathy.

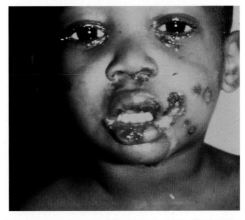

Image 96.3
Staphylococcus aureus hordeolum (sebaceous gland abscess) in an adolescent girl.

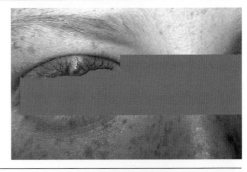

Image 96.4
An infant with orbital cellulitis and ethmoid sinusitis caused by *Staphylococcus aureus*.

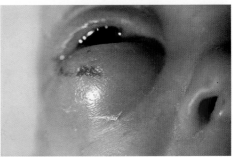

Image 96.5
Periorbital cellulitis caused by *Staphylococcus aureus.*

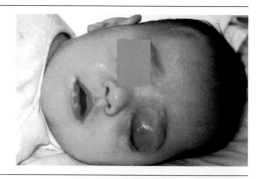

Image 96.6
Orbital abscess with proptosis of the globe due to *Staphylococcus aureus* in a 12-year-old boy. Delayed surgical drainage contributed to permanent visual impairment due to central retinal vascular involvement. The patient also had left ethmoid and maxillary sinusitis.

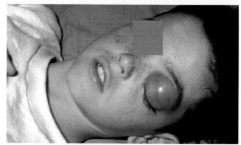

Image 96.7
Abscess of the face caused by *Staphylococcus aureus* in an 8-year-old girl.

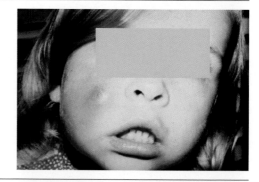

Image 96.8
Staphylococcus aureus abscess of the lobe of the left ear secondary to ear piercing in an adolescent girl.

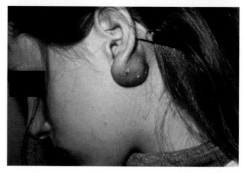

Image 96.9

Cervical adenitis with abscess formation due to *Staphylococcus aureus.* Delay in seeking medical care resulted in spontaneous drainage of the abscess.

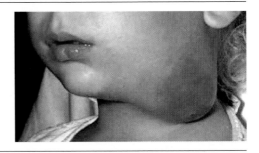

Image 96.10

Abscess of axillary lymph node caused by *Staphylococcus aureus.*

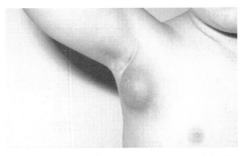

Image 96.11

Perionychia in a 4-year-old girl with acute lymphocytic leukemia in relapse. Purulent drainage grew group A streptococcus and *Staphylococcus aureus.*

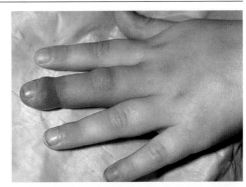

Image 96.12

Infected finger-stick site with cellulitis. *Micrococcus* species isolated from blood. The girl also had chronic myelogenous leukemia/ acute myelogenous leukemia in relapse.

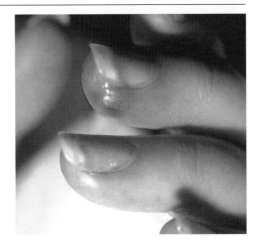

Image 96.13

Chronic osteomyelitis of the right tibia caused by *Staphylococcus aureus*.

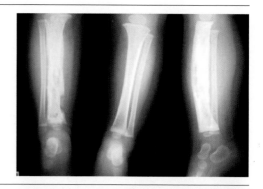

Image 96.14

Osteomyelitis of the calcaneus due to *Staphylococcus aureus* with no history of injury.

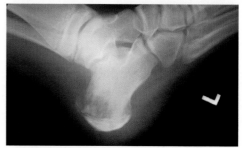

Image 96.15

Vertebral osteomyelitis in a 13-year-old child with a 6-week history of back pain. MRI revealed osteolytic changes of the anterior segments of the first and second lumbar vertebrae. A culture of the biopsy specimen grew methicillin-resistant *Staphylococcus aureus*.

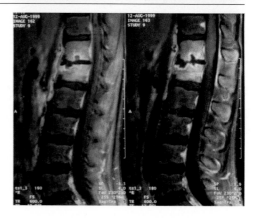

Image 96.16

Cerebral infarct in a patient with bacterial endocarditis.

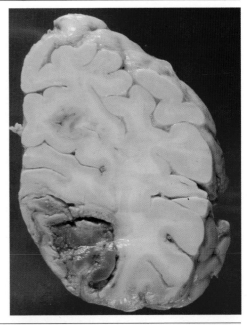

Image 96.17

Infant with staphylococcal scalded skin syndrome with sheets of skin desquamation.

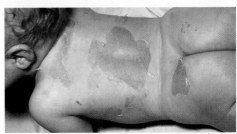

Image 96.18

Staphylococcal scalded skin syndrome. Epidermolytic exotoxin results in superficial, generalized desquamation.

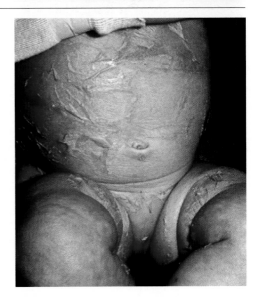

Image 96.19

A 9-month-old white male infant with erythro-
dermal and crusted lesions about the eyes,
nose, and mouth characteristic of staphylococcal
scalded skin syndrome. No residual skin
scarring occurred.

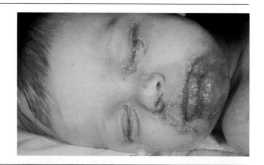

Image 96.20

Staphylococcal pneumonia, primary, with rapid
progression and empyema. The infant had only
mild respiratory distress and paralytic ileus without fever when first examined.

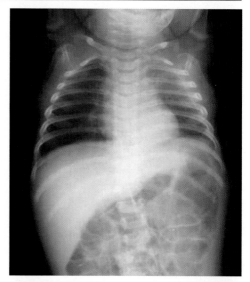

Image 96.21

Staphylococcal pneumonia, primary, with
rapid progression and empyema. This is
the same patient as in Image 96.20.

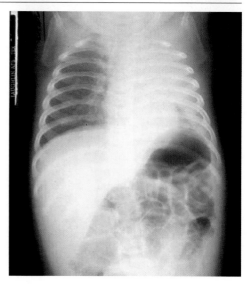

97

Group A Streptococcal Infections

Clinical Manifestations

The most common group A streptococcal (GAS) infection is acute pharyngotonsillitis. Purulent complications, including otitis media, sinusitis, peritonsillar and retropharyngeal abscesses, and suppurative cervical adenitis develop in some patients, usually people who are untreated. The significance of GAS upper respiratory tract disease is related to acute morbidity and to nonsuppurative sequela (acute rheumatic fever).

Scarlet fever occurs most often in association with pharyngitis and, rarely, with pyoderma or an infected wound. Scarlet fever has a characteristic confluent erythematous sandpaper-like rash, which is caused by one or more of several erythrogenic exotoxins produced by GAS strains. Severe scarlet fever occurs rarely. Other than the occurrence of rash, the epidemiologic features, symptoms, signs, sequelae, and treatment of scarlet fever are the same as those of streptococcal pharyngitis.

Toddlers (1–3 years of age) with GAS respiratory tract infection initially have serous rhinitis and develop a protracted illness with moderate fever, irritability, anorexia, and lymphadenopathy (streptococcal fever). The classic presentation of streptococcal upper respiratory tract infection as acute pharyngitis is uncommon in children younger than 3 years. Rheumatic fever also is rare in children younger than 3 years.

The second most common site of GAS infection is the skin. Streptococcal skin infections (ie, pyoderma or impetigo) can result in acute glomerulonephritis, which occasionally occurs in epidemics. The nonsuppurative sequela of GAS skin infection is acute glomerulonephritis. Acute rheumatic fever is not a proven sequela of streptococcal skin infection.

Other GAS infections include erysipelas, perianal cellulitis, vaginitis, bacteremia, pneumonia, endocarditis, pericarditis, septic arthritis, cellulitis, necrotizing fasciitis, osteomyelitis, myositis, puerperal sepsis, surgical wound infection, and neonatal omphalitis. Necrotizing fasciitis and other invasive GAS infections in children can occur as complications of varicella. Invasive GAS infections can be severe, with or without an identified focus of local infection, and can be associated with streptococcal toxic shock syndrome. The portal of entry of invasive infections often is the skin but often is not identified. Infection can follow minor or unrecognized trauma. An association between GAS infection and sudden onset of obsessive-compulsive and/or tic disorders has been proposed. This condition has been described as pediatric autoimmune neuropsychiatric disorders associated with streptococcal infection (PANDAS). The hypothesized association between PANDAS and GAS infections is unproven.

Etiology

More than 100 distinct M-protein types of group A beta-hemolytic streptococci *(Streptococcus pyogenes)* have been identified. Typing based on the M-protein sequence *(emm* typing) also is performed and is more discriminating than M serotyping. Epidemiologic studies suggest an association between certain M types (eg, types 1, 3, 5, 6, 18, 19, and 24) and rheumatic fever, but a specific rheumatogenic factor has not been identified. Several M types (eg, types 49, 55, 57, and 59) are associated with pyoderma and acute glomerulonephritis. Other M types (eg, types 1, 6, and 12) are associated with pharyngitis and acute glomerulonephritis.

Epidemiology

Pharyngitis usually results from contact with a person who has GAS pharyngitis. Transmission of GAS infection, including school outbreaks of pharyngitis, almost always follows contact with respiratory tract secretions. Pharyngitis and impetigo (and their nonsuppurative complications) can be associated with crowding, which often is present in socioeconomically disadvantaged populations. The close contact that occurs in schools, child care centers, and military installations facilitates transmission. Food-borne outbreaks of pharyngitis have occurred and are a consequence of human contamination of food in conjunction with improper food preparation or improper refrigeration procedures.

Streptococcal pharyngitis occurs at all ages but is most common among school-aged children and adolescents. GAS pharyngitis and pyoderma are less common in adults than in children.

Geographically, GAS pharyngitis and pyoderma are ubiquitous. Pyoderma is more common in tropical climates and warm seasons, presumably because of antecedent insect bites and other minor skin trauma. Streptococcal pharyngitis is more common during late autumn, winter, and spring in temperate climates, presumably because of close person-to-person contact in schools. Communicability of patients with streptococcal pharyngitis is highest during the acute infection and, in untreated people, gradually diminishes over a period of weeks. Patients no longer are contagious within 24 hours after initiation of appropriate antimicrobial therapy.

Throat culture surveys of healthy children during school outbreaks of pharyngitis have yielded GAS prevalence rates as high as 15% to 50%. These surveys include children who were pharyngeal carriers with no subsequent immune response to GAS cellular or extracellular antigens. Carriage of GAS can persist for many months, but the risk of transmission to others is minimal.

The incidence of acute rheumatic fever in the United States has decreased sharply over several decades, but focal outbreaks of rheumatic fever in school-aged children occurred throughout the 1990s. Although the reason(s) for these local outbreaks is not clear, their occurrence reemphasizes the importance of diagnosing GAS pharyngitis and of adherence to recommended antimicrobial regimens.

In streptococcal impetigo, the organism usually is acquired from another person with impetigo by direct contact. GAS colonization of healthy skin usually precedes development of skin infection. Impetiginous lesions occur at the site of breaks in skin (insect bites, burns, traumatic wounds). GAS organisms

do not penetrate intact skin. After development of impetiginous lesions, the upper respiratory tract often becomes colonized with GAS. Infection of surgical wounds and postpartum (puerperal) sepsis usually result from contact transmission by hands. Anal or vaginal carriers and people with pyoderma or local suppurative infections can transmit GAS to surgical and obstetrical patients, resulting in nosocomial outbreaks. Infections in neonates can result from intrapartum or contact transmission; in the latter situation, infection can begin as omphalitis, cellulitis, or necrotizing fasciitis.

The incidence of invasive GAS infections is highest in infants and older people. Varicella is the most commonly identified risk factor in children. Other risk factors include intravenous drug use, HIV infection, diabetes mellitus, and chronic cardiac or pulmonary disease. The portal of entry is unknown in almost 50% of invasive GAS infections; in most cases, the entry site is believed to be the skin or mucous membranes. Such infections rarely follow GAS pharyngitis. Although case reports have described a temporal association between use of nonsteroidal anti-inflammatory drugs and invasive GAS infections in children with varicella, a causal relationship has not been established.

Incubation Period

Pharyngitis, 2 to 5 days; impetigo, 7 to 10 days.

Diagnostic Tests

Laboratory confirmation of GAS is recommended for children with pharyngitis because accurate clinical differentiation of viral and GAS pharyngitis is not possible. A specimen should be obtained by vigorous swabbing of both tonsils and the posterior pharynx. Culture on sheep blood agar can confirm GAS infection, and latex agglutination, fluorescent antibody, coagglutination, or precipitation techniques performed on colonies growing on an agar plate can differentiate group A from other beta-hemolytic streptococci. False-negative culture results occur in fewer than 10% of symptomatic patients when an adequate throat swab specimen is obtained. Recovery of GAS from the pharynx or the number of colonies on an agar plate does not distinguish patients with true streptococcal infection (defined by a serologic antibody response) from streptococcal carriers who have an intercurrent viral pharyngitis. Cultures that are negative for GAS after 24 hours should be incubated for a second day to optimize recovery of GAS.

Several rapid diagnostic tests for GAS pharyngitis are available. Most are based on nitrous acid extraction of group A carbohydrate antigen from organisms obtained by throat swab. The specificities of these tests generally are high, but the reported sensitivities vary considerably. As with throat cultures, the sensitivity of these tests is highly dependent on the quality of the throat swab specimen, the experience of the person performing the test, and the rigor of the culture standard used for comparison. Therefore, when a patient suspected of having GAS pharyngitis has a negative rapid streptococcal test, a throat culture should be obtained to ensure that the patient does not have GAS infection. Because of the high specificity of these rapid tests, a positive test result generally does not require throat culture confirmation. Rapid diagnostic tests using techniques such as optical immunoassay and chemiluminescent DNA probes have been developed. These tests may be as sensitive as standard throat cultures on sheep blood agar. Physicians who use any of these rapid tests without culture backup may wish to compare their results with those of culture to validate adequate sensitivity in their practice.

Indications for GAS Testing. Factors to be considered in the decision to obtain a throat swab specimen for testing in children with pharyngitis are the patient's age; clinical signs and symptoms; the season; and family and community epidemiology, including contact with a case of GAS infection or presence in the family of a person with a history of acute rheumatic fever or with poststreptococcal glomerulonephritis. GAS pharyngitis is uncommon in children younger than 3 years, but outbreaks of GAS pharyngitis have been reported in young children in child care settings. The risk of acute rheumatic fever is so remote in resource-rich countries in such young children that diagnostic studies for

GAS pharyngitis are indicated considerably less often for children younger than 3 years than for older children. Children with manifestations highly suggestive of viral infection, such as coryza, conjunctivitis, hoarseness, cough, anterior stomatitis, discrete ulcerative lesions, or diarrhea, are unlikely to have GAS as the cause of their pharyngitis and generally should not be tested for GAS. Children with acute onset of sore throat and clinical signs and symptoms such as pharyngeal exudate, pain on swallowing, fever, and enlarged tender anterior cervical lymph nodes or exposure to a person with GAS pharyngitis are more likely to have GAS as the cause of their pharyngitis and should have a rapid antigen test and/or throat culture performed.

Indications for testing contacts for GAS vary according to circumstances. Testing asymptomatic household contacts for GAS is not recommended except when contacts are at increased risk of developing sequelae of GAS infection. Throat swab specimens should be obtained from siblings and all other household contacts of a child who has acute rheumatic fever or poststreptococcal glomerulonephritis, and if test results are positive, contacts should be treated regardless of whether they currently are or recently were symptomatic. Household contacts of an index case with streptococcal pharyngitis who have recent or current symptoms suggestive of streptococcal infection also should be tested. Pyoderma lesions should be cultured in families with one case or more of acute nephritis or streptococcal toxic shock syndrome so that antimicrobial therapy can be administered to eradicate GAS.

Posttreatment throat swab cultures are indicated only for patients at particularly high risk of acute rheumatic fever or who remain symptomatic at that time. Repeated courses of antimicrobial therapy are not indicated for asymptomatic patients who remain GAS positive after appropriate antimicrobial therapy; the exceptions are people who have had, or whose family members have had, acute rheumatic fever or other uncommon epidemiologic circumstances, such as outbreaks of rheumatic fever or acute poststreptococcal glomerulonephritis.

Patients in whom repeated episodes of GAS pharyngitis occur at short intervals documented by culture or antigen detection test present a special problem. Often these people are chronic GAS carriers who are experiencing frequent viral illnesses. In assessing such patients, inadequate adherence to oral treatment also should be considered. Although uncommon, in some areas erythromycin resistance among GAS strains does occur, resulting in erythromycin treatment failures. Such strains also are resistant to other macrolides, such as clarithromycin and azithromycin. Testing asymptomatic household contacts usually is not helpful. However, if multiple household members have pharyngitis or other GAS infections, such as pyoderma, simultaneous cultures of all household members and treatment of all people with positive cultures or rapid antigen test results may be of value.

In schools, child care centers, or other environments in which a large number of people are in close contact, the prevalence of GAS pharyngeal carriage in healthy children can be as high as 15% even in the absence of an outbreak of streptococcal disease. Therefore classroom or more widespread culture surveys are not indicated and should be considered only if more than one case of acute rheumatic fever, glomerulonephritis, or severe invasive GAS disease has occurred.

Cultures of impetiginous lesions are not indicated routinely because lesions often yield both streptococci and staphylococci, and determination of the primary pathogen is not possible.

In suspected invasive GAS infections, cultures of blood and focal sites of possible infection are indicated. In necrotizing fasciitis, imaging studies often delay, rather than facilitate, the diagnosis. Clinical suspicion of necrotizing fasciitis should prompt surgical inspection of the deep tissues with Gram stain and culture of surgical specimens.

Treatment

Pharyngitis. Penicillin V is the drug of choice for treatment of GAS pharyngitis, except in people who are severely allergic to penicillin. A clinical isolate of GAS resistant to penicillin never has been documented. Ampicillin or amoxicillin often is used, but these drugs have no microbiologic advantage over penicillin. Penicillin therapy prevents acute rheumatic fever even when therapy is started 9 days after onset of the acute illness, shortens the clinical course, decreases risk of transmission, and decreases risk of suppurative sequelae. For all patients with acute rheumatic fever, a complete course of penicillin or other appropriate antimicrobial agents for GAS pharyngitis should be given to eradicate GAS from the throat, even though the organism may not be recovered in the initial throat culture.

Intramuscular penicillin G benzathine is appropriate therapy. It ensures adequate blood concentrations and avoids the problem of adherence, but administration is painful. Discomfort is less if the preparation of penicillin G benzathine is brought to room temperature before intramuscular injection. Mixtures containing shorter-acting penicillins (eg, penicillin G procaine) in addition to penicillin G benzathine have not been demonstrated to be more effective than penicillin G benzathine alone but are less painful when administered.

Orally administered erythromycin is indicated for patients who are allergic to penicillin unless GAS strains resistant to erythromycin are prevalent in the community. Other macrolides, such as clarithromycin or azithromycin, also are effective.

A narrow-spectrum (first-generation) oral cephalosporin is an acceptable alternative, particularly for people who are allergic to penicillin. However, as many as 5% of penicillin-allergic people also are allergic to cephalosporins. Patients with immediate or type I hypersensitivity to penicillin should not be treated with a cephalosporin. The additional cost of many cephalosporins and their wider range of antibacterial activity compared with penicillin preclude recommending them for routine use in people with GAS pharyngitis who are not allergic to penicillin. Tetracyclines and sulfonamides should not be used for treating GAS pharyngitis.

Management of a patient who has repeated and frequent episodes of acute pharyngitis associated with a positive laboratory test for GAS is problematic. To determine whether the patient is a long-term streptococcal pharyngeal carrier who is experiencing repeated episodes of intercurrent viral pharyngitis (which is the situation in most cases), the following should be determined: (1) whether the clinical findings are more suggestive of a GAS or a viral cause, (2) whether epidemiologic factors in the community are more suggestive of a GAS or a viral cause, (3) the nature of the clinical response to the antimicrobial therapy (in true GAS pharyngitis, response to therapy usually is rapid), (4) whether laboratory tests are positive for GAS between episodes of acute pharyngitis, and (5) whether a serologic response to GAS extracellular antigens (eg, antistreptolysin O) has occurred.

Pharyngeal Carriers. Antimicrobial therapy is not indicated for most GAS pharyngeal carriers. Exceptions (ie, specific situations in which eradication of carriage may be indicated) include the following: (1) an outbreak of acute rheumatic fever or poststreptococcal glomerulonephritis occurs, (2) an outbreak of GAS pharyngitis in a closed or semiclosed community occurs, (3) a family history of acute rheumatic fever exists, (4) multiple episodes of documented symptomatic GAS pharyngitis continue to occur within a family during a period of many weeks despite appropriate therapy, (5) a family has excessive anxiety about GAS infections, or (6) tonsillectomy is considered only because of chronic GAS carriage.

Streptococcal carriage can be difficult to eradicate with conventional antimicrobial therapy. A number of antimicrobial agents, including clindamycin, amoxicillin-clavulanate, azithromycin, and a combination of rifampin for the last 4 days of treatment with either penicillin V or penicillin G benzathine, have been demonstrated to be more effective than penicillin in eliminating chronic streptococcal carriage. Of these drugs, oral clindamycin has been reported to be the most effective.

Streptococcal Impetigo. Local mupirocin ointment may be useful for limiting person-to-person spread of GAS impetigo and for eradicating localized disease. With multiple lesions or with impetigo in multiple family members, child care groups, or athletic teams, impetigo should be treated with antimicrobial regimens administered systemically. Because episodes of impetigo may be caused by *Staphylococcus aureus* or *Streptococcus pyogenes,* children with impetigo usually should be treated with an antimicrobial agent active against both GAS and *S aureus.*

Other Infections. Parenteral antimicrobial therapy is required for severe infections, such as endocarditis, pneumonia, septicemia, meningitis, arthritis, osteomyelitis, erysipelas, necrotizing fasciitis, neonatal omphalitis, and streptococcal toxic shock syndrome.

Image 97.1

Inflammation of the oropharynx with petechiae on the soft palate caused by group A streptococcal pharyngitis.

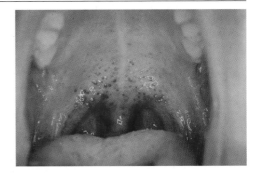

Image 97.2
Erythematous tonsils in a child with group A streptococcal pharyngitis.

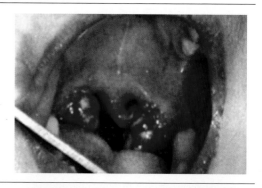

Image 97.3
Protracted nasopharyngitis is the most common presentation of group A streptococcal infection in toddlers. Inflammation of the skin beneath the nares often is present, as in this child.

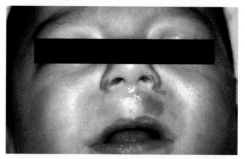

Image 97.4
Cervical lymphadenitis, unilateral, caused by group A streptococci.

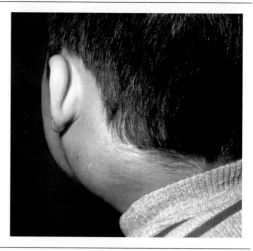

Image 97.5
Posterior cervical lymph node aspiration specimen grew group A streptococci.

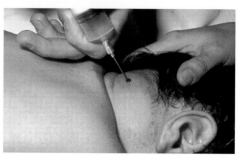

Image 97.6
A 13-year-old white male with group A strepto-coccal erysipelas of the left cheek. Erysipelas is characterized by a palpable margin at the edge of the cellulitis.

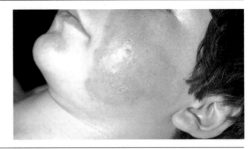

Image 97.7
Group A streptococcal arthritis of the left ankle in a 4-year-old white female.

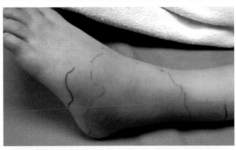

Image 97.8
Group A streptococcal necrotizing fasciitis com-plicating varicella in a 3-year-old white female.

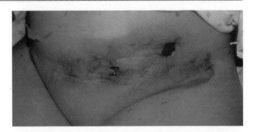

Image 97.9
Perianal group A streptococcal cellulitis in an 18-month-old white male.

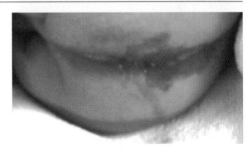

Image 97.10
Pastia lines in the antecubital space of a 2-year-old white male with scarlet fever.

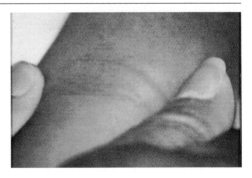

Image 97.11
The characteristic inflammatory changes in the tongue (ie, the "strawberry tongue") of scarlet fever.

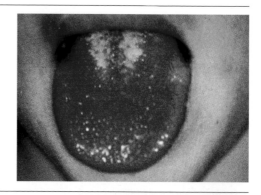

Image 97.12
Erythema marginatum in a 12-year-old white female. Although a characteristic rash of rheumatic fever, it is noted in fewer than 3% of cases. Its serpiginous border and evanescent nature serve to distinguish it from erythema migrans lesions of Lyme disease.

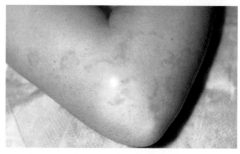

Image 97.13
Beau lines involving the thumbnail of a child in the post-recovery stage of a severe group A streptococcal infection. Beau lines may occur following wasting diseases of varying causes, including HIV infection and malabsorption syndromes.

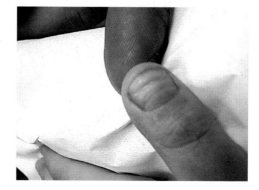

98

Group B Streptococcal Infections

Clinical Manifestations

Group B streptococci are a major cause of perinatal bacterial infections, including bacteremia, endometritis, chorioamnionitis, urinary tract infections in pregnant women, and systemic and focal infections in infants from birth until 3 months of age or, rarely, older. Invasive disease in young infants is categorized on the basis of chronologic age at onset. Early-onset disease usually occurs within the first 24 hours of life (range, 0–6 days) and is characterized by signs of systemic infection, respiratory distress, apnea, shock, pneumonia and, less often, meningitis (5%–10% of cases). Late-onset disease, which typically occurs at 3 to 4 weeks of age (range, 7 days–3 months), commonly manifests as occult bacteremia or meningitis; other focal infections, such as osteomyelitis, septic arthritis, adenitis, and cellulitis, can occur. Late-onset disease has onset beyond age 3 months in very preterm infants requiring prolonged hospitalization. Group B streptococci also cause systemic infections in nonpregnant adults with underlying medical conditions, such as diabetes mellitus, chronic liver or renal disease, malignancy, or other immunocompromising conditions, and adults 65 years of age and older.

Etiology

Group B streptococci (*Streptococcus agalactiae*) are gram-positive, aerobic diplococci that typically produce a narrow zone of beta hemolysis on 5% sheep blood agar. These organisms are divided into 9 serotypes on the basis of capsular polysaccharides (Ia, Ib, II, and III through VIII). Serotypes Ia, Ib, II, III, and V account for approximately 95% of cases in the United States. Serotype III is the predominant cause of early-onset meningitis and most late-onset infections in infants.

Epidemiology

Group B streptococci are common inhabitants of the gastrointestinal and genitourinary tracts. Less commonly, they colonize the pharynx. The colonization rate in pregnant women and newborn infants ranges from 15% to 40%. Colonization during pregnancy can be constant or intermittent. Before recommendations for prevention of early-onset group B streptococcal (GBS) disease by maternal intrapartum antimicrobial prophylaxis were made, the incidence was 1 to 4 cases per 1000 live births; early-onset disease accounted for approximately 75% of infant cases and occurred in approximately 1 infant per 100 to 200 colonized women. Associated with implementation of widespread maternal intrapartum antimicrobial prophylaxis, the incidence of early-onset disease has decreased by approximately 81% to approximately 0.3 cases per 1000 live births in 2005 and now equals that of late-onset disease. Case fatality rates in term infants range from 3% to 5% but are higher in preterm neonates. Transmission from mother to infant occurs shortly before or during delivery. After delivery, person-to-person transmission can occur. Although uncommon, GBS can be acquired in the nursery from hospital personnel (probably via hand contamination) or more commonly in the community from healthy colonized people. The risk of early-onset disease is increased in preterm infants born at less than 37 weeks of gestation, in infants born after the amniotic membranes have been ruptured 18 hours or more, and in infants born to women with high genital GBS inoculum, intrapartum fever (temperature ≥38°C [≥100.4°F]), chorioamnionitis, GBS bacteriuria during the pregnancy, or a previous infant with invasive GBS disease. A low concentration of serotype-specific serum antibody also is a predisposing factor. Other risk factors are intrauterine fetal monitoring, maternal age younger than 20 years, and black or Hispanic ethnic origin. The period of communicability is unknown but may extend throughout the duration of colonization or disease. Infants can remain colonized for several months after birth and after treatment for systemic infection. Recurrent GBS disease affects an estimated 1% of appropriately treated infants.

Incubation Period

Fewer than 7 days; late-onset and very late-onset disease, unknown.

Diagnostic Tests

Gram-positive cocci in body fluids that typically are sterile (such as CSF, pleural fluid, or joint fluid) provide presumptive evidence of infection. Cultures of blood, other typically sterile body fluids, or a suppurative focus are necessary to establish the diagnosis. Rapid tests that identify group B streptococcal antigen in body fluids other than CSF are not recommended because of poor specificity.

Treatment

Ampicillin plus an aminoglycoside is the initial treatment of choice for a newborn infant with presumptive invasive GBS infection. Penicillin G alone can be given when GBS has been identified as the cause of the infection and when clinical and microbiologic responses have been documented. For meningitis, some experts believe that a second lumbar puncture approximately 24 to 48 hours after initiation of therapy assists in management and prognosis. If CSF sterility is not achieved, a complicated course (eg, cerebral infarcts) can be expected; also an increasing protein concentration suggests an intracranial complication (eg, infarction, ventricular obstruction). Additional lumbar punctures and diagnostic imaging studies are indicated if response to therapy is in doubt, neurologic abnormalities persist, or focal neurologic deficits occur. Consultation with a specialist in pediatric infectious diseases often is useful.

Because of the reported increased risk of infection, the twin or any multiples of an index case with early- or late-onset disease should be observed carefully and evaluated and treated empirically for suspected systemic infection if any signs of illness occur.

Image 98.1
Bilateral, severe group B streptococcal pneumonia in a neonate.

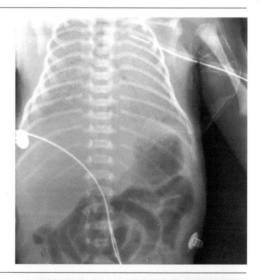

Image 98.2
MRI after group B streptococcal meningitis showing extensive destructive changes in the cerebrum.

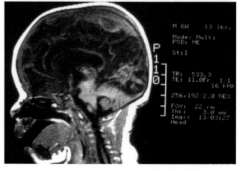

Image 98.3
Neonatal group B streptococcal osteomyelitis of the right proximal humerus.

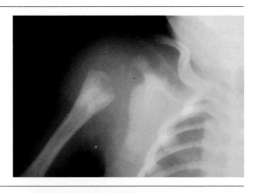

Image 98.4
Necrotizing fasciitis of the periumbilical area. Group B streptococcus, *Staphylococcus aureus,* and anaerobic streptococci were isolated at the time of surgical debridement.

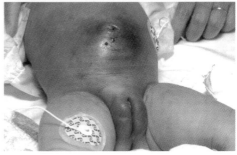

99

Non–Group A or B Streptococcal and Enterococcal Infections

Clinical Manifestations

Streptococci of groups other than A or B can be associated with invasive disease in infants, children, adolescents, and adults. Urinary tract infection, endocarditis, upper and lower respiratory tract infections, skin and soft tissue infections, pharyngitis, and meningitis are the principal clinical syndromes. Viridans streptococci are associated with endocarditis in patients with congenital or valvular heart disease and bacteremia in neonates and neutropenic patients with cancer. Enterococci are associated with bacteremia in neonates and bacteremia, device-associated infections, intra-abdominal abscesses, and urinary tract infections in older children and adults.

Etiology

Changes in taxonomy and nomenclature of the *Streptococcus* genus have evolved as a result of application of molecular technology. Among gram-positive organisms that are catalase negative and that display chains in Gram stains, the 2 genera associated most often with human disease are *Streptococcus* and *Enterococcus*. The *Streptococcus* genus contains organisms that are (a) beta-hemolytic on blood agar plates *(Streptococcus pyogenes; Streptococcus agalactiae;* and groups C, G, and F streptococci); (b) non–beta-hemolytic on blood agar plates *(Streptococcus pneumoniae, Streptococcus bovis* group, and 26 species of viridans streptococci, which are divided into 6 groups by phenotypic characteristics); (c) nutritionally variant streptococci (now referred to as *Abiotrophia* and *Granulicatella*); and (d) unusual streptococcal species that do not fit into any of the other *Streptococcus* species groups.

The genus *Enterococcus* (previously included with group D streptococci) contains more than 20 species, with *Enterococcus faecalis* and *Enterococcus faecium* accounting for most human enterococcal infections.

Epidemiology

The habitats that streptococci and enterococci occupy in humans include skin (groups C, F, and G streptococci), oropharynx (groups B, C, F, and G streptococci and the mutans group streptococci), gastrointestinal tract (groups B, C, F, and G and the bovis group streptococci and *Enterococcus* species), and vagina (groups B, C, D, F, and G streptococci and *Enterococcus* species). The typical human habitats of different species of viridans streptococci include the oropharynx, epithelial surfaces of the oral cavity, teeth, skin, and genitourinary tract. Intrapartum transmission probably is responsible for most cases of early-onset neonatal infection. Vertical colonization of viridans streptococci and cariogenic mutans streptococcus from mother to infant is well documented. Environmental contamination or transmission via hands of health care professionals can lead to colonization of patients.

Incubation Period

Unknown.

Diagnostic Tests

Microscopic examination of fluids that ordinarily are sterile can yield presumptive evidence of infections by streptococci and enterococci. Diagnosis is established by culture and serogrouping of the isolate, using group-specific antisera. Antimicrobial susceptibility testing of enterococci isolated from sterile sites is important to determine ampicillin and vancomycin susceptibility as well as high-level gentamicin and streptomycin resistance to assess potential for synergy when used in combination with a cell wall active agent (ampicillin or vancomycin). Some susceptibility testing methods may not reliably detect vancomycin resistance; the addition of testing on vancomycin screening agar increases reliability.

Treatment

For most streptococcal infections, treatment with penicillin G alone is adequate. However, for penicillin-resistant isolates, options include penicillin with gentamicin, other beta-lactam agents, and vancomycin. Enterococci and some streptococcal strains (especially viridans streptococci and nutritionally variant streptococci requiring growth media additives) are resistant to penicillin. Enterococci uniformly are resistant to cephalosporins and can be resistant to ampicillin and vancomycin as well, making treatment challenging. Invasive enterococcal infections such as endocarditis should be treated with ampicillin or vancomycin (if penicillin allergy is documented) in combination with an aminoglycoside (usually gentamicin) to achieve bactericidal activity. However, the aminoglycoside should be discontinued if in vitro susceptibility testing demonstrates high-level resistance, in which case synergy cannot be achieved. Quinupristin-dalfopristin has been licensed for use in adults for treatment of infections attributable to vancomycin-resistant *E faecium*. Linezolid is approved for use for treatment of vancomycin-resistant enterococcal infections, including *E faecium* and *E fecalis*.

Image 99.1
A patient with Osler nodes from viridans streptococci bacterial endocarditis.

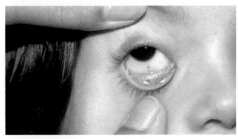

Image 99.2
Conjunctival (palpebral) petechiae in an adolescent girl with viridans streptococci subacute bacterial endocarditis.

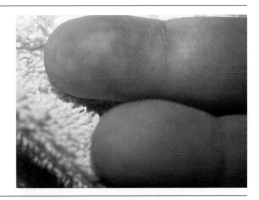

Image 99.3
A conjunctival hemorrhage in an adolescent female with enterococcal endocarditis.

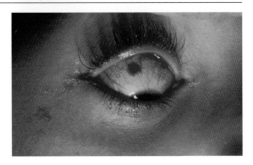

Image 99.4
Osler nodes on the fingers and a Janeway lesion on the palm of a patient with enterococcal endocarditis.

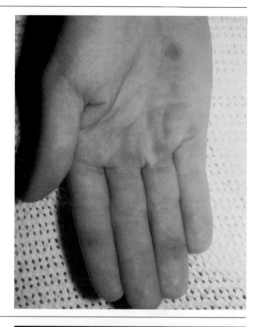

Image 99.5
Hemorrhagic retinitis with Roth spots in an adolescent female with enterococcal endocarditis.

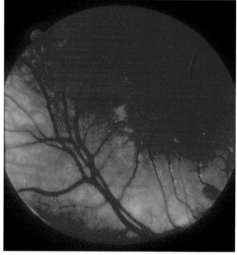

100

Strongyloidiasis
(Strongyloides stercoralis)

Clinical Manifestations

Asymptomatic infection accompanied by peripheral blood eosinophilia can be the only manifestation of infection. Strongyloidiasis should be considered in any patient with unexplained eosinophilia. When symptoms occur, they are related to the 3 stages of infection: skin invasion, migration of larvae, and penetration of the intestinal mucosa by adult worms. Infective larvae typically are acquired from soil and enter the body through the skin, producing transient pruritic papules at the site of penetration, usually on the feet. Larvae then migrate to the lungs and can cause pneumonitis or a Löffler-like syndrome. Larvae then ascend the tracheobronchial tree and are swallowed; once they are in the gastrointestinal tract, they mature into adults and can cause vague abdominal pain, malabsorption, vomiting, and diarrhea. Larval migration from defecated stool can result in pruritic skin lesions in the perianal area, buttocks, and upper thighs, which can present as serpiginous, erythematous tracks called larva currens. Because of the ability of a *Strongyloides* organism to complete its life cycle entirely in humans (autoinfection), a disseminated (hyperinfection) syndrome can occur in immunocompromised people, characterized by abdominal pain, rapidly changing or diffuse pulmonary infiltrates, and septicemia or meningitis from enteric gram-negative bacilli.

Etiology

Strongyloides stercoralis is a nematode (roundworm).

Epidemiology

Strongyloidiasis is endemic in the tropics and subtropics, including the southeastern United States, wherever suitable moist soil and improper disposal of human waste coexist. Humans are the principal hosts, but dogs, cats, and other animals also can be reservoirs. Transmission involves penetration of skin by infective (filariform) larvae from contact with infected soil. Infections rarely can be acquired from intimate skin contact or from inadvertent coprophagy, such as from ingestion of contaminated food scavenged from garbage. In addition, because some larvae mature into infective forms in the colon, autoinfection can occur. Adult females lodge in the gut wall, where they lay eggs that become free-living rhabditiform larvae that generally pass into the external environment in feces but also can be swallowed or penetrate the perianal skin of the same host. Because of this cycle of autoinfection, patients can remain infected for decades.

Incubation Period

Unknown.

Diagnostic Tests

Strongyloidiasis can be difficult to diagnose because the parasite burden often is low. Stool examination can disclose characteristic larvae, but several fresh stool specimens may need to be examined, and stool concentration procedures may be required. Examination of duodenal contents obtained by a commercially available string test (Entero-Test) or a direct aspirate through a flexible endoscope can demonstrate larvae. Serodiagnosis can be helpful but is available only at the CDC and in a few reference laboratories. Results of enzyme immunoassay for antibodies to *Strongyloides* are positive in approximately 90% of infected people. However, serologic cross-reaction with other helminths limits specificity of serodiagnosis. Eosinophilia (blood eosinophil count >500/μL) is common. In disseminated strongyloidiasis, larvae can be found in the sputum.

Treatment

Treatment with ivermectin is preferred and is curative in most people. Albendazole or thiabendazole also can be used, but both drugs are associated with slightly lower cure rates. Prolonged or repeated treatment may be necessary in the hyperinfection syndrome or immunocompromised patients. Relapses occur and should be treated with the same drugs.

Figure 100.1
Strongyloides Life Cycle

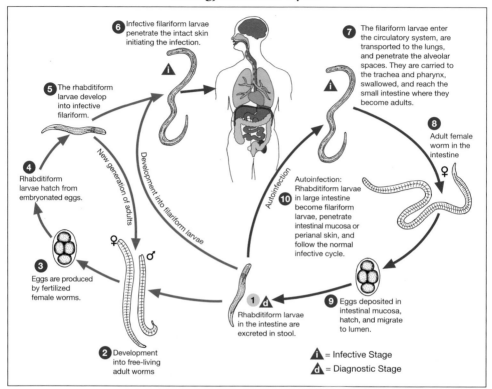

6 Infective filariform larvae penetrate the intact skin initiating the infection.

7 The filariform larvae enter the circulatory system, are transported to the lungs, and penetrate the alveolar spaces. They are carried to the trachea and pharynx, swallowed, and reach the small intestine where they become adults.

5 The rhabditiform larvae develop into infective filariform.

8 Adult female worm in the intestine ♀

4 Rhabditiform larvae hatch from embryonated eggs.

New generation of adults

Development into filariform larvae

Autoinfection

10 Autoinfection: Rhabditiform larvae in large intestine become filariform larvae, penetrate intestinal mucosa or perianal skin, and follow the normal infective cycle.

3 Eggs are produced by fertilized female worms.

♀ ♂

1 **d** Rhabditiform larvae in the intestine are excreted in stool.

9 Eggs deposited in intestinal mucosa, hatch, and migrate to lumen.

2 Development into free-living adult worms

i = Infective Stage

d = Diagnostic Stage

The *Strongyloides* life cycle is complex among helminths with its alternation between free-living and parasitic cycles, and its potential for autoinfection and multiplication within the host. Two types of cycles exist: Free-living cycle: The rhabditiform larvae passed in the stool (1) (see Parasitic cycle below) can either molt twice and become infective filariform larvae (direct development) (6) or molt 4 times and become free-living adult males and females (2) that mate and produce eggs (3) from which rhabditiform larvae hatch (4). The latter in turn can either develop (5) into a new generation of free-living adults (2) or into infective filariform larvae (6). The filariform larvae penetrate the human host skin to initiate the parasitic cycle. Parasitic cycle: Filariform larvae in contaminated soil penetrate the human skin (6) and are transported to the lungs where they penetrate the alveolar spaces; they are carried through the bronchial tree to the pharynx, are swallowed, and then reach the small intestine (7). In the small intestine they molt twice and become adult female worms (8). The females live threaded in the epithelium of the small intestine and by parthenogenesis produce eggs (9), which yield rhabditiform larvae. The rhabditiform larvae can either be passed in the stool (1) (see Free-living cycle above) or can cause autoinfection (10). In autoinfection, the rhabditiform larvae become infective filariform larvae, which can penetrate either the intestinal mucosa (internal autoinfection) or the skin of the perianal area (external autoinfection); in either case, the filariform larvae may follow the previously described route, being carried successively to the lungs, the bronchial tree, the pharynx, and the small intestine where they mature into adults; or they may disseminate widely in the body. To date, occurrence of autoinfection in humans with helminthic infections is recognized only in *Strongyloides stercoralis* and *Capillaria philippinensis* infections. In the case of *Strongyloides,* autoinfection may explain the possibility of persistent infections for many years in persons who have not been in an endemic area and of hyperinfections in immunodepressed individuals.

Courtesy of the Centers for Disease Control and Prevention.

Image 100.1
Strongyloides stercoralis larvae (oil-immersion magnification).

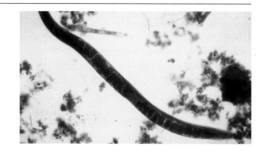

Image 100.2
Strongyloides stercoralis larvae (low-power magnification).

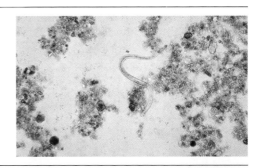

Image 100.3
Cutaneous migration sites of *Strongyloides stercoralis* over the left shoulder area.

101

Syphilis

Clinical Manifestations

Congenital Syphilis. Intrauterine infection can result in stillbirth, hydrops fetalis, or preterm birth. Infants can have hepatosplenomegaly, snuffles, lymphadenopathy, mucocutaneous lesions, osteochondritis and pseudoparalysis, edema, rash, hemolytic anemia, or thrombocytopenia at birth or within the first 4 to 8 weeks of life. Untreated infants, regardless of whether they have manifestations in early infancy, can develop late manifestations, which usually appear after 2 years of age and involve the CNS, bones and joints, teeth, eyes, and skin. Some consequences of intrauterine infection may not become apparent until many years after birth, such as interstitial keratitis (5–20 years of age), eighth cranial nerve deafness (10–40 years of age), Hutchinson teeth (peg-shaped, notched central incisors), anterior bowing of the shins, frontal bossing, mulberry molars, saddle nose, rhagades, and Clutton joints (symmetric, painless swelling of the knees). The first 3 manifestations are referred to as the Hutchinson triad.

Acquired Syphilis. Infection can be divided into 3 stages. The **primary stage** appears as one or more painless indurated ulcers (chancres) of the skin or mucous membranes at the site of inoculation, but chancres may not be recognized. These lesions most commonly appear on the genitalia. The **secondary stage,** beginning 1 to 2 months later, is characterized by rash, mucocutaneous lesions, and lymphadenopathy. The polymorphic maculopapular rash is generalized and typically includes the palms and soles. In moist areas around the vulva or anus, hypertrophic papular lesions (condylomata lata) can occur and can be confused with condyloma acuminata secondary to HPV. Generalized lymphadenopathy, fever, malaise, splenomegaly, sore throat, headache, and arthralgia can be present. A variable latent period follows but sometimes is interrupted during the first few years by recurrences of symptoms of secondary syphilis. **Latent** syphilis is defined as the period after infection when patients are seroreactive but demonstrate no clinical manifestations of disease. Latent syphilis acquired within the preceding year is referred to as *early latent syphilis;* all other cases of latent syphilis are *late latent syphilis* or *syphilis of unknown duration.* The tertiary stage of infection refers to gumma formation and cardiovascular involvement but not neurosyphilis. The tertiary stage can be marked by aortitis or gummatous changes of the skin, bone, or viscera, occurring from years to decades after the primary infection. Neurosyphilis is defined as infection of the CNS with *Treponema pallidum.* Manifestations of neurosyphilis can occur at any stage of infection, especially in people infected with HIV.

Etiology

T pallidum is a thin, motile spirochete that is extremely fastidious, surviving only briefly outside the host. The organism has not been cultivated successfully on artificial media.

Epidemiology

Syphilis, which is rare in much of the industrialized world, persists in the United States and in developing countries. The incidence of acquired and congenital syphilis increased dramatically in the United States during the late 1980s and early 1990s, but subsequently decreased. Rates of infection remain disproportionately high in large urban areas, in the southern United States, and among men who have sex with men. In adults, syphilis is more common among people with HIV infection.

Congenital syphilis is contracted from an infected mother via transplacental transmission of *T pallidum* at any time during pregnancy or at birth. Among women with untreated early syphilis, as many as 40% of pregnancies result in spontaneous abortion, stillbirth, or perinatal death. Infection can be transmitted to the fetus at any stage of disease; the rate of transmission is 60% to 100% during primary and secondary syphilis and slowly decreases with later stages of maternal infection (approximately 40% with early latent infection and 8% with late latent infection). Skin lesions or moist nasal secretions of congenital syphilis are highly infectious. However, organisms rarely are found in lesions more than 24 hours after treatment has begun.

Acquired syphilis almost always is contracted through direct sexual contact with ulcerative lesions of the skin or mucous membranes of infected people. Sexual abuse must be suspected in any young child with acquired syphilis. Open, moist lesions of the primary or secondary stages are highly infectious. Relapses of secondary syphilis with infectious mucocutaneous lesions can occur up to 4 years after primary infection.

Incubation Period

Primary syphilis, 3 weeks (range, 10–90 days).

Diagnostic Tests

Definitive diagnosis is made when spirochetes are identified by microscopic darkfield examination or direct fluorescent antibody tests of lesion exudate or tissue, such as placenta or umbilical cord. Specimens should be scraped from moist mucocutaneous lesions or aspirated from a regional lymph node. Specimens from mouth lesions require direct fluorescent antibody techniques to distinguish *T pallidum* from nonpathogenic treponemes. Because false-negative microscopic results are common, serologic testing often is necessary. PCR tests and IgM immunoblotting have been developed but are not yet available commercially.

Presumptive diagnosis is possible using nontreponemal and treponemal tests. The use of only 1 type of test is insufficient for diagnosis because false-positive nontreponemal test results occur with various medical conditions, and false-positive treponemal test results occur with other spirochetal diseases.

The standard nontreponemal tests for syphilis include the Venereal Disease Research Laboratory (VDRL) slide test, the rapid plasma reagin (RPR) test, and the automated reagin test (ART). These tests measure antibody directed against lipoidal antigen from *T pallidum,* antibody interaction with host tissues, or both. These tests are inexpensive, rapidly performed, and provide quantitative results. Quantitative results help define disease activity and monitor response to therapy. Nontreponemal test results can be falsely negative (ie, nonreactive) with early primary syphilis, latent acquired syphilis of long duration, and late congenital syphilis. Occasionally, a nontre-

ponemal test performed on serum samples containing high concentrations of antibody against *T pallidum* will be weakly reactive or falsely negative, a reaction termed the *prozone* phenomenon. Diluting the serum results in a positive test. When nontreponemal tests are used to monitor treatment response, the same specific test (eg, VDRL, RPR, or ART) must be used throughout the follow-up period, preferably by the same laboratory, to ensure comparability of results.

A reactive nontreponemal test result from a patient with typical lesions indicates the need for treatment. However, any reactive nontreponemal test result must be confirmed by one of the specific treponemal tests to exclude a false-positive test result. False-positive results can be caused by certain viral infections (eg, Epstein Barr virus infection, hepatitis, varicella, and measles), lymphoma, tuberculosis, malaria, endocarditis, connective tissue disease, pregnancy, abuse of injection drugs, laboratory or technical error, or Wharton jelly contamination when cord blood specimens are used. Treatment should not be delayed while awaiting the results of the treponemal test if the patient is symptomatic or at high risk of infection. A sustained 4-fold decrease in titer of the nontreponemal test result after treatment demonstrates adequate response to therapy; a 4-fold increase in titer after treatment suggests reinfection or treatment failure. The quantitative nontreponemal test usually decreases 4-fold within 6 months after therapy for primary or secondary syphilis and usually becomes nonreactive within 1 year after successful therapy if the infection (primary or secondary syphilis) was treated early. The patient usually becomes seronegative within 2 years even if the initial titer was high or the infection was congenital. Some people will continue to have low nontreponemal antibody titers despite effective therapy. This serofast state is more common in patients treated for latent or tertiary syphilis.

Treponemal tests in use are fluorescent treponemal antibody absorption (FTA-ABS) and *T pallidum* particle agglutination (TP-PA) tests. People who have positive FTA-ABS and TP-PA test results usually remain reactive for life, even after successful therapy. Treponemal test antibody titers correlate poorly with disease activity and should not be used to assess response to therapy.

Treponemal tests also are not 100% specific for syphilis; positive reactions variably occur in patients with other spirochetal diseases, such as yaws, pinta, leptospirosis, rat-bite fever, relapsing fever, and Lyme disease. Nontreponemal tests can be used to differentiate Lyme disease from syphilis because the VDRL test is nonreactive in Lyme disease.

Usually, a serum nontreponemal test is obtained initially, and if it is reactive, a treponemal test is performed. The probability of syphilis is high in a sexually active person whose serum is reactive on both nontreponemal and treponemal tests. Differentiating syphilis treated in the past from reinfection often is difficult unless the nontreponemal titer is increasing. Some clinical laboratories and blood banks have begun to screen samples using treponemal enzyme immunoassay (EIA) tests.

In summary, nontreponemal antibody tests (VDRL, RPR, and ART) are used for screening, and treponemal tests (FTA-ABS and TP-PA) are used to establish a presumptive diagnosis. Quantitative nontreponemal antibody tests are useful in assessing the adequacy of therapy and in detecting reinfection and relapse. All patients who have syphilis should be tested for HIV infection.

CSF Tests. For evaluation of possible neurosyphilis, the VDRL test should be performed on CSF. In addition to VDRL testing of CSF, evaluation of CSF protein and white blood cell count is used to assess the likelihood of CNS involvement. Although the FTA-ABS test of CSF is less specific than the VDRL test, some experts recommend using the FTA-ABS test, believing it to be more sensitive than the VDRL test. Results from the VDRL test should be interpreted cautiously because a negative result on a VDRL test of CSF does not exclude a diagnosis of neurosyphilis.

Testing During Pregnancy. All women should be screened serologically for syphilis early in pregnancy with a nontreponemal test (eg, VDRL or RPR) and preferably again at delivery. In areas of high prevalence of syphilis and in patients considered at high risk of syphilis, a nontreponemal serum test at the beginning of the third trimester (28 weeks of gestation and at delivery) is indicated. For women treated during pregnancy, follow-up serologic testing is necessary to assess the efficacy of therapy. Low-titer false-positive nontreponemal antibody test results occasionally occur in pregnancy. The result of a positive nontreponemal antibody test should be confirmed with a treponemal antibody test (eg, FTA-ABS). When a pregnant woman has a reactive nontreponemal test result and a persistently negative treponemal test result, a false-positive test result is confirmed. Some laboratories are screening pregnant women using an EIA treponemal test. Pregnant women with reactive treponemal screening tests should have confirmatory testing with a nontreponemal test with titers. Any woman who delivers a stillborn infant after 20 weeks' gestation should be tested for syphilis.

Evaluation of Newborn Infants for Congenital Infection. No newborn infant should be discharged from the hospital without determination of the mother's serologic status for syphilis. Testing of cord blood or an infant serum sample is inadequate for screening because these test results can be nonreactive even when the mother is seropositive. All infants born to seropositive mothers require a careful examination and a quantitative nontreponemal syphilis test. The test performed on the infant should be the same as that performed on the mother to enable comparison of titer results.

An infant should be evaluated further for congenital syphilis if the maternal titer has increased 4-fold, if the infant titer is 4-fold greater than the mother's titer, or if the infant has clinical manifestations of syphilis. In addition, an infant should be evaluated further if born to a mother with positive nontreponemal and treponemal test results if the mother has one or more of the following conditions:

- Syphilis untreated or inadequately treated or treatment is not documented
- Syphilis during pregnancy treated with a nonpenicillin regimen (including erythromycin)
- Syphilis treated less than 1 month before delivery (because treatment failures occur and the efficacy of treatment cannot be assumed)
- Syphilis treated before pregnancy but with insufficient serologic follow-up to assess the response to treatment and current infection status

Evaluation for syphilis in an infant should include the following:

- Physical examination
- Quantitative nontreponemal serologic test of serum from the infant for syphilis (not cord blood, because false-positive and false-negative results can occur)
- A VDRL test of CSF and analysis of CSF for cells and protein concentration
- Long-bone radiographs (unless the diagnosis has been established otherwise)
- Complete blood cell and platelet count
- Other clinically indicated tests (eg, chest radiography, liver function tests, ultrasonography, ophthalmologic examination, and auditory brainstem response test)

Pathologic examination of the placenta or umbilical cord using specific fluorescent antitreponemal antibody staining, if available, also is recommended.

A guide for interpretation of the results of nontreponemal and treponemal serologic tests is given in Table 101.1. An infected infant's test can be reactive or nonreactive, depending on the timing of maternal and fetal infection; thus the emphasis on screening maternal blood. Conversely, transplacental transmission of nontreponemal and treponemal antibodies to the fetus can occur in a mother who has been treated appropriately for syphilis during pregnancy, resulting in false-positive test results in the uninfected newborn infant.

The neonate's nontreponemal test titer in these circumstances usually reverts to negative in 4 to 6 months, whereas a positive FTA-ABS or TP-PA test result from passively acquired antibody may not become negative for 1 year or longer.

In an infant with clinical or tissue findings suggestive of congenital syphilis, a positive serum nontreponemal test result strongly supports the diagnosis regardless of therapy the mother received during the pregnancy. Infants who have a nonreactive nontreponemal test and normal physical examination do not require evaluation, although treatment depends on maternal history.

CSF Testing. CSF should be examined in all infants who are evaluated for congenital syphilis if the infant has any of the following: (1) abnormal physical examination findings consistent with congenital syphilis, (2) a serum quantitative nontreponemal titer that is 4-fold greater than the mother's titer, or (3) a positive darkfield or fluorescent antibody test result on body fluid(s). Testing of CSF can be indicated in other situations to help determine appropriate treatment. CSF should be examined in all patients with suspected neurosyphilis or with acquired untreated syphilis of more than 1 year's duration. Abnormalities in CSF in patients with neurosyphilis include increased protein concentration, increased white blood cell count, and a reactive VDRL test result. Some experts also recommend performing the FTA-ABS test on CSF, believing it to be more sensitive but less specific than VDRL testing of CSF for neurosyphilis. Because of the wide range of normal values for CSF white blood cell counts and protein concentrations in the newborn infant, interpretation can be difficult. A white blood cell count as high as 25 cells/µL and a protein concentration greater than 150 mg/dL might be normal. A negative result on VDRL or FTA-ABS testing of CSF does not exclude congenital neurosyphilis, and that is one of the reasons why infants with proven or probable congenital syphilis require 10 days of parenteral treatment with penicillin G regardless of CSF test results.

Treatment

Parenteral penicillin G remains the preferred drug for treatment of syphilis at any stage. Recommendations for penicillin G and duration of therapy vary depending on the stage of disease and clinical manifestations. Parenteral penicillin G is the only documented effective therapy for patients who have neurosyphilis, congenital syphilis, or syphilis during pregnancy and is recommended for HIV-infected patients. Such patients always should be treated with penicillin, even if desensitization for penicillin allergy is necessary.

Congenital Syphilis: Newborn Infants
(Table 101.2.) Infants should be treated for congenital syphilis if they have proven or probable disease demonstrated by one or more of the following: (1) physical, laboratory, or radiographic evidence of active disease; (2) positive placenta or umbilical cord test results for treponemes using direct fluorescent antibody–T pallidum staining or darkfield test; (3) a reactive result on VDRL testing of CSF; or (4) a serum quantitative nontreponemal titer that is at least 4-fold higher than the mother's titer using the same test and preferably the same laboratory. If the infant's titer is less than 4 times higher than that of the mother, congenital syphilis still can be present. When an infant warrants evaluation for congenital syphilis, the infant should be treated if test results cannot exclude infection, if the infant cannot be evaluated completely, or if adequate follow-up cannot be ensured.

In infants with proven or probable disease, aqueous crystalline penicillin G is preferred. The dosage should be based on chronologic, not gestational, age. Alternatively, some experts recommend penicillin G procaine for treatment of congenital syphilis; however, adequate CSF concentrations may not be achieved by this regimen. If more than 1 day of therapy is missed, the entire course should be restarted.

Healthy-appearing infants are at minimal risk of syphilis if (1) they are born to mothers who completed appropriate penicillin treatment for syphilis more than 4 weeks before delivery, (2) the mother had an appropriate serologic response to treatment (in early or high-titer syphilis, a documented 4-fold or greater decrease in VDRL, RPR, or ART titer or in latent low-titer syphilis, titers remained stable and low), (3) infants have a serum quantitative nontreponemal serologic titer the same as or less than 4-fold the maternal titer, and (4) the mother had no evidence of reinfection or relapse. Although a full evaluation may be unnecessary, these infants should be treated with a single injection of penicillin G benzathine. Alternatively, these infants can be examined carefully, preferably monthly, until their nontreponemal serologic test results are negative.

Infants whose mothers received no treatment or inadequate treatment for syphilis require special consideration. Maternal treatment for syphilis is deemed inadequate if (1) the mother's penicillin dose is unknown, undocumented, or inadequate; (2) the mother received erythromycin or any other nonpenicillin regimen during pregnancy for syphilis; or (3) treatment was given within 28 days of the infant's birth.

Healthy infants whose quantitative nontreponemal serologic titer is the same or less than 4-fold their mother's titer and born to women who received no treatment or inadequate treatment (as defined by one or more of these criteria) should be evaluated fully, including CSF examination. Some experts would treat all such infants with aqueous crystalline penicillin G (or aqueous penicillin G procaine) for 10 days because physical examination and laboratory test results cannot reliably exclude the diagnosis in all cases. However, if the infant's physical examination, including ophthalmologic examination, CSF findings, radiographs of long bones and chest, and complete blood cell and platelet counts all are normal, some experts would treat infants in the specific circumstances given in Table 101.2 with a single dose of penicillin G benzathine. In the case in which maternal response to treatment has not been demonstrated but the mother received an appropriate regimen of penicillin therapy more than 1 month before delivery, the infant's evaluation is normal, and clinical and serologic follow-up can be ensured, some experts would give a single dose of penicillin G benzathine and continue to observe the infant.

Congenital Syphilis: Older Infants and Children. Because establishing the diagnosis of neurosyphilis is difficult, infants older than 4 weeks who possibly have congenital syphilis or who have neurologic involvement should be treated with aqueous crystalline penicillin (Table 101.3). This regimen also should be used to treat children older than 1 year who have late and previously untreated congenital syphilis. Some experts also suggest giving such patients penicillin G benzathine intramuscularly, in 3 weekly doses after the 10-day course of intravenous aqueous crystalline penicillin. If the patient has minimal clinical manifestations of disease, the CSF examination is normal, and the result of the VDRL test of CSF is negative, some experts would treat with 3 weekly doses of penicillin G benzathine.

Syphilis in Pregnancy. Regardless of the stage of pregnancy, patients should be treated with penicillin according to the dosage schedules appropriate for the stage of syphilis as recommended for nonpregnant patients. For penicillin-allergic patients, no proven alternative therapy has been established. A pregnant woman with a history of penicillin allergy should be treated with penicillin after desensitization. In some patients, skin testing may be helpful. Desensitization should be performed in consultation with a specialist and only in facilities in which emergency assistance is available.

Erythromycin, azithromycin, or any other nonpenicillin treatment of syphilis during pregnancy cannot be considered reliable to cure infection in the fetus. Tetracycline is not recommended for pregnant women because of potential adverse effects on the fetus.

Early Acquired Syphilis (Primary, Secondary, Early Latent Syphilis). A single intramuscular dose of penicillin G benzathine is the preferred treatment for children and adults (Table 101.3). All children should have a CSF examination before treatment to exclude a diagnosis of neurosyphilis. Evaluation of CSF in adolescents and adults is necessary only if clinical signs or symptoms of neurologic or ophthalmic

involvement are present. Neurosyphilis should be considered in the differential diagnosis of neurologic disease in HIV-infected people.

For nonpregnant patients who are allergic to penicillin, doxycycline or tetracycline should be given. Children younger than 8 years should not be given tetracycline or doxycycline unless the benefits of therapy are greater than the risks of dental staining. Drugs other than penicillin and tetracycline do not have proven efficacy in the treatment of syphilis. Clinical studies, along with biologic and pharmacologic considerations, suggest ceftriaxone should be effective for early-acquired syphilis. Because efficacy of ceftriaxone is not well documented, close follow-up is essential. Single-dose therapy with ceftriaxone is not effective. When follow-up cannot be ensured, especially for children younger than 8 years, consideration must be given to hospitalization and desensitization followed by administration of penicillin G.

Syphilis of More Than 1 Year's Duration (Except Neurosyphilis). Penicillin G benzathine should be given intramuscularly weekly for 3 successive weeks (Table 101.3). In patients who are allergic to penicillin, doxycycline or tetracycline for 4 weeks should be given only if a CSF examination has excluded neurosyphilis. Patients who have syphilis and who demonstrate any of the following criteria should have a prompt CSF examination:

- Neurologic or ophthalmic signs or symptoms
- Evidence of active tertiary syphilis (eg, aortitis, gumma)
- Treatment failure
- HIV infection with late latent syphilis or syphilis of unknown duration

If dictated by circumstances and patient preferences, a CSF examination may be performed for patients who do not meet these criteria. Some specialists recommend performing a CSF examination on all patients who have latent syphilis and a nontreponemal serologic test result of 1:32 or higher or, if the patient is HIV infected, a serum CD4+ T-lymphocyte count of 350 or lower. The risk of neurosyphilis in this circumstance is unknown. If a CSF examination is performed and the results indicate abnormalities consistent with neurosyphilis, the patient should be treated for neurosyphilis. Children younger than 8 years should not be given tetracycline or doxycycline unless the benefits of therapy are greater than the risks of dental staining. Performing a VDRL test of CSF, protein concentration test, and leukocyte cell count is mandatory for people with suspected neurosyphilis, people who have concurrent HIV infection, people who have failed treatment, and people receiving antimicrobial agents other than penicillin.

Neurosyphilis. The recommended regimen for adults is aqueous crystalline penicillin G, intravenously (Table 101.3). If adherence to therapy can be ensured, patients may be treated with an alternative regimen of intramuscular penicillin G procaine plus oral probenecid.

Other Considerations.
- Mothers of infants with congenital syphilis should be tested for other STIs, including gonorrhea and *Chlamydia trachomatis,* HIV, and hepatitis B virus infection. If injection drug use is suspected, the mother also may be at risk of hepatitis C virus infection.
- All recent sexual contacts of people with acquired syphilis should be evaluated for other STIs as well as syphilis.
- All patients with syphilis should be tested for other STIs, including HIV and hepatitis B virus infection. Patients who have primary syphilis should be retested for HIV after 3 months if the first HIV test result is negative.
- For HIV-infected patients with syphilis, careful follow-up is essential. Patients infected with HIV who have early syphilis may be at increased risk of neurologic complications and higher rates of treatment failure with currently recommended regimens.

Follow-up and Management.

Congenital syphilis. Treated infants should have careful follow-up evaluations during regularly scheduled visits at 1, 2, 4, 6, and 12 months of age. Serologic nontreponemal tests should be performed 2 to 4, 6, and 12 months after conclusion of treatment or until results become nonreactive or the titer has decreased 4-fold. Nontreponemal antibody titers should decrease by 3 months of age and should be nonreactive by 6 months of age if the infant was infected and adequately treated or was not infected and initially seropositive because of transplacentally acquired maternal antibody. The serologic response after therapy may be slower for infants treated after the neonatal period. Patients with increasing titers or with persistent stable titers 6 to 12 months after initial treatment should be evaluated, including a CSF examination, and treated with a 10-day course of parenteral penicillin G, even if they were treated previously.

Treated infants with congenital neurosyphilis and initially positive results of VDRL tests of CSF or abnormal or uninterpretable CSF cell counts and/or protein concentrations should undergo repeated clinical evaluation and CSF examination at 6-month intervals until their CSF examination is normal. A reactive result of VDRL testing of CSF at the 6-month interval is an indication for re-treatment. If white blood cell counts still are abnormal at 2 years or are not decreasing at each examination, re-treatment is indicated.

Acquired syphilis. Treated pregnant women with syphilis should have quantitative nontreponemal serologic tests repeated at 28 to 32 weeks of gestation, at delivery, and following the recommendations for the stage of disease. Serologic titers may be repeated monthly in women at high risk of reinfection or in geographic areas where the prevalence of syphilis is high. The clinical and antibody response should be appropriate for stage of disease. Most women will deliver before their serologic response to treatment can be assessed definitively. Therapy should not be judged inadequate if the maternal antibody titer has not decreased 4-fold by delivery. Inadequate maternal treatment is likely if delivery occurs within 30 days of therapy, if clinical signs of infection are present at delivery, or if the maternal antibody titer is 4-fold higher than the pretreatment titer.

Indications for Re-treatment.

Primary/secondary syphilis:

- If clinical signs or symptoms persist or recur or if a 4-fold increase in titer of a nontreponemal test occurs, evaluate CSF and HIV status and re-treat.
- If the nontreponemal titer fails to decrease 4-fold within 6 months after therapy, evaluate for HIV; re-treat unless follow-up for continued clinical and serologic assessment can be ensured. Some experts recommend CSF evaluation.

Latent syphilis: In the following situations, CSF examination should be performed and re-treatment should be provided:

- Titers increase 4-fold.
- An initially high titer (>1:32) fails to decrease at least 4-fold within 12 to 24 months.
- Signs or symptoms attributable to syphilis develop.

In these instances, re-treatment, when indicated, should be performed with 3 weekly injections of penicillin G benzathine, 2.4 million U, intramuscularly, unless CSF examination indicates that neurosyphilis is present, at which time treatment for neurosyphilis should be initiated. Re-treated patients should be treated with the schedules recommended for patients with syphilis for more than 1 year. In general, only 1 re-treatment course is indicated. The possibility of reinfection or concurrent HIV infection always should be considered when re-treating patients with early syphilis.

Patients with neurosyphilis must have periodic serologic testing, clinical evaluation at 6-month intervals, and repeated CSF examinations. If the CSF cell count has not decreased after 6 months or CSF is not entirely normal after 2 years, re-treatment should be considered. CSF abnormalities may persist for extended periods in HIV-infected people with neurosyphilis. Close follow-up is warranted.

Table 101.1

Guide for Interpretation of Syphilis Serologic Test Results of Mothers and Their Infants[1]

Nontreponemal Test Result (eg, VDRL, RPR, ART)		Treponemal Test Result (eg,TP-PA, FTA-ABS)		Interpretation[2]
Mother	Infant	Mother	Infant	
-	-	-	-	No syphilis or incubating syphilis in the mother or infant or prozone phenomenon
+	+	-	-	No syphilis in mother or infant (false-positive result of nontreponemal test with passive transfer to infant)
+	+ or -	+	+	Maternal syphilis with possible infant infection; mother treated for syphilis during pregnancy; or mother with latent syphilis and possible infant infection[3]
+	+	+	+	Recent or previous syphilis in the mother; possible infant infection
-	-	+	+	Mother successfully treated for syphilis before or early in pregnancy; or mother with Lyme disease (ie, false-positive serologic test result); infant syphilis unlikely

[1] VDRL indicates Venereal Disease Research Laboratory; RPR, rapid plasma reagin; ART, automated reagin test; TP-PA, *Treponema pallidum* particle agglutination test; FTA-ABS, fluorescent treponemal antibody absorption; +, reactive; -, nonreactive.

[2] Table presents a guide and not a definitive interpretation of serologic test results for syphilis in mothers and their newborn infants. Maternal history is the most important aspect for interpretation of test results. Factors that should be considered include timing of maternal infection, nature and timing of maternal treatment, quantitative maternal and infant titers, and serial determination of nontreponemal test titers in both mother and infant.

[3] Mothers with latent syphilis may have nonreactive nontreponemal test results.

Table 101.2

Recommended Treatment of Neonates (≤4 Weeks of Age) With Proven or Possible Congenital Syphilis[1]

Clinical Status	Evaluation	Antimicrobial Therapy[2]
Proven or highly probable disease[3]	CSF analysis for VDRL, cell count, and protein CBC and platelet count Other tests as clinically indicated (eg, long-bone radiography, liver function tests, ophthalmologic examination)	Aqueous crystalline penicillin G, 100 000–150 000 U/kg per day, administered as 50 000 U/kg per dose, IV, every 12 h during the first 7 days of life and every 8 h thereafter for a total of 10 days OR Penicillin G procaine,[4] 50 000 U/kg per day, IM, in a single dose for 10 days
Normal physical examination and serum quantitative nontreponemal titer the same or less than 4-fold the maternal titer		
(a) (i) Mother was not treated, inadequately treated, or has no documented treatment; (ii) mother was treated with erythromycin or other nonpenicillin regimen; (iii) mother received treatment ≤4 weeks before delivery	CSF analysis for VDRL, cell count, and protein CBC and platelet count Long-bone radiography	Aqueous crystalline penicillin G, IV, for 10 days[5] OR Penicillin G procaine,[4] 50 000 U/kg per day, IM, in a single dose for 10 days[5] OR Penicillin G benzathine,[4] 50 000 U/kg, IM, in a single dose[5]
(b) (i) Adequate maternal therapy given >4 wk before delivery; (ii) mother has no evidence of reinfection or relapse	None	Clinical, serologic follow-up, and penicillin G benzathine, 50 000 U/kg, IM, in a single dose[6]
(c) Adequate therapy before pregnancy and mother's nontreponemal serologic titer remained low and stable during pregnancy and at delivery	None	None[7]

[1] CSF indicates cerebrospinal fluid; VDRL, Venereal Disease Research Laboratory; CBC, complete blood cell; IV, intravenously; and IM, intramuscularly.

[2] If more than 1 day of therapy is missed, the entire course should be restarted.

[3] Abnormal physical examination, serum quantitative nontreponemal titer that is 4-fold greater than the mother's titer, or positive result of darkfield or fluorescent antibody test of body fluid(s).

[4] Penicillin G benzathine and penicillin G procaine are approved for IM administration only.

[5] A complete evaluation (CSF analysis, bone radiography, CBC) is not necessary if 10 days of parenteral therapy is administered but may be useful to support a diagnosis of congenital syphilis. If a single dose of penicillin G benzathine is used, then the infant must be evaluated fully, the full evaluation must be normal, and follow-up must be certain. If any part of the infant's evaluation is abnormal or not performed or if the CSF analysis is uninterpretable, the 10-day course of penicillin is required.

[6] Some experts would not treat the infant but would provide close serologic follow-up.

[7] Some experts would treat with penicillin G benzathine, 50 000 U/kg, as a single IM injection if follow-up is uncertain.

Table 101.3
Recommended Treatment for Syphilis in People >4 Weeks of Age[1]

	Children	Adults
Congenital syphilis	Aqueous crystalline penicillin G, 200 000–300 000 U/kg per day, IV, administered as 50 000 U/kg every 4–6 h for 10 days[2]	
Primary, secondary, and early latent syphilis[3]	Penicillin G benzathine,[4] 50 000 U/kg, IM, up to the adult dose of 2.4 million U in a single dose	Penicillin G benzathine, 2.4 million U, IM, in a single dose *OR* *If allergic to penicillin and not pregnant,* doxycycline, 100 mg, orally, twice a day for 14 days *OR* Tetracycline, 500 mg, orally, 4 times/day for 14 days
Late latent syphilis[5] or latent syphilis of unknown duration	Penicillin G benzathine, 50 000 U/kg, IM, up to the adult dose of 2.4 million U, administered as 3 single doses at 1-wk intervals (total 150 000 U/kg, up to the adult dose of 7.2 million U)	Penicillin G benzathine, 7.2 million U total, administered as 3 doses of 2.4 million U, IM, each at 1-wk intervals *OR* *If allergic to penicillin and not pregnant,* doxycycline, 100 mg, orally, twice a day for 4 wk *OR* Tetracycline, 500 mg, orally, 4 times/day for 4 wk
Tertiary		Penicillin G benzathine, 7.2 million U total, administered as 3 doses of 2.4 million U, IM, at 1-wk intervals *If allergic to penicillin and not pregnant, same as for late latent syphilis*
Neurosyphilis[6]	Aqueous crystalline penicillin G, 200 000 to 300 000 U/kg per day, given every 4–6 h for 10–14 days in doses not to exceed the adult dose	Aqueous crystalline penicillin G, 18–24 million U per day, administered as 3–4 million U, IV, every 4 h for 10–14 days[7] *OR* Penicillin G procaine,[3] 2.4 million U, IM, once daily **PLUS** probenecid, 500 mg, orally, 4 times/day, both for 10–14 days[7]

[1] IV, indicates intravenously; IM, intramuscularly.

[2] If the patient has no clinical manifestations of disease, the cerebrospinal fluid (CSF) examination is normal, and the CSF VDRL result is negative, some experts would treat with up to 3 weekly doses of penicillin G benzathine, 50 000 U/kg, IM. Some experts also suggest giving these patients a single dose of penicillin G benzathine, 50 000 U/kg, IM, after the 10-day course of IV aqueous penicillin.

[3] Early latent syphilis is defined as being acquired within the preceding year.

[4] Penicillin G benzathine and penicillin G procaine are approved for IM administration only.

[5] Late latent syphilis is defined as syphilis beyond 1 year's duration.

[6] Patients who are allergic to penicillin should be desensitized.

[7] Some experts administer penicillin G benzathine, 2.4 million U, IM, once per week for up to 3 weeks after completion of these neurosyphilis treatment regimens.

Image 101.1

An electron photomicrograph of 2 spiral-shaped *Treponema pallidum* bacteria (36 000x).

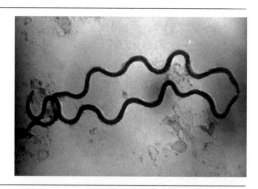

Image 101.2

Cutaneous syphilis in a 6-month-old infant.

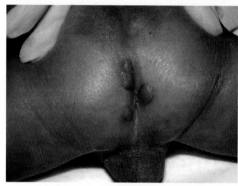

Image 101.3

Newborn with congenital syphilis. Note the marked generalized desquamation.

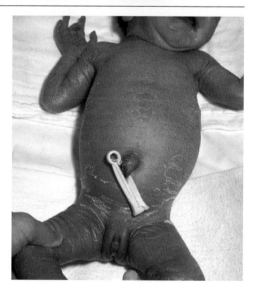

Image 101.4
The face of a newborn infant with congenital syphilis displaying striking mucous membrane involvement.

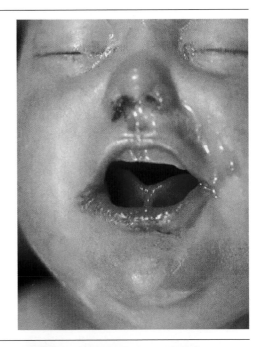

Image 101.5
Congenital syphilis in a 2-week-old infant boy with marked hepatosplenomegaly. The infant kept his upper extremities in a flail-like position because of painful periostitis.

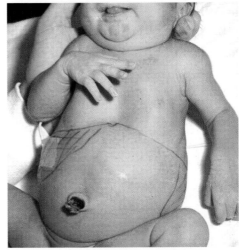

Image 101.6
Newborn with congenital syphilis with bleeding from the nares and tender swelling of the wrists and elbows secondary to luetic periostitis.

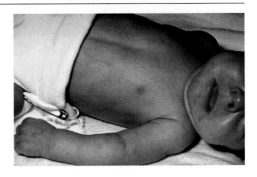

Image 101.7
Congenital syphilis with a pathologic fracture
of the proximal humerus and the distal femur.

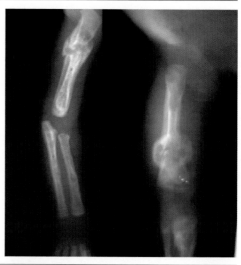

Image 101.8
Congenital syphilis with pneumonia alba.
The infant survived with penicillin treatment.

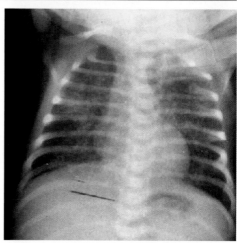

Image 101.9
Congenital syphilis with desquamation over
the hand.

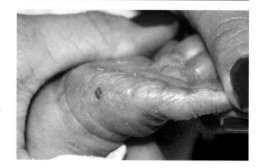

Image 101.10
Hutchinson teeth, a late manifestation of
congenital syphilis. Changes occur in secondary
dentition. The central incisors are smaller than
normal and have sloping sides.

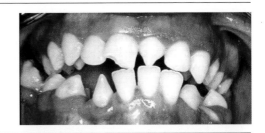

Image 101.11
A 4-year-old child with diaphyseal cortical
thickening secondary to congenital syphilis
(a late finding).

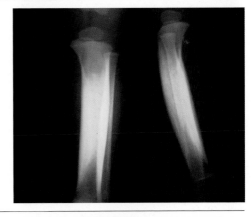

Image 101.12
Syphilis with penile chancre.

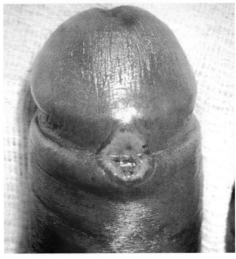

Image 101.13
Condylomata lata in a 7-year-old girl who was sexually abused. These moist lesions are whitish gray, are caused by *Treponema pallidum,* and are highly contagious.

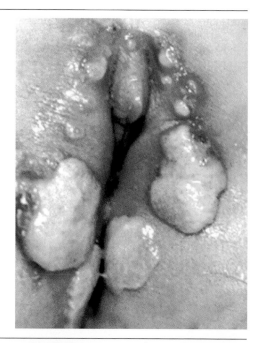

Image 101.14
This photograph depicts the presence of a diffuse stromal haze in the cornea of a female patient, known as interstitial keratitis (IK), which was due to her late-stage congenital syphilitic condition. IK, which is an inflammation of the cornea's connective tissue elements and usually affects both eyes, can occur as a complication brought on by congenital or acquired syphilis. IK usually occurs in children older than 2 years.

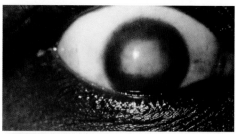

Image 101.15
A 16-year-old girl with the rash of secondary syphilis noticed at 3 months' gestation of her pregnancy. The signs and symptoms of secondary syphilis generally occur 6 to 8 weeks after the primary infection, when primary lesions have healed.

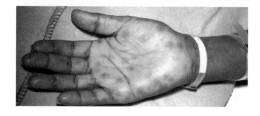

Image 101.16

This patient presented with a papular rash on the sole of the foot due to secondary syphilis. The second stage of syphilis starts when one or more areas of the skin break into a rash that appears as rough, red, or reddish brown spots both on the palms of hands and on the bottoms of feet. Even without treatment, the rash resolves spontaneously.

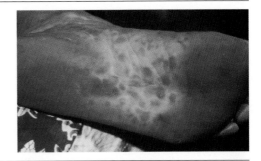

Image 101.17

This image depicts a lingual mucous patch on the tongue of a patient who was subsequently diagnosed with secondary syphilis. Secondary syphilis is the most contagious of all the stages of this disease and is characterized by a systemic spread of *Treponema pallidum* bacterial spirochetes. Skin rash and mucous membrane lesions characterize the secondary stage.

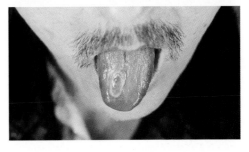

102

Tapeworm Diseases
(Taeniasis and Cysticercosis)

Clinical Manifestations

Taeniasis. Infection often is asymptomatic; however, mild gastrointestinal tract symptoms, such as nausea, diarrhea, and pain, can occur. Tapeworm segments can be seen migrating from the anus or feces.

Cysticercosis. Manifestations depend on the location and numbers of pork tapeworm cysts (cysticerci) and the host response. Cysts can be found anywhere in the body. The most common and serious manifestations are caused by cysts in the CNS. Cysts of *Taenia solium* in the brain (neurocysticercosis) can cause seizures, behavioral disturbances, obstructive hydrocephalus, and other neurologic signs and symptoms. In some countries, neurocysticercosis is a leading cause of epilepsy. The host reaction to degenerating cysts can produce signs and symptoms of meningitis. Cysts in the spinal column can cause gait disturbance, pain, or transverse myelitis. Subcutaneous cysts produce palpable nodules, and ocular involvement can cause visual impairment.

Etiology

Taeniasis is caused by intestinal infection by the adult tapeworm: *Taenia saginata* (beef tapeworm) or *T solium* (pork tapeworm). *Taenia asiatica* causes taeniasis in Asia. Human cysticercosis is caused only by the larvae of *T solium (Cysticercus cellulosae).*

Epidemiology

These tapeworm diseases have worldwide distribution. Prevalence is high in areas with poor sanitation and human fecal contamination in areas where cattle graze or swine are fed. Most cases of *T solium* infection in the United States are imported from Latin America or Asia. High rates of *T saginata* infection occur in Mexico, parts of South America, East Africa, and central Europe. *T asiatica* is common in China, Taiwan, and Southeast Asia. Taeniasis is acquired by eating undercooked beef *(T saginata)* or pork *(T solium). T asiatica* is acquired by eating viscera of infected pigs that contain encysted larvae. Infection often is asymptomatic.

Cysticercosis in humans is acquired by ingesting eggs of the pork tapeworm *(T solium),* through fecal-oral contact with a person harboring the adult tapeworm, or by autoinfection. The eggs are found only in human feces because humans are the obligate definitive host. The eggs liberate oncospheres in the intestine that migrate through the blood and lymphatics to tissues throughout the body, including the CNS, where cysts form. Although most cases of cysticercosis in the United States have been imported, cysticercosis can be acquired in the United States from tapeworm carriers who emigrated from an area with endemic infection and still have *T solium* intestinal stage infection.

Incubation Period

Taeniasis, 2 to 3 months; cysticercosis, several years.

Diagnosis

Diagnosis of taeniasis (adult tapeworm infection) is based on demonstration of the proglottids or ova in feces or the perianal region. However, these techniques are insensitive. Species identification of the parasite is based on the different structures of the terminal gravid segments. Diagnosis of neurocysticercosis is made primarily on the basis of CT scanning or MRI of the brain or spinal cord. Antibody assays that detect specific antibody to larval *T solium* in serum and CSF are the antibody tests of choice. In the United States, this test is available through the CDC and several commercial laboratories. The test is more sensitive with serum specimens than with CSF specimens. Serum antibody assay results often are negative in children with solitary parenchymal lesions but usually are positive in patients with multiple lesions.

Treatment

Taeniasis. Praziquantel is highly effective for eradicating infection with the adult tapeworm, and niclosamide and nitazoxanide are alternatives.

Cysticercosis. Neurocysticercosis treatment should be individualized on the basis of the number and viability of cysticerci as assessed by neuroimaging studies (MRI or CT scan) and where they are located. For patients with only nonviable cysts (eg, only calcifications on CT scan), management should be aimed at symptoms and should include anticonvulsants for patients with seizures and insertion of shunts for patients with hydrocephalus. Two antiparasitic drugs, albendazole and praziquantel, are available. Although both drugs are cysticercidal and hasten radiologic resolution of cysts, most symptoms result from the host inflammatory response and can be exacerbated by treatment. Most experts recommend therapy for patients with non-enhancing or multiple cysticerci. Coadministration of corticosteroids for the first 2 to 3 days of therapy may decrease adverse effects. Arachnoiditis, vasculitis, or diffuse cerebral edema (cysticercal encephalitis) is treated with corticosteroid therapy, until cerebral edema is controlled, and albendazole or praziquantel.

Seizures may recur for months or years. Anticonvulsant therapy is recommended until there is neuroradiologic evidence of resolution and seizures have not occurred for 1 to 2 years. Calcification of cysts may require indefinite use of anticonvulsants. Intraventricular cysts and hydrocephalus usually require surgical therapy. Intraventricular cysts often can be removed by endoscopic surgery, which is the treatment of choice. If cysts cannot be removed easily, hydrocephalus should be corrected with placement of intraventricular shunts. Ocular cysticercosis is treated by surgical excision of the cysts. Ocular and spinal cysts generally are not treated with anthelmintic drugs. An ophthalmic examination should be performed before treatment to rule out intraocular cysts.

Image 102.1
Taenia saginata ova (high-power magnification).

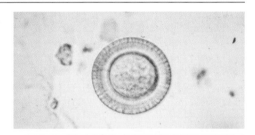

Image 102.2
Taenia solium. Gravid proglottid.

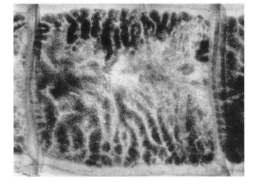

Image 102.3

Neurocysticercosis on CT scan of brain (*Taenia solium,* pork tapeworm).

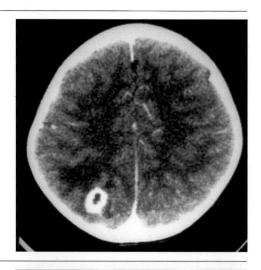

Image 102.4

Cerebral neurocysticercosis with diffuse, scattered, ring-enhancing lesions throughout the brain parenchyma with focal edema.

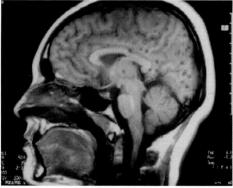

103

Other Tapeworm Infections
(Including Hydatid Disease)

Clinical Manifestations

Most infections are asymptomatic, but nausea, abdominal pain, and diarrhea have been observed in people who are heavily infected.

Hymenolepis nana. This tapeworm, also called dwarf tapeworm because it is the smallest of the adult tapeworms, has its entire cycle within humans. Direct person-to-person transmission is possible. More problematic is autoinfection, which tends to perpetuate infection in the host because eggs can hatch within the intestine and reinitiate the cycle, leading to development of new worms and a large worm burden. If infection persists after treatment, re-treatment with praziquantel is indicated. Nitazoxanide is an alternative drug.

Dipylidium caninum. This tapeworm is the most common and widespread adult tapeworm of dogs and cats. *D caninum* infects children when they inadvertently swallow a dog or cat flea, which serves as the intermediate host. Diagnosis is made by finding the characteristic eggs or motile proglottids in stool. Proglottids resemble rice kernels. Therapy with praziquantel is effective. Niclosamide is an alternative therapeutic option.

Diphyllobothrium latum *(and related species).* This tapeworm, also called fish tapeworm, has fish as one of its intermediate hosts. Consumption of infected, raw freshwater fish (including salmon) leads to infection. Three to 5 weeks are needed for the adult tapeworm to mature and begin to lay eggs. The worm sometimes causes mechanical obstruction of the bowel or diarrhea, abdominal pain or, rarely, megaloblastic anemia secondary to vitamin B12 deficiency. Diagnosis is made by recognition of the characteristic eggs or proglottids passed in stool. Therapy with praziquantel is effective; niclosamide is an alternative.

Echinococcus granulosus *and* Echinococcus multilocularis. The larval forms of these tapeworms are the causes of hydatid disease. The distribution of *E granulosus* is related to sheep or cattle herding. Areas of high prevalence include parts of South America, East Africa, eastern Europe, the Middle East, the Mediterranean region, China, and central Asia. Disease also is endemic in Australia and New Zealand. In the United States, small foci of endemic infection exist in Arizona, California, New Mexico, and Utah, and a strain adapted to wolves, moose, and caribou occurs in Alaska and Canada. Dogs, coyotes, wolves, dingoes, and jackals can become infected by swallowing protoscolices of the parasite within hydatid cysts in the organs of sheep or other intermediate hosts. Dogs pass embryonated eggs in their stools, and sheep become infected by swallowing the eggs. If humans swallow *Echinococcus* eggs, they can become inadvertent intermediate hosts, and cysts can develop in various organs, such as the liver, lungs, kidney, and spleen. These cysts usually grow slowly (1 cm in diameter per year) and eventually can contain several liters of fluid. If a cyst ruptures, anaphylaxis and multiple secondary cysts from seeding of protoscolices can result. Clinical diagnosis often is difficult. A history of contact with dogs in an area with endemic infection is helpful. Cystic lesions can be demonstrated by radiography, ultrasonography, or CT of various organs. Serologic tests, available at the CDC, are helpful, but false-negative results occur. In uncomplicated cases, the treatment of choice is percutaneous aspiration, infusion of scolicidal agents, and re-aspiration (PAIR). This should be performed at least a few days after initiation of albendazole chemotherapy. Contraindications to PAIR include communication of the cyst with the biliary tract (eg, bile staining after initial aspiration), superficial cysts, and heavily septated cysts. Surgical therapy is indicated for complicated cases and requires meticulous care to prevent spillage. Surgical drapes should be soaked in hypertonic saline. In general, the cyst should be removed intact because leakage of contents is associated with a higher rate of complications. Treatment with albendazole generally should be initiated days to weeks before surgery and continued for several months afterward.

E multilocularis, a species whose life cycle involves foxes, dogs, and rodents, causes the alveolar form of hydatid disease, which is characterized by invasive growth of the larvae in the liver with occasional metastatic spread. The alveolar form of hydatid disease is limited to the northern hemisphere and usually is diagnosed in people 50 years of age or older. The preferred treatment is surgical removal of the entire larval mass. In nonresectable cases, continuous treatment with albendazole has been associated with clinical improvement.

Image 103.1

Proglottids of *Dipylidium caninum.* Such proglottids (average mature size 12 mm x 3 mm) have 2 genital pores, one in the middle of each lateral margin. Proglottids may be passed singly or in chains, and occasionally may be seen dangling from the anus. They are pumpkin seed–shaped when passed and often resemble rice grains when dried. The genital pores are clearly visible in the carmine-stained proglottid shown in A. The proglottid shown in B (size 15 mm x 3 mm, preserved in formalin) was passed by a 9-month-old boy in the state of Oregon.

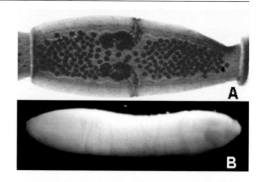

Image 103.2

Fluid-filled echinococcus cyst in the lung of an adolescent male.

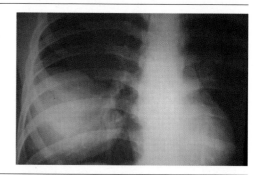

Image 103.3

Hydatid sand. Fluid aspirated from a hydatid cyst will show multiple protoscolices (size approximately 100 µm), each of which has typical hooklets. The protoscolices are normally invaginated (left), and evaginate (middle, then right) when put in saline.

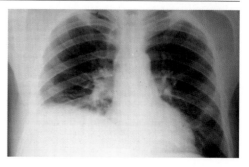

Image 103.4

Echinococcus cyst in the right lower lobe of the liver in a 27-year-old male. Note the striking elevation of the right hemidiaphragm.

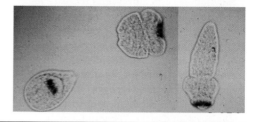

104

Tetanus
(Lockjaw)

Clinical Manifestations

Generalized tetanus (lockjaw) is a neurologic disease manifesting as trismus and severe muscular spasms. Tetanus is caused by neurotoxin produced by the anaerobic bacterium *Clostridium tetani* in a contaminated wound. Onset is gradual, occurring over 1 to 7 days, and symptoms progress to severe generalized muscle spasms, which often are aggravated by any external stimulus. Severe spasms persist for 1 week or more and subside over several weeks in people who recover.

Localized tetanus manifests as local muscle spasms in areas contiguous to a wound. Cephalic tetanus is a dysfunction of cranial nerves associated with infected wounds on the head and neck. Both conditions can precede generalized tetanus.

Etiology

C tetani is a spore-forming, anaerobic, gram-positive bacillus. This organism is a wound contaminant that causes neither tissue destruction nor an inflammatory response. The vegetative form of *C tetani* produces a potent plasmid-encoded exotoxin (tetanospasmin), which binds to gangliosides at the myoneural junction of skeletal muscle and on neuronal membranes in the spinal cord, blocking inhibitory pulses to motor neurons.

Epidemiology

Tetanus occurs worldwide and is more common in warmer climates and during warmer months, in part because of the higher frequency of contaminated wounds associated with those locations and seasons. The organism, a normal inhabitant of soil and animal and human intestines, is ubiquitous in the environment, especially where contamination by excreta is common. Wounds, recognized or unrecognized, are the sites at which the organism multiplies and elaborates toxin. Contaminated wounds, especially wounds with devitalized tissue and deep-puncture trauma, are at greatest risk. Neonatal tetanus is common in many developing countries where women are not immunized appropriately against tetanus and nonsterile umbilical cord care practices are followed. Widespread active immunization against tetanus has modified the epidemiology of disease in the United States, where 40 or fewer cases have been reported annually since 1999. Tetanus is not transmissible from person to person.

Incubation Period

Usually within 5 to 14 days (range, 2 days to months).

Diagnostic Tests

The diagnosis of tetanus is made clinically by excluding other causes of tetanic spasms, such as hypocalcemic tetany, phenothiazine reaction, strychnine poisoning, and hysteria. Attempts to culture *C tetani* are associated with poor yield, and a negative culture does not exclude the diagnosis.

Treatment

- Human tetanus immune globulin (TIG) given in a single dose intramuscularly is recommended. Infiltration of part of the dose locally around the wound is recommended, although the efficacy of this approach has not been proven.
- In countries where TIG is not available, equine tetanus antitoxin may be available. Equine antitoxin is administered after appropriate testing for sensitivity and desensitization if necessary.
- IGIV contains antibodies to tetanus and can be considered for treatment in a dose of 200 to 400 mg/kg if TIG is not available.
- All wounds should be cleaned and debrided properly, especially if extensive necrosis is present. In neonatal tetanus, wide excision of the umbilical stump is not indicated.
- Supportive care and pharmacotherapy to control tetanic spasms are of major importance.
- Oral (or intravenous) metronidazole is effective in decreasing the number of vegetative forms of *C tetani* and is the antimicrobial agent of choice. Parenteral penicillin G is an alternative treatment.

Image 104.1

This infant with tetanus has spasm of the facial muscles with trismus.

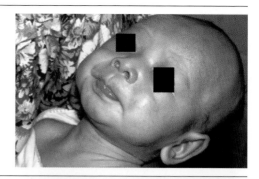

Image 104.2

Severe muscular spasms with trismus in an infant who acquired neonatal tetanus from contamination of the umbilical stump.

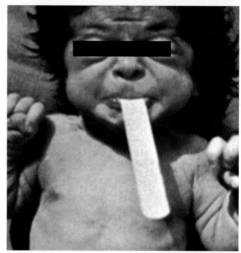

Image 104.3

Face of infant with neonatal tetanus with risus sardonicus.

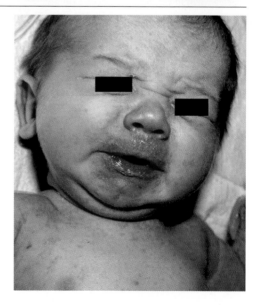

Image 104.4

This patient has opisthotonos secondary to severe tetanus, in which the head and heels are bent backward and the body is bowed forward.

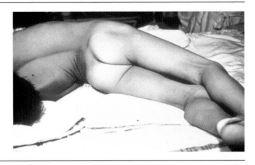

Image 104.5

This neonate is displaying body rigidity produced by *Clostridium tetani* exotoxin.

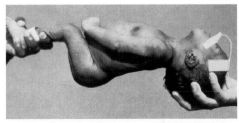

Image 104.6

A preschool-aged boy with tetanus with severe muscle generalized contractions caused by tetanospasmin action in the CNS.

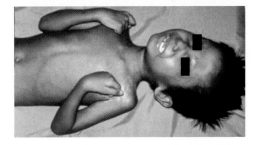

105

Tinea Capitis
(Ringworm of the Scalp)

Clinical Manifestations

Fungal infection of the scalp manifests as one of the following distinct clinical syndromes:
- Patchy areas of dandruff-like scaling, with subtle or extensive hair loss, which easily is confused with dandruff, seborrheic dermatitis, or atopic dermatitis
- Discrete areas of hair loss studded by stubs of broken hairs, which is referred to as *black-dot ringworm*
- Numerous discrete pustules or excoriations with little hair loss or scaling
- Kerion, a boggy inflammatory mass surrounded by follicular pustules, which is a hypersensitivity reaction to the fungal infection (can be accompanied by fever and local lymphadenopathy and commonly is misdiagnosed as impetigo, cellulitis, or an abscess of the scalp)

A pruritic, fine, papulovesicular eruption (dermatophytid or id reaction) involving the trunk, hands, or face, caused by a hypersensitivity response to the infecting fungus, can accompany scalp lesions.

Tinea capitis may be confused with many other diseases, including seborrheic dermatitis, atopic dermatitis, psoriasis, alopecia areata, trichotillomania, folliculitis, impetigo, and lupus erythematosus.

Etiology

Trichophyton tonsurans is the cause of tinea capitis in more than 90% of cases in North and Central America. *Microsporum canis, Microsporum audouinii,* and *Trichophyton mentagrophytes* are less common. The causative agents vary in different geographic areas.

Epidemiology

Infection of the scalp with *T tonsurans* results from person-to-person transmission. Although the organism remains viable on combs, hairbrushes, and other fomites for long periods, the role of fomites in transmission has not been defined. Occasionally, *T tonsurans* is cultured from the scalp of asymptomatic children or family members of an index case. Asymptomatic carriers are thought to have a significant role as reservoirs for infection and reinfection within families, schools, and communities. Tinea capitis attributable to *T tonsurans* occurs most commonly in children between the ages of 3 and 9 years and seems to be more common in African American children.

M canis infection results from animal-to-human transmission. Infection often is the result of contact with household pets.

Incubation Period

Unknown.

Diagnostic Tests

Potassium hydroxide wet mount, cultures, and/or Wood light examination may be used to confirm the diagnosis before treatment. Hairs obtained by gentle scraping of a moistened area of the scalp with a blunt scalpel, toothbrush, tweezers, or a moistened cotton swab are used for potassium hydroxide wet mount examination and culture. In black-dot ringworm, broken hairs should be obtained for diagnosis. In cases of *T tonsurans* infection, microscopic examination of a potassium hydroxide wet mount preparation will disclose numerous arthroconidia within the hair shaft. In *Microsporum* infection, spores surround the hair shaft. Use of dermatophyte test medium also is a reliable, simple, and inexpensive method of diagnosing tinea capitis. Skin scrapings, brushings, or hairs from lesions are inoculated directly onto culture medium and incubated at room temperature. After 1 to 2 weeks, a phenol red indicator in the agar will turn from yellow to red in the area surrounding a dermatophyte colony. When necessary, the diagnosis also may be confirmed by culture on Sabouraud dextrose agar by direct plating technique, moistened cotton-tipped applicators, or Culturettes transported to reference laboratories.

Examination of hair of patients with *Microsporum* infection using Wood light results in brilliant green fluorescence. However, because *T tonsurans* does not fluoresce under Wood light, this diagnostic test is not helpful for most patients with tinea capitis.

Treatment

Because topical antifungal medications are not effective for treatment of tinea capitis, systemic antifungal therapy is required. Micro-size or ultramicrosize griseofulvin is given orally once daily. Optimally, griseofulvin is given after a meal containing fat (eg, peanut butter or ice cream). Griseofulvin is approved for children older than 2 years. Terbinafine has been shown to be as effective as a course of griseofulvin for treatment of *Trichophyton* infection but may not be as effective against *Microsporum* species. Terbinafine is not approved by the FDA for this condition.

Treatment with oral itraconazole or flucon-azole may be effective for tinea capitis, but these products have not been approved by the FDA for this indication. In addition, itra-conazole and terbinafine are not approved for use in children. Selenium sulfide shampoo, either 1% or 2.5%, decreases fungal shedding and may help curb the spread of infection.

Kerion is treated with griseofulvin. Cortico-steroid therapy consisting of prednisone or prednisolone may be used in addition. Anti-bacterial agents generally are not needed, except if there is suspected secondary infec-tion. Surgery is not indicated.

Image 105.1
Tinea capitis can cause hair loss. Remnants of infected hairs (black dots) that have broken at the scalp line may be noted within areas of alopecia.

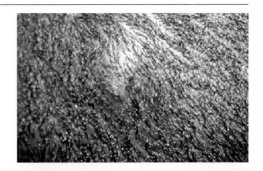

Image 105.2
Three-year-old male with a *Tinea* lesion on the occiput for 1 month. The mother had been applying a topical antifungal agent but the lesion became progressively larger. The patient was treated successfully with griseofulvin.

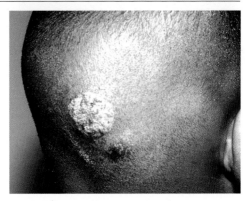

Image 105.3
An 8-year-old boy with a bald spot, hair loss, and enlarging posterior cervical lymph node for 2 weeks. The node was described as tender, not fluctuant, and without erythema of the overlying scalp. The area of hair loss was boggy and fluctuant. The patient responded well to treatment with griseofulvin.

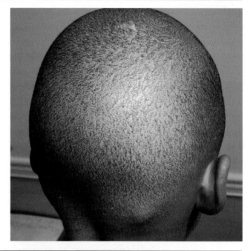

Image 105.4
Tinea capitis in the hairline of an 8-year-old boy.

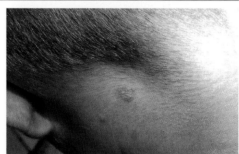

Image 105.5
A 2½-year-old boy with a kerion secondary to chronic, progressive tinea capitis.

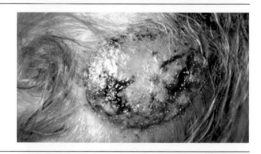

Image 105.6
Tinea capitis, close-up *(Microsporum audouinii)*.

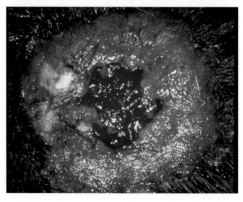

106

Tinea Corporis
(Ringworm of the Body)

Clinical Manifestations

Superficial tinea infections of the nonhairy (glabrous) skin can involve the face, trunk, or limbs but not the scalp, beard, groin, hands, or feet. The lesion generally is circular (hence the term "ringworm"), slightly erythematous, and well demarcated with a scaly, vesicular, or pustular border. Pruritus is common. Lesions often are mistaken for atopic, seborrheic, or contact dermatitis. A frequent source of confusion is an alteration in the appearance of lesions as a result of application of a topical corticosteroid preparation, termed *tinea incognito*. In patients with diminished T-lymphocyte function (eg, HIV infection), the rash may appear as grouped papules or pustules unaccompanied by scaling or erythema.

A pruritic, fine, papulovesicular eruption (dermatophytic or id reaction) involving the trunk, hands, or face, caused by a hypersensitivity response to infecting fungus, may accompany the rash.

Etiology

The primary causes of tinea corporis are fungi of the genus *Trichophyton,* especially *Trichophyton rubrum, Trichophyton mentagrophytes,* and *Trichophyton tonsurans;* the genus *Microsporum,* especially *Microsporum canis;* and *Epidermophyton floccosum.*

Epidemiology

These causative fungi occur worldwide and are transmissible by direct contact with infected humans, animals, or fomites. Fungi in lesions are communicable.

Incubation Period

Unknown.

Diagnosis

The fungi responsible for tinea corporis can be detected by microscopic examination of a potassium hydroxide wet mount of skin scrapings. Use of dermatophyte test medium also is a reliable, simple, and inexpensive method of diagnosis. Skin scrapings from lesions are inoculated directly onto culture medium and incubated at room temperature. After 1 to 2 weeks, a phenol red indicator in the agar will turn from yellow to red in the area surrounding a dermatophyte colony. When necessary, the diagnosis also can be confirmed by culture on Sabouraud dextrose agar.

Treatment

Topical application of a miconazole, clotrimazole, terbinafine, tolnaftate, naftifine, or ciclopirox preparation twice a day or of a ketoconazole, econazole, oxiconazole, butenafine, or sulconazole preparation once a day is recommended. Topical preparations of antifungal medication mixed with high-potency corticosteroids should not be used because of the potential for local and systemic adverse events.

If lesions are extensive or unresponsive to topical therapy, griseofulvin is administered orally. Oral itraconazole, fluconazole, and terbinafine may be effective alternative therapies for tinea corporis, but these products are not approved by the FDA for this indication.

Image 106.1
This is the bottom or "reverse" view of a Sabouraud dextrose plate culture growing the fungus *Microsporum persicolor.*

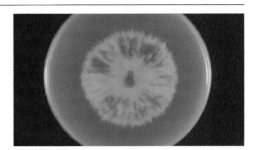

Image 106.2
Generalized tinea corporis in a 5-year-old female.

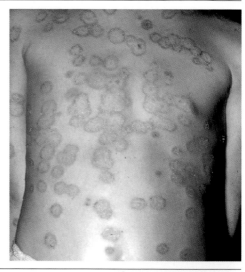

Image 106.3
Tinea corporis of the face. These annular
erythematous lesions have a scaly center.

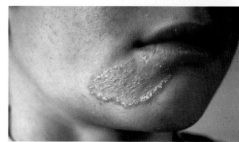

Image 106.4
Tinea corporis of the arm. This 6-year-old girl
had an enlarging skin lesion of 1-week duration.

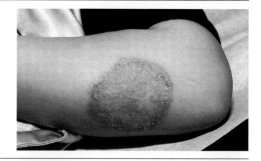

Image 106.5
Tinea corporis of the chin on a 6-year-old girl,
with enlarging lesions. The patient was successfully treated with clotrimazole.

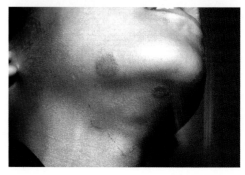

107

Tinea Cruris

(Jock Itch)

Clinical Manifestations

Tinea cruris is a common superficial fungal disorder of the groin and upper thighs. The eruption is marginated sharply and usually is bilaterally symmetric. Involved skin is erythematous and scaly and varies from red to brown; occasionally, the eruption is accompanied by central clearing and a vesiculopapular border. In chronic infections, the margin can be subtle and lichenification can be present. Tinea cruris skin lesions can be extremely pruritic. These lesions should be differentiated from intertrigo, seborrheic dermatitis, psoriasis, primary irritant dermatitis, allergic contact dermatitis (generally caused by the therapeutic agents applied to the area), or erythrasma, which is a superficial bacterial infection of the skin caused by *Corynebacterium minutissimum.*

Etiology

The fungi *Epidermophyton floccosum, Trichophyton rubrum,* and *Trichophyton mentagrophytes* are the most common causes.

Epidemiology

Tinea cruris occurs predominantly in adolescent and adult males, mainly via indirect contact from desquamated epithelium or hair. Moisture, close-fitting garments, friction, and obesity are predisposing factors. Direct or indirect person-to-person transmission can occur. This infection commonly occurs in association with tinea pedis.

Incubation Period

Unknown.

Diagnostic Tests

The fungi responsible for tinea cruris can be detected by microscopic examination of a potassium hydroxide wet mount of scales. Use of dermatophyte test medium also is a reliable, simple, and inexpensive method of diagnosing tinea cruris. Skin scrapings from lesions are inoculated directly onto culture medium and incubated at room temperature. After 1 to 2 weeks, a phenol red indicator in the agar will turn from yellow to red in the area surrounding a dermatophyte colony. When necessary, the diagnosis also can be confirmed by culture on Sabouraud dextrose agar. A characteristic coral-red fluorescence under Wood light can identify the presence of erythrasma and, thus, exclude tinea cruris.

Treatment

Twice-daily topical application of a clotrimazole, miconazole, terbinafine, tolnaftate, or ciclopirox preparation rubbed or sprayed onto the affected areas and surrounding skin is effective. Once-daily therapy with topical econazole, ketoconazole, naftifine, oxiconazole, butenafine, or sulconazole preparation also is effective.

Topical preparations of antifungal medication mixed with high-potency corticosteroids should be avoided because of the potential for local and systemic adverse events. Loose-fitting, washed, cotton underclothes to decrease chafing as well as the use of a bland absorbent powder can be helpful adjuvants to therapy. Griseofulvin, given orally, may be effective in unresponsive cases. Oral itraconazole, fluconazole, or terbinafine may be effective alternative therapies. Because many conditions mimic tinea cruris, a differential diagnosis should be considered if primary treatments fail.

Image 107.1
Symmetric, confluent, annular, scaly red, and hyperpigmented plaques. This 10-year-old girl developed a chronic itchy eruption on the groin that spread to the anterior thighs. A potassium hydroxide preparation showed hyphae, and she was treated successfully with topical antifungal cream.

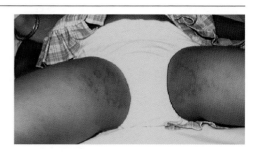

108

Tinea Pedis and Tinea Unguium

(Athlete's Foot, Ringworm of the Feet)

Clinical Manifestations

Tinea pedis manifests as fine vesiculopustular or scaly lesions that commonly are pruritic. The lesions can involve all areas of the foot, but usually lesions are patchy in distribution, with a predisposition to fissures and scaling between toes, particularly in the third and fourth interdigital spaces. Toenails can be infected and can be dystrophic (tinea unguium). Tinea pedis must be differentiated from dyshidrotic eczema, atopic dermatitis, contact dermatitis, juvenile plantar dermatosis, and erythrasma (a superficial bacterial infection caused by *Corynebacterium minutissimum*). Tinea pedis commonly occurs in association with tinea cruris.

Tinea pedis and many other fungal infections can be accompanied by a hypersensitivity reaction to the fungi (the dermatophytid or id reaction), with resulting vesicular eruptions on the palms and the sides of fingers and, occasionally, by an erythematous vesicular eruption on the extremities and trunk.

Etiology

The fungi *Trichophyton rubrum, Trichophyton mentagrophytes,* and *Epidermophyton floccosum* are the most common causes.

Epidemiology

Tinea pedis is a common infection worldwide in adolescents and adults but is relatively uncommon in young children. The fungi are acquired by contact with skin scales containing fungi or with fungi in damp areas, such as swimming pools, locker rooms, and shower rooms. Tinea pedis can spread throughout the household among family members and is communicable for as long as infection is present.

Incubation Period

Unknown.

Diagnosis

Tinea pedis usually is diagnosed by clinical manifestations and can be confirmed by microscopic examination of a potassium hydroxide wet mount of the cutaneous scrapings. Use of dermatophyte test medium is a reliable, simple, and inexpensive method of diagnosis in complicated or unresponsive cases. Skin scrapings are inoculated directly onto the culture medium and incubated at room temperature. After 1 to 2 weeks, a phenol red indicator in the agar will turn from yellow to red in the area surrounding a dermatophyte colony. When necessary, the diagnosis also can be confirmed by culture on Sabouraud dextrose agar. Infection of the nail can be verified by direct microscopic examination and fungal culture of desquamated subungual material.

Treatment

Topical application of terbinafine, or an azole agent (clotrimazole, miconazole, econazole) usually is adequate for milder cases. Fluconazole administered orally once per week can be an effective alternative therapy, but fluconazole has not been approved for this use. Acute vesicular lesions may be treated with intermittent use of open wet compresses (eg, with Burrow solution, 1:80). Tinea cruris, if present, should be treated concurrently.

Tinea pedis that is severe, chronic, or refractory to topical treatment may be treated with oral griseofulvin. Oral itraconazole or terbinafine may be effective alternative therapies for tinea pedis unresponsive to topical therapy. Id (hypersensitivity response) reactions are treated by wet compresses, topical corticosteroids, occasionally systemic corticosteroids, and eradication of the primary source of infection.

Recurrence is prevented by proper foot hygiene, which includes keeping the feet dry and cool, gentle cleaning, drying between the toes, use of absorbent antifungal foot powder, frequent airing of affected areas, and avoidance of occlusive footwear and nylon socks or other fabrics that interfere with dissipation of moisture.

In the past, most nail infections (tinea unguium), particularly toenail infections, have been highly resistant to oral griseofulvin therapy. Recurrences are common. Removal of the nail plate followed by use of oral therapy during the period of regrowth can help to effect a cure in resistant cases.

Image 108.1
This patient had ringworm or tinea pedis of the toes (also known as athlete's foot) when first examined. Tinea pedis is a fungal infection of the feet, principally involving the toe webs and soles. Athlete's foot can be caused by the fungi *Epidermophyton floccosum* or by numerous members of the *Trichophyton* genus.

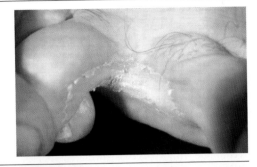

Image 108.2
Tinea pedis and tinea unguium.

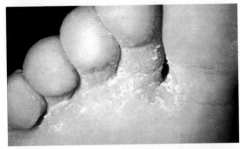

Image 108.3
Tinea pedis and tinea unguium.

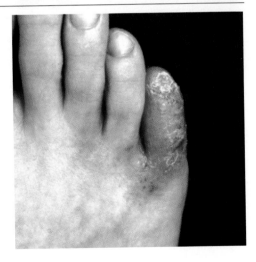

109

Toxic Shock Syndrome

Clinical Manifestations

Toxic shock syndrome (TSS) is caused by toxin-producing *Staphylococcus aureus* or *Streptococcus pyogenes* (group A streptococci). TSS is an acute illness characterized by fever, generalized erythroderma, rapid-onset hypotension, and symptoms of multisystem organ involvement that can include profuse watery diarrhea, vomiting, conjunctival injection, and severe myalgias (Tables 109.1 and 109.2). Evidence of local soft tissue infection (eg, cellulitis, abscess, myositis, or necrotizing fasciitis) associated with severe increasing pain is common with *S pyogenes*–mediated TSS. *S aureus*–mediated TSS commonly occurs in menstruating females using tampons but also occurs in males and females with focal *S aureus* infection (eg, abscess, sinusitis). Both forms of TSS can occur without a readily identifiable focus of infection. Each form of TSS also can be associated with invasive infections, such as pneumonia, osteomyelitis, bacteremia, pyarthrosis, or endocarditis. Patients with *S aureus*–mediated TSS, especially menses associated, are at risk of a recurrent episode of TSS. Toxic shock can be confused with many infectious and noninfectious causes of fever with mucocutaneous manifestations. The mortality rate is less than 5% overall and is highest in men and women older than 45 years.

Etiology

S aureus–mediated TSS usually is caused by strains producing TSS toxin-1 (TSST-1) or possibly other related staphylococcal enterotoxins. Most cases of *S pyogenes*–mediated TSS are caused by strains producing at least 1 of several different pyrogenic exotoxins. These toxins act as superantigens that stimulate production of tumor necrosis factor and other mediators that cause capillary leakage leading to hypotension and organ damage.

Epidemiology

S aureus–Mediated TSS. This syndrome was first recognized in 1978, occurring in children and adults, male and female; many early cases frequently were associated with tampon use in menstruating women, with a predilection for adolescents and young women with no circulating antibody to TSST-1. Although changes in tampon composition and use may have resulted in some decrease in the proportion of cases associated with menstruation, both menstrual and nonmenstrual cases of TSS continue to occur. Risk factors for TSS include lack of antibody to TSST-1 and a focal *S aureus* infection with a TSST-1–producing strain.

In adults, TSST-1–producing strains of *S aureus* may be part of the normal flora of the anterior nares or the vagina. Colonization is believed to produce protective antibody, and more than 90% of adults have antibodies to TSST-1. People in whom *S aureus*–mediated TSS with TSST-1–producing strains develops usually do not have antibodies to TSST-1. Nosocomial cases can occur and most often have followed surgical procedures. In postoperative cases, the organism generally originates from the patient's own flora. The incubation period may be as short as 12 hours.

S pyogenes–Mediated TSS. The incidence of *S pyogenes*–mediated TSS seems to be highest among young children, particularly children with concomitant varicella, and the elderly, although it can occur in people of any age. Of all cases of severe invasive streptococcal infections in children, fewer than 10% are associated with TSS. Other people at increased risk include people with diabetes mellitus, chronic cardiac or pulmonary disease, and HIV infection, and intravenous drug and alcohol users. The risk of severe invasive infection in contacts is greater than for the general population but still is rare.

Mortality rates are higher for adults than for children and depend on whether the *S pyogenes*–mediated TSS is associated only with bacteremia or with a specific focal infection (eg, necrotizing fasciitis, myositis, or pneumonia). The incubation period is not defined clearly, but may be as short as 14 hours after penetrating trauma.

Diagnostic Tests

S aureus-Mediated TSS. *S aureus*–mediated TSS remains a clinical diagnosis (Table 109.1). Blood culture results are positive for *S aureus* in fewer than 5% of patients. Specimens for culture should be obtained from an identified site of infection because these sites usually will be positive and susceptibility testing of isolated organisms can be performed. Because approximately one third of isolates of *S aureus* from nonmenstrual cases produce toxins other than TSST-1, and TSST-1–producing organisms can be present as part of the normal flora of the anterior nares and vagina, production of TSST-1 by an isolate of *S aureus* is not helpful diagnostically.

S pyogenes-Mediated TSS. Blood culture results are positive for *S pyogenes* in more than 50% of patients with *S pyogenes*–mediated TSS. Culture results from the site of infection usually are positive and can remain positive for several days after appropriate antimicrobial agents have been initiated. A significant increase in antibody titers to antistreptolysin O, antideoxyribonuclease B, or other streptococcal extracellular products 4 to 6 weeks after infection can help confirm the diagnosis if culture results were negative.

For both forms of TSS, laboratory studies can reflect multisystem organ involvement and disseminated intravascular coagulation.

Treatment

Most aspects of management are the same for TSS caused by *S aureus* and *S pyogenes* (Tables 109.3 and 109.4). The first priority is aggressive fluid replacement as well as management of respiratory or cardiac failure or arrhythmias if present. Because distinguishing between the 2 forms of TSS may not be possible, initial empiric antimicrobial therapy should include an antistaphylococcal antimicrobial agent and a protein synthesis-inhibiting antimicrobial

drug, such as clindamycin. Vancomycin should be substituted for the beta-lactamase–resistant penicillin or cephalosporin in areas where community-acquired methicillin-resistant *S aureus* infections are common. Both should be given parenterally at maximal doses. The addition of clindamycin is more effective than penicillin alone for treating well-established *S pyogenes* infections because the antimicrobial activity of clindamycin is not affected by inoculum size, has a long postantimicrobial effect, and acts on bacteria by inhibiting protein synthesis. Inhibition of protein synthesis results in suppression of synthesis of the *S pyogenes* antiphagocytic M protein and bacterial toxins. Clindamycin should not be used alone as initial empiric therapy.

Once the organism has been identified, antimicrobial therapy can be changed to penicillin and clindamycin for *S pyogenes*–mediated TSS. For *S aureus*–mediated TSS, the most appropriate antimicrobial agent on the basis of susceptibility testing should be given with clindamycin.

Aggressive drainage and irrigation of accessible sites of infection should be performed as soon as possible. Concerted efforts should be made to identify a foreign body at the site of infection, and all foreign bodies, including those recently inserted during surgery, should be removed if possible. If necrotizing fasciitis is suspected, immediate surgical exploration or biopsy is crucial to identify a deep soft tissue infection that should be debrided immediately.

The use of IGIV may be considered in treatment of either form of TSS. The mechanism of action of IGIV is unclear but may be neutralization of circulating bacterial toxins. For *S aureus*–mediated TSS, IGIV may be considered for patients who remain unresponsive to all other therapeutic measures and for patients with infection in an area that cannot be drained.

Table 109.1
Staphylococcal Toxic Shock Syndrome: Clinical Case Definition

- Fever: temperature ≥38.9°C (≥102.0°F)
- Rash: diffuse macular erythroderma
- Desquamation: 1–2 wk after onset, particularly on palms, soles, fingers, and toes
- Hypotension: systolic pressure ≤90 mm Hg for adults; lower than fifth percentile for age for children younger than 16 years; orthostatic drop in diastolic pressure of ≥15 mm Hg from lying to sitting; orthostatic syncope or orthostatic dizziness
- Multisystem organ involvement: 3 or more of the following:
  - Gastrointestinal: vomiting or diarrhea at onset of illness
  - Muscular: severe myalgia or creatinine phosphokinase concentration greater than twice the upper limit of normal
  - Mucous membrane: vaginal, oropharyngeal, or conjunctival hyperemia
  - Renal: serum urea nitrogen or serum creatinine concentration greater than twice the upper limit of normal or urinary sediment with ≥5 white blood cells per high-power field in the absence of urinary tract infection
  - Hepatic: total bilirubin, aspartate transaminase, or alanine transaminase concentration greater than twice the upper limit of normal
  - Hematologic: platelet count ≤100 000/mm³
  - Central nervous system: disorientation or alterations in consciousness without focal neurologic signs when fever and hypotension are absent
- Negative results on the following tests, if obtained:
  - Blood, throat, or cerebrospinal fluid cultures; blood culture may be positive for *Staphylococcus aureus*
  - Serologic tests for Rocky Mountain spotted fever, leptospirosis, or measles

Case Classification
Probable: A case with 5 of the 6 clinical findings.
Confirmed: A case with all 6 of the clinical findings, including desquamation. If the patient dies before desquamation could have occurred, the other 5 criteria constitute a definitive case.

Adapted from Wharton M, Chorba TL, Vogt RL, Morse DL, Buehler JW. Case definitions for public health surveillance. *MMWR Recomm Rep.* 1990;39(RR-13):1–43.

Table 109.2
Streptococcal Toxic Shock Syndrome: Clinical Case Definition[1]

I. Isolation of group A streptococcus *(Streptococcus pyogenes)*
  A. From a normally sterile site (eg, blood, cerebrospinal fluid, peritoneal fluid, or tissue biopsy specimen)
  B. From a nonsterile site (eg, throat, sputum, vagina, surgical wound, or superficial skin lesion)
II. Clinical signs of severity
  A. Hypotension: systolic pressure ≤90 mm Hg in adults or lower than the fifth percentile for age in children
AND
  B. Two or more of the following signs:
    - Renal impairment: creatinine concentration ≥177 μmol/L (≥2 mg/dL) for adults or 2 times or more the upper limit of normal for age
    - Coagulopathy: platelet count ≤100 000/mm³ or disseminated intravascular coagulation
    - Hepatic involvement: alanine transaminase, aspartate transaminase, or total bilirubin concentrations 2 times or more the upper limit of normal for age
    - Adult respiratory distress syndrome
    - A generalized erythematous macular rash that may desquamate
    - Soft tissue necrosis, including necrotizing fasciitis or myositis, or gangrene

[1] An illness fulfilling criteria IA and IIA and IIB can be defined as a *definite* case. An illness fulfilling criteria IB and IIA and IIB can be defined as a *probable* case if no other cause for the illness is identified.

Adapted from The Working Group on Severe Streptococcal Infections. Defining the group A streptococcal toxic shock syndrome: rationale and consensus definition. *JAMA.* 1993;269:390–391.

Table 109.3

Management of Staphylococcal or Streptococcal Toxic Shock Syndrome *Without* Necrotizing Fasciitis

- Fluid management to maintain adequate venous return and cardiac filling pressures to prevent end-organ damage
- Anticipatory management of multisystem organ failure
- Parenteral antimicrobial therapy at maximum doses
  - Kill organism with bactericidal cell wall inhibitor (eg, beta-lactamase–resistant antistaphylococcal antimicrobial agent)
  - Stop enzyme, toxin, or cytokine production with protein synthesis inhibitor (eg, clindamycin)
- Immune globulin intravenous may be considered for infection refractory to several hours of aggressive therapy, or in the presence of an undrainable focus, or persistent oliguria with pulmonary edema

Table 109.4

Management of Streptococcal Toxic Shock Syndrome *With* Necrotizing Fasciitis

- Principles outlined in Table 109.3
- Immediate surgical evaluation
  - Exploration or incisional biopsy for diagnosis and culture
  - Resection of all necrotic tissue
- Repeated resection of tissue may be needed if infection persists or progresses

Image 109.1
Facial erythroderma secondary to *Staphylococcus aureus* toxic shock syndrome in a woman who was obtunded and hypotensive on admission.

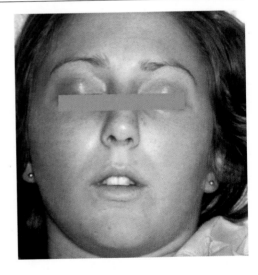

Image 109.2
Erythroderma that blanches on pressure in
a patient with toxic shock syndrome. The
mortality rate for staphylococcal toxic shock
syndrome is lower than that of streptococcal
toxic shock syndrome.

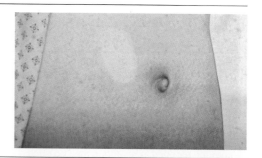

Image 109.3
Characteristic erythroderma of the hand.

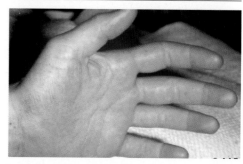

Image 109.4
A woman with toxic shock syndrome shows
characteristic erythroderma of the feet.

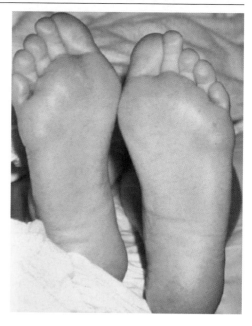

Image 109.5

This patient displayed marked desquamation of right thumb and palm due to toxic shock syndrome.

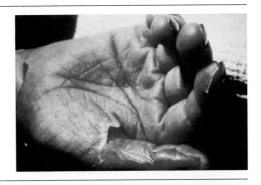

Image 109.6

Staphylococcal pustules on the cheek of a patient with toxic shock syndrome.

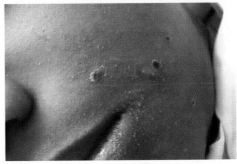

110

Toxocariasis

(Visceral Larva Migrans, Ocular Larva Migrans)

Clinical Manifestations

The severity of symptoms depends on the number of larvae ingested and the degree of allergic response. Most people who are infected lightly are asymptomatic. Visceral larva migrans typically occurs in children 1 to 4 years of age with a history of pica but can occur in older children and adults. Characteristic manifestations include fever, leukocytosis, eosinophilia, hypergammaglobulinemia, and hepatomegaly. Other manifestations include malaise, anemia, cough and, in rare instances, pneumonia, myocarditis, and encephalitis. When ocular invasion (endophthalmitis or retinal granulomas) occurs, other evidence of infection usually is lacking, suggesting that the visceral and ocular manifestations are distinct syndromes. Atypical manifestations include hemorrhagic rash and seizures. In some cases, so-called covert toxocariasis may manifest only as asymptomatic eosinophilia or wheezing.

Etiology

Toxocariasis is caused by *Toxocara* species, which are common roundworms of dogs and cats (especially puppies or kittens), specifically *Toxocara canis* and *Toxocara cati* in the United States; most cases are caused by *T canis*. Other nematodes of animals also can cause this syndrome, although rarely.

Epidemiology

Humans are infected by ingestion of soil containing infective eggs of the parasite. A history of pica, particularly eating soil, is common. Direct contact with dogs is of secondary importance because eggs are not infective immediately when shed in the feces. Most reported cases involve children. Toxocariasis is endemic wherever dogs are present. Infection risk is highest in hot, humid regions where eggs persist in soil. The infection is endemic in many underserved urban areas. Eggs may be found wherever dogs and cats defecate.

Incubation Period

Unknown.

Diagnostic Tests

Hypereosinophilia and hypergammaglobulinemia associated with increased titers of isohemagglutinin to the A and B blood group antigens are presumptive evidence of infection. Microscopic identification of larvae in a liver biopsy specimen is diagnostic, but this finding is rare. A liver biopsy negative for larvae does not exclude the diagnosis. An enzyme immunoassay for *Toxocara* antibodies in serum, available at the CDC and some commercial laboratories, can provide confirmatory evidence of toxocariasis. This assay is specific and sensitive for diagnosis of visceral larva migrans but is less sensitive for diagnosis of ocular larva migrans.

Treatment

Albendazole or mebendazole is the recommended drug for treatment of toxocariasis. In severe cases with myocarditis or involvement of the CNS, corticosteroid therapy is indicated. Correcting the underlying causes of pica helps prevent reinfection.

Anthelmintic treatment of ocular larva migrans may not be effective. Inflammation may be decreased by injection of corticosteroids, and secondary damage may be aided by surgery.

Image 110.1

Toxocariasis (visceral larva migrans) with *Toxocara canis* larvae on liver biopsy.

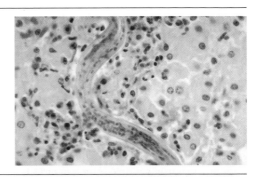

Image 110.2

Fundus damage from *Toxocara canis* larval invasion.

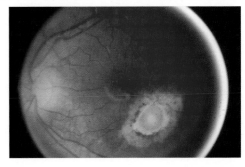

111

Toxoplasma gondii Infections
(Toxoplasmosis)

Clinical Manifestations

Infants with congenital infection are asymptomatic at birth in 70% to 90% of cases, although visual impairment, learning disabilities, or mental retardation will become apparent in a large proportion of children several months to years later. Signs of congenital toxoplasmosis at birth can include a maculopapular rash, generalized lymphadenopathy, hepatomegaly, splenomegaly, jaundice, and thrombocytopenia. As a consequence of intrauterine meningoencephalitis, CSF abnormalities, hydrocephalus, microcephaly, chorioretinitis, seizures, and deafness can develop. Some of the severely affected infants die in utero or within a few days of birth. Cerebral calcifications can be demonstrated by radiography, ultrasonography, or CT of the head.

Toxoplasma gondii infection acquired after birth usually is asymptomatic. When symptoms develop, they are nonspecific and include malaise, fever, sore throat, and myalgia. Lymphadenopathy, frequently cervical, is the most common sign. Occasionally patients may have a mononucleosis-like illness associated with a macular rash and hepatosplenomegaly. The clinical course usually is benign and self-limited. Myocarditis, pericarditis, and pneumonitis are rare complications.

Isolated ocular toxoplasmosis most commonly results from congenital infection but also occurs in a small percentage of people with acquired infection. Characteristic retinal infiltrates develop in up to 85% of young adults after congenital infection. Acute ocular involvement manifests as blurred vision. Ocular disease can become reactivated years after the initial infection in healthy and immunocompromised people.

In chronically infected immunodeficient patients, including people with HIV infection, reactivated infection can result in encephalitis, pneumonitis or, less commonly, systemic toxoplasmosis. Rarely, infants who are born to HIV-infected mothers or mothers who are immunocompromised for other reasons who have chronic infection with *T gondii* may have acquired congenital toxoplasmosis in utero as a result of reactivated maternal parasitemia.

Etiology

T gondii, a protozoan parasite, is the only known species of *Toxoplasma*.

Epidemiology

T gondii is worldwide in distribution and infects most species of warm-blooded animals. Members of the cat family are definitive hosts. Cats generally acquire the infection by feeding on infected animals, such as mice or uncooked household meats. The parasite replicates sexually in the feline small intestine. Cats may begin to excrete oocysts in their stools 3 to 30 days after primary infection and can shed oocysts for 7 to 14 days. After excretion, oocysts require a maturation phase (sporulation) of 24 to 48 hours in temperate climates before they are infective by the oral route. Intermediate hosts (including sheep, pigs, and cattle) can have tissue cysts in the brain, myocardium, skeletal muscle, and other organs. These cysts remain viable for the lifetime of the host. Humans usually become infected by consumption of raw or undercooked meat that contains cysts or by accidental ingestion of sporulated oocysts from soil or in contaminated food. A large outbreak linked epidemiologically to contamination of a municipal water supply also has been reported. Transmission of *T gondii* has been documented to result from blood or blood product transfusion and organ (eg, heart) or stem cell transplantation from a seropositive donor with latent infection. Rarely, infection has occurred as a result of a laboratory accident. In most cases, congenital transmission occurs as a result of primary maternal infection during pregnancy. The incidence of congenital toxoplasmosis in the United States has been estimated to be 1 in 1000 to 1 in 10 000 live births.

Incubation Period

Estimated to be 7 days (range, 4–21).

Diagnostic Tests

Serologic tests are the primary means of diagnosis, but results must be interpreted carefully. Laboratories with special expertise in *Toxoplasma* serologic assays are preferred. IgG-specific antibodies achieve a peak concentration 1 to 2 months after infection and remain positive indefinitely. To determine the approximate time of infection in IgG-positive adults, specific IgM antibody determinations should be performed. The lack of *T gondii*–specific IgM antibodies indicates infection more than 6 months ago. The presence of *T gondii*–specific IgM antibodies can indicate recent infection or can result from a false-positive reaction. Enzyme immunoassay tests are the more sensitive assays for IgM, and indirect fluorescent antibody tests are the least sensitive in detecting IgM. IgM-specific antibodies can be detected 2 weeks after infection, achieve peak concentrations in 1 month, decrease thereafter, and usually become undetectable within 6 to 9 months but uncommonly persist for as long as 2 years. In adults, when determining the timing of infection is clinically important (eg, in a pregnant woman), a positive IgM test should be followed by an IgG avidity test. The presence of high IgG avidity antibodies indicates that infection occurred at least 12 to 16 weeks previously. However, the presence of low avidity antibodies is not a reliable indication of recent infection. Tests to detect IgA and IgE antibodies, which decrease to undetectable concentrations sooner than IgM antibodies, are useful for diagnosis of congenital infections and infections in other patients, such as pregnant women, for whom more precise information about the duration of infection is needed. *T gondii*–specific IgA and IgE antibody tests are available in *Toxoplasma* reference laboratories but not generally in other laboratories.

Special Situations

Prenatal. A definitive diagnosis of congenital toxoplasmosis can be made prenatally by detecting parasite DNA in amniotic fluid or fetal blood or by isolating the parasite by mouse or tissue culture inoculation. Serial fetal ultrasonographic examinations can be performed in cases of suspected congenital infection to detect any increase in size of the lateral ventricles of the CNS or other signs of fetal infection.

Postnatal. Infants who are born to women who have evidence of primary *T gondii* infection during gestation or women who are infected with HIV and have serologic evidence of past infection with *T gondii* should be assessed for congenital toxoplasmosis.

If the diagnosis for an infant is unclear at the time of delivery, *Toxoplasma*-specific laboratory tests for IgG, IgM, IgA, and IgE on newborn and maternal serum samples should be performed. Peripheral white blood cells, CSF, and amniotic fluid specimens should be assayed for *T gondii* by PCR in a reference laboratory. Evaluation of the infant should include ophthalmologic, auditory, and neurologic examinations; lumbar puncture; and CT of the head. An attempt may be made to isolate *T gondii* from the placenta, umbilical cord, or blood specimen from the infant by mouse inoculation.

Congenital infection is confirmed serologically by persistently positive IgG titers beyond the first 12 months of life. Before 12 months of age, a persistently positive or increasing IgG antibody concentration in the infant compared with the mother, or a positive *Toxoplasma*-specific IgM or IgA assay, indicate congenital infection. The sensitivity of *T gondii*–specific IgM by the double-sandwich enzyme immunoassay or an immunosorbent assay is 75% to 80%. IgA antibodies are found more frequently than IgM antibodies; some infants may have only IgA or only IgM antibodies. The indirect fluorescent assay for IgM should not be relied on to diagnose congenital infection. In an uninfected infant, a continuous decrease in IgG titer without detection of IgM or IgA antibodies will occur. Transplacentally transmitted IgG antibody usually will become undetectable by 6 to 12 months of age.

HIV Infection. Patients with HIV infection who are infected latently with *T gondii* have variable titers of IgG antibody to *T gondii* but rarely have IgM antibody. Although seroconversion and 4-fold increases in IgG antibody titers may occur, the ability to diagnose active disease in patients with AIDS commonly is impaired by immunosuppression. In HIV-infected patients who are seropositive for *T gondii* IgG, *T gondii* encephalitis is diagnosed presumptively on the basis of the presence of characteristic clinical and radiographic findings. If the infection does not respond to an empiric trial of anti–*T gondii* therapy, demonstration of *T gondii* organisms, antigen, or DNA in sites such as blood, CSF, or bronchoalveolar fluid, where the organism would not be expected to reside in the chronic cyst form, may be necessary to confirm the diagnosis.

Infants born to women who are infected simultaneously with HIV and *T gondii* should be evaluated for congenital toxoplasmosis because of an increased likelihood of maternal reactivation and congenital transmission in this setting.

Ocular toxoplasmosis usually is diagnosed on the basis of observation of characteristic retinal lesions in conjunction with serum *T gondii*–specific IgG or IgM antibodies.

Treatment

Most cases of acquired infection in an immunocompetent host do not require specific antimicrobial therapy. When indicated (eg, chorioretinitis or significant organ damage), the combination of pyrimethamine and sulfadiazine, with supplemental leucovorin (folinic acid) to minimize pyrimethamine-associated hematologic toxicity, is the most widely accepted regimen for children and adults with acute symptomatic disease. Alternatively, pyrimethamine can be used in combination with clindamycin if the patient does not tolerate sulfadiazine. Corticosteroids seem to be useful in the management of ocular complications and CNS disease in certain patients.

Patients infected with HIV who have had toxoplasmic encephalitis should receive lifelong suppressive therapy to prevent recurrence. Regimens for primary treatment also are effective for suppressive therapy.

For HIV-infected adults, primary chemoprophylaxis with trimethoprim-sulfamethoxazole against toxoplasmosis is the preferred regimen for people who are *T gondii*–seropositive and have CD4+ T-lymphocyte counts less than 100 × 10^6/L (<100/μL). Prophylaxis to prevent the first episode of toxoplasmosis generally is recommended for children. The safety of discontinuing primary or secondary prophylaxis in HIV-infected children receiving highly active antiretroviral therapy has not been studied extensively.

For symptomatic and asymptomatic congenital infections, pyrimethamine combined with sulfadiazine (supplemented with folinic acid) is recommended as initial therapy. However, the optimal dosage and duration are not established definitively and should be determined in consultation with appropriate specialists.

Treatment of primary *T gondii* infection in pregnant women, including women with HIV infection, is recommended. Appropriate specialists should be consulted for management. Spiramycin treatment of primary infection during gestation is used in an attempt to decrease transmission of *T gondii* from the mother to the fetus.

Image 111.1
Infant girl with congenital toxoplasmosis and hepatosplenomegaly.

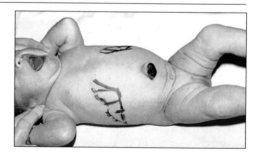

Image 111.2
Extensive chorioretinitis in an infant with congenital toxoplasmosis.

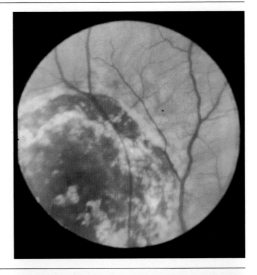

Image 111.3
Toxoplasma gondii retinitis. Note well-defined areas of choroidoretinitis with pigmentation and irregular scarring.

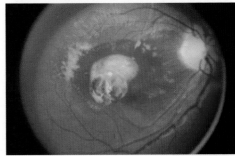

Image 111.4
Congenital infection evident on a CT scan of the head that shows diffuse calcifications and hydrocephaly.

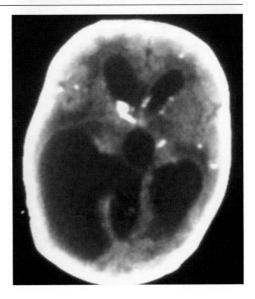

Image 111.5

A CT scan of the brain of a child with leukemia infected with HIV through a blood transfusion (before routine screening of blood for HIV). A brain biopsy revealed *Toxoplasma gondii*.

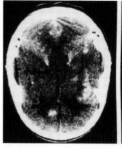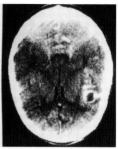

Image 111.6

The brain biopsy shows multiple *Toxoplasma gondii* organisms (Giemsa stain, 400x).

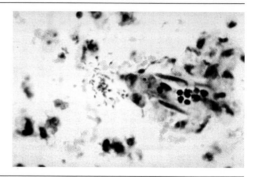

Image 111.7

Histopathology of toxoplasmosis of brain in fatal AIDS. Pseudocyst contains numerous tachyzoites of *Toxoplasma gondii*.

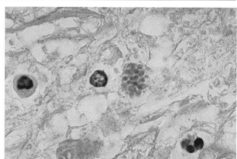

Image 111.8

Toxoplasmosis of the heart in AIDS. Histopathology of active toxoplasmosis of myocardium. Numerous tachyzoites of *Toxoplasma gondii* are visible within a pseudocyst in a myocyte.

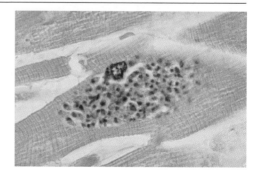

112

Trichinellosis
(Trichinella spiralis)

Clinical Manifestations

The clinical spectrum of infection ranges from inapparent to fulminant and fatal illness, but most infections are inapparent. The severity of the disease is proportional to the infective dose. During the first week after ingesting infected meat, a person can be asymptomatic or experience abdominal discomfort, nausea, vomiting, or diarrhea. Two to 8 weeks later, as larvae migrate into tissues, fever, myalgia, periorbital edema, urticarial rash, and conjunctival and subungual hemorrhages can develop. Larvae can remain viable in tissues for years; calcification of some larvae in skeletal muscle usually occurs within 6 to 24 months and may be detected on radiographs. In severe infections, myocarditis, neurologic involvement, and pneumonitis can follow in 1 to 2 months.

Etiology

Infection is caused by nematodes (roundworms) of the genus *Trichinella*. At least 5 species capable of infecting only warm-blooded animals have been identified. Worldwide, *Trichinella spiralis* is the most common cause of human infection.

Epidemiology

The infection is enzootic worldwide in many carnivores, especially scavengers. Infection occurs as a result of ingestion of raw or insufficiently cooked meat containing encysted larvae of *T spiralis*. The usual source of human infection is pork, but horse meat and wild carnivorous game, such as bear, seal, and walrus meat in North America, can be sources. *Trichinella nativa* is the causative organism in most of these arctic sources. Feeding pigs uncooked garbage perpetuates the cycle of infection. In the United States, the incidence of infection in humans has decreased considerably, but infection occurs sporadically, often within a family or among friends who have prepared uncooked sausage from fresh pork. The disease is not transmitted from person to person.

Incubation Period

1 to 2 weeks.

Diagnostic Tests

Eosinophilia approaching 70%, with compatible symptoms and dietary history, suggests the diagnosis. Increases in concentrations of muscle enzymes, such as creatinine phosphokinase and lactic dehydrogenase, also occur. Encapsulated larvae in a skeletal muscle biopsy specimen (particularly deltoid and gastrocnemius) can be visualized microscopically beginning 2 weeks after infection. Fresh tissue, compressed between 2 microscope slides, should be examined. Digestion of muscle tissue in artificial gastric juice followed by examination of the sediment for larvae is more sensitive. Identification of larvae in suspect meat can be the most rapid source of diagnostic information. Serologic tests are available through some state laboratories and the CDC. Serum antibody titers rarely become positive before the second week of illness. Testing paired acute and convalescent serum specimens usually is diagnostic.

Treatment

Mebendazole and albendazole have comparable efficacy for treatment of trichinosis. Neither drug is very effective for *Trichinella* larvae already in the muscles. Coadministration of corticosteroids with mebendazole or albendazole often is recommended when symptoms are severe. Corticosteroids alleviate symptoms of the inflammatory reaction and can be lifesaving when the CNS or heart is involved.

Image 112.1
Striking edema of the face of a 22-year-old woman with trichinellosis. A history of ingestion of poorly cooked hogs head was obtained. Periorbital edema and conjunctivitis are commonly seen in patients with trichinosis.

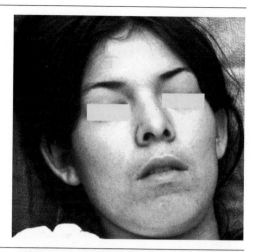

Image 112.2
Striking edema of the feet of the same patient as in Image 112.1.

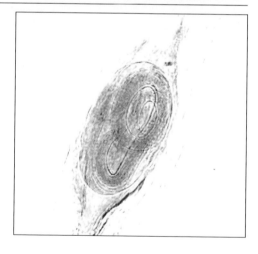

Image 112.3
Larvae of *Trichinella spiralis* in skeletal muscle biopsy.

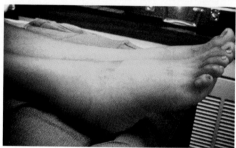

Image 112.4

This patient with trichinellosis had periorbital swelling, muscle pain, diarrhea, and 28% (0.28) eosinophils in her peripheral CBC.

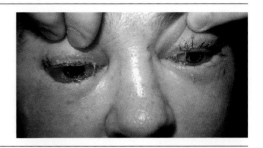

Image 112.5

Here the parasitic disease trichinellosis is manifested by splinter hemorrhages under the finger nails.

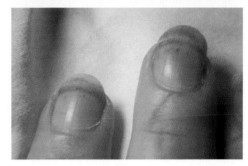

[113]

Trichomonas vaginalis Infections
(Trichomoniasis)

Clinical Manifestations

Infection with *Trichomonas vaginalis* is asymptomatic in 90% of men and 50% of women infected with this organism. Clinical manifestations in symptomatic postmenarcheal female patients consist of a frothy vaginal discharge and mild vulvovaginal itching and burning. Dysuria and, rarely, lower abdominal pain can occur. The vaginal discharge usually is pale yellow to gray-green and has a musty or fishy odor. Symptoms commonly are more severe just before or after menstruation. The vaginal mucosa often is deeply erythematous, and the cervix is friable and diffusely inflamed, sometimes covered with numerous petechiae ("strawberry cervix"). Urethritis and, more rarely, epididymitis or prostatitis can develop in infected males, but most are asymptomatic. Reinfection is common. *T vaginalis* is considered an important cofactor in amplifying HIV transmission.

Etiology

T vaginalis is a flagellated protozoan that is slightly larger than a granulocyte. It depends on adherence to host cells for survival.

Epidemiology

T vaginalis infection is the second most common STI in the United States and commonly coexists with other conditions, particularly infection with *Neisseria gonorrhoeae* and *Chlamydia trachomatis* and bacterial vaginitis. The presence of *T vaginalis* in a prepubertal child should raise suspicion of sexual abuse. *T vaginalis* acquired during birth by newborn infants can cause a vaginal discharge during the first weeks of life.

Incubation Period

Average, 1 week (range, 4–28 days).

Diagnostic Tests

Diagnosis usually is established by examination of a wet-mount preparation of the vaginal discharge. Lashing of the flagella and jerky motility of the organism are distinctive. Positive preparation results, found more commonly in women who have symptoms, are related directly to the number of organisms but are identified only in 50% to 60% of cases. Culture of the organism and tests using enzyme immunoassay and immunofluorescent techniques are more sensitive than wet-mount preparations but generally are not required for diagnosis. Culture for *T vaginalis* is positive in more than 80% of cases. Fecal contamination of specimens makes microscopic diagnosis difficult because of the somewhat similar morphology of *Trichomonas hominis*. Motile trichomonads also can be identified by microscopic examination of centrifuged urine.

Treatment

Treatment with metronidazole or tinidazole results in cure rates of approximately 95%. Sexual partners should be treated concurrently because reinfection often occurs. Patients should abstain from alcohol for 48 hours after treatment with either medication because of the disulfiram-like effects of the drugs. During pregnancy, patients can be treated with a single or multiple dose regimen of metronidazole or with tinidazole. Use of metronidazole or tinidazole is contraindicated during the first trimester of pregnancy.

Patients whose infections do not respond to treatment should be re-treated with metronidazole. Patients who repeatedly fail to respond to this regimen should be treated with high-dose metronidazole. In the event of continued treatment failure, consultation with an expert is advised.

People infected with *T vaginalis* should be evaluated for the presence of other STIs, including syphilis and *N gonorrhoeae*, *C trachomatis,* hepatitis B virus, and HIV infection. Newborn infection is self-limited and treatment generally is not recommended.

Image 113.1
Wet mount showing the presence of motile trichomonads in vaginal secretions. This indicates an infection caused by *Trichomonas vaginalis*.

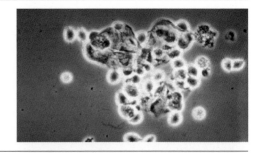

Image 113.2
A case of *Trichomonas* vaginitis revealing a copious purulent discharge emanating from the cervical os. *Trichomonas vaginalis,* a flagellate, is the most common pathogenic protozoan of humans in industrialized countries. This protozoan resides in the female lower genital tract and the male urethra and prostate, where it replicates by binary fission.

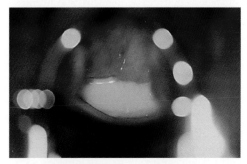

Image 113.3
This patient presented with a "strawberry cervix" due to a *Trichomonas vaginalis* infection, or trichomoniasis. The term "strawberry cervix" is used to describe the appearance of the cervix caused by the presence of *T vaginalis* protozoa. The cervical mucosa reveals punctate hemorrhages along with accompanying vesicles or papules.

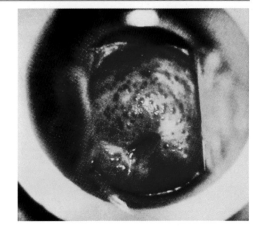

114

Trichuriasis
(Whipworm Infection)

Clinical Manifestations

Most infected children harbor only small numbers of the organism and are asymptomatic. Children with heavy infestations can develop a *Trichuris trichiura* dysentery syndrome consisting of abdominal pain, tenesmus, and bloody diarrhea with mucus or a chronic *T trichiura* colitis. *T trichiura* colitis can mimic other forms of inflammatory bowel disease and lead to physical growth retardation. Even otherwise asymptomatic infections can have adverse effects on nutritional status. Chronic illness associated with heavy infestation also can be associated with rectal prolapse.

Etiology

T trichiura, the whipworm, is the causative agent. Adult worms are 30 to 50 mm long with a large, thread-like anterior end that is embedded in the mucosa of the large intestine.

Epidemiology

The parasite has a worldwide distribution but is more common in the tropics and in areas of poor sanitation. In some areas of Asia, the prevalence of infection is 50%. In the United States, trichuriasis generally has been limited to rural areas of the southeast and no longer is a serious public health problem. Migrants from tropical areas also may be infected. Eggs require a minimum of 10 days of incubation in the soil before they are infectious. The disease is not communicable from person to person.

Incubation Period

Unknown; time required for mature worms to begin laying eggs that are passed in feces is approximately 90 days after ingestion of eggs.

Diagnostic Tests

Eggs may be found on direct examination of stool or by using concentration techniques.

Treatment

Mebendazole or alternatively albendazole or ivermectin usually is effective in eradicating most of the worms. In mass treatment efforts involving entire communities, a single dose of either mebendazole or albendazole will reduce worm burdens.

Image 114.1
Trichuris trichiura ova. A, B, C: Atypical *Trichuris* species eggs.

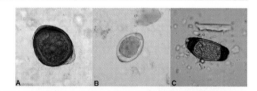

Image 114.2
This micrograph of an adult *Trichuris* female human whipworm reveals that its size is approximately 4 cm. The female *Trichuris trichiura* worms begin to oviposit in the cecum and ascending colon 60 to 70 days after infection. Female worms in the cecum shed between 3 000 and 20 000 eggs per day. The life span of the adults is about 1 year.

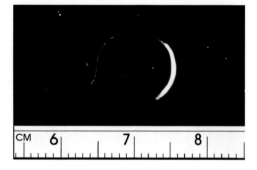

115

African Trypanosomiasis

(African Sleeping Sickness)

Clinical Manifestations

The rapidity and severity of clinical manifestations vary with the infecting subspecies. With *Trypanosoma brucei gambiense* (West African) infection, a cutaneous nodule or chancre can appear at the site of parasite inoculation within a few days of a bite by an infected tsetse fly. Systemic illness is chronic, occurring months to years later, and is characterized by intermittent fever, posterior cervical lymphadenopathy (Winterbottom sign), and multiple nonspecific complaints, including malaise, weight loss, arthralgia, rash, pruritus, and edema. If the CNS is involved, chronic meningoencephalitis with behavioral changes, cachexia, headache, hallucinations, delusions, and somnolence can occur. In contrast, *Trypanosoma brucei rhodesiense* (East African) infection is an acute, generalized illness that develops days to weeks after parasite inoculation, with manifestations including high fever, cutaneous chancre, myocarditis, hepatitis, anemia, thrombocytopenia, and laboratory evidence of disseminated intravascular coagulopathy. Clinical meningoencephalitis can develop as early as 3 weeks after onset of the untreated systemic illness. *T brucei rhodesiense* infection has a high fatality rate; without treatment, infected patients usually die within days to months after clinical onset of disease.

Etiology

The West African (Gambian) form of sleeping sickness is caused by *T brucei gambiense,* whereas the East African (Rhodesian) form is caused by *T brucei rhodesiense.* Both are extracellular protozoan hemoflagellates that live in blood and tissue of the human host.

Epidemiology

Approximately 30 000 human cases are reported annually worldwide, although only a few cases, acquired in Africa, are reported every year in the United States. There has been a recent increase of trypanosomiasis in travelers after short visits to game parks in Tanzania. Transmission is confined to an area in Africa between the latitudes of 15° north and 20° south, corresponding precisely with the distribution of the tsetse fly vector (*Glossina* species). In East Africa, wild animals, such as antelope, constitute the major reservoirs for *T brucei rhodesiense,* although cattle serve as reservoir hosts in local outbreaks. Domestic pigs and dogs have been found as incidental reservoirs of *T brucei gambiense;* however, humans are the only important reservoir in West and Central Africa.

Incubation Period

T brucei rhodesiense, 3 to 21 days (usually 5–14); *T brucei gambiense,* variable, ranging from several months to years.

Diagnostic Tests

Diagnosis is made by identification of trypomastigotes in specimens of blood, CSF, or fluid aspirated from a chancre or lymph node or by inoculation of susceptible laboratory animals (mice) with heparinized blood. Examination of the CSF is critical to management and should be performed using the double-centrifugation technique. Concentration and Giemsa staining of the buffy coat layer of peripheral blood also can be helpful. *T brucei gambiense* is more likely to be found in lymph node aspirates. Although an increased concentration of IgM in serum or CSF is considered characteristic of African trypanosomiasis, polyclonal hyperglobulinemia is common.

Treatment

When no evidence of CNS involvement is present (including absence of trypanosomes and CSF pleocytosis), the drug of choice for the acute hemolymphatic stage of infection is pentamidine for *T brucei gambiense* infection and suramin for *T brucei rhodesiense* infection. Because of the risk of relapse, patients who have had CNS involvement should undergo repeated CSF examinations every 6 months for 2 years.

Image 115.1

Trypanosoma forms in blood smear from patient with African trypanosomiasis (hemotoxylin-eosin stain).

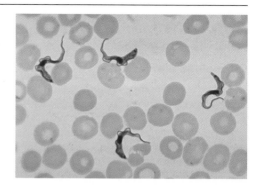

116

American Trypanosomiasis
(Chagas Disease)

Clinical Manifestations

Patients can have acute or chronic disease. The early phase of this disease commonly is asymptomatic. However, children are more likely to exhibit symptoms than are adults. In some patients, a red nodule known as a *chagoma* develops at the site of the original inoculation, usually on the face or arms. The surrounding skin becomes indurated and, later, hypopigmented. Unilateral firm edema of the eyelids, known as Romaña sign, is the earliest indication of the infection when the portal of entry is the conjunctiva; it is not always present. The edematous skin is violaceous and associated with conjunctivitis and enlargement of the ipsilateral preauricular lymph node. A few days after appearance of Romaña sign, fever, generalized lymphadenopathy, and malaise can develop. Acute myocarditis, hepatosplenomegaly, edema, and meningoencephalitis can follow. In nearly all cases, acute Chagas disease resolves after 1 to 3 months, and an asymptomatic or indeterminate period follows. In 20% to 30% of cases, serious sequelae, consisting of cardiomyopathy and heart failure (the major cause of death), megaesophagus, or megacolon, develop many years after the initial infection (chronic phase). Congenital disease is characterized by low birth weight, hepatomegaly, and meningoencephalitis with seizures and tremors, but most infants infected in utero have no signs or symptoms of disease. Reactivation can occur, especially in immunocompromised people, including people infected with HIV.

Etiology

Trypanosoma cruzi, a protozoan hemoflagellate, is the causative agent.

Epidemiology

Parasites are transmitted through feces of the insects of the triatomine family, usually an infected reduviid (cone-nose or kissing) bug. These insects defecate during or after taking blood. The bitten person is inoculated by inadvertently rubbing the insect feces containing the parasite into the site of the bite or mucous membranes of the eye or the mouth. The parasite also can be transmitted congenitally, during organ transplantation, through blood transfusion, and by consumption of the vector or the vector's excretion. Accidental laboratory infections can result from handling blood from infected people or laboratory animals. The disease is limited to the Western hemisphere, predominantly Mexico and Central and South America. Although some small mammals in the southern and southwestern United States harbor *T cruzi,* vector-borne transmission to humans is rare in the United States. Several transfusion- and transplantation-associated cases have been documented in the United States. Infection is common in immigrants from Central and South America. The disease is an important cause of death in South America, where between 7 and 15 million people are infected.

Incubation Period

Acute phase, 1 to 2 weeks or longer; chronic manifestations, years to decades.

Diagnostic Tests

During the acute phase of disease, the parasite is demonstrable in blood specimens by Giemsa staining after a concentration technique or by direct wet-mount or buffy coat preparation. During the indeterminate and chronic phases, which are characterized by low-level parasitemia, recovery of the parasite requires culture on special media (available at the CDC) but this can be negative because of a low parasite burden. Xenodiagnosis (isolation of trypanosomes from the intestine of a reduviid bug that has fed on patient blood) is available in Central and South America. Serologic tests include indirect hemagglutination, indirect immunofluorescence, and enzyme immunoassay, which are especially useful in chronic disease. The diagnosis of congenital Chagas disease is difficult and often is not made until 6 to 9 months of age, when IgG measurements reflect infant rather than maternal infection.

Treatment

The acute phase of Chagas disease is treated with benznidazole or nifurtimox. Although treatment of children during the latent and chronic phases of infection is routine in most Latin American countries, the effectiveness of this approach has not been established.

Image 116.1

A photomicrograph of *Trypanosoma cruzi* in a blood smear using Giemsa staining technique. This protozoan parasite is the causative agent for Chagas disease, also known as American trypanosomiasis. It is estimated that 16 million to 18 million people are infected with Chagas disease and, of those infected, 50 000 will die each year.

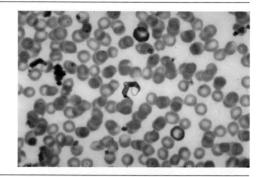

Image 116.2

Triatomine bug *(Trypanosoma cruzi)* defecating on the wound after taking a blood meal.

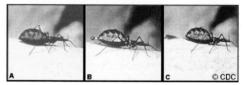

117

Tuberculosis

Clinical Manifestations

Most infections caused by *Mycobacterium tuberculosis* and *Mycobacterium bovis* in children and adolescents are asymptomatic. When tuberculosis disease does occur, clinical manifestations most often appear 1 to 6 months after infection and include fever, growth delay, weight loss or poor weight gain, cough, night sweats, and chills. Radiographic findings in *M tuberculosis* infection range from normal to diverse abnormalities, such as lymphadenopathy of the hilar, subcarinal, paratracheal, or mediastinal nodes; atelectasis or infiltrate of a segment or lobe; pleural effusion; cavitary lesions; or miliary disease. Radiographic findings in *M bovis* infection can include the same pulmonary manifestations as *M tuberculosis,* extensive cervical and mesenteric lymphadenopathy, bowel wall thickening, and multiple enteric fistulae. Extrapulmonary manifestations of *M tuberculosis* disease include meningitis and granulomatous inflammation of the lymph nodes, bones, joints, skin, and middle ear and mastoid. Renal tuberculosis and progression to disease from latent tuberculosis infection or adult-type pulmonary tuberculosis are rare in young children but can occur in adolescents. In addition, chronic abdominal pain with intermittent partial intestinal obstruction can be present in disease caused by *M bovis.* Clinical findings in patients with drug-resistant tuberculosis disease are indistinguishable from manifestations in patients with drug-susceptible disease.

Etiology

M tuberculosis is an acid-fast bacillus (AFB) that requires special media for optimal growth. Human disease caused by *M bovis,* the cause of bovine tuberculosis, occurs in the United States in children who have ingested unpasteurized milk or milk products.

Definitions

- **Positive tuberculin skin test (TST).** A positive TST result (Table 117.1) indicates possible infection with *M tuberculosis* or *M bovis.* Tuberculin reactivity appears 2 to 12 weeks after initial infection; the median interval is 3 to 4 weeks.

- **Exposed person.** A patient who has had recent contact with a person with suspected or confirmed contagious pulmonary tuberculosis disease and who has a negative TST result, normal physical examination findings, and chest radiographic findings that are not compatible with tuberculosis. Some exposed people become infected (and subsequently have a positive TST result) and some people do not become infected; the 2 groups cannot be distinguished initially.

- **Source case.** The person who has transmitted *M tuberculosis* to a child who subsequently develops either latent tuberculosis infection or tuberculosis disease.

- **Latent tuberculosis infection (LTBI).** *M tuberculosis* or *M bovis* infection in a person who has a positive TST result, no physical findings of disease, and chest radiograph findings that are normal or reveal evidence of healed infection (eg, granulomas or calcification in the lung, hilar lymph nodes, or both).

- **Tuberculosis disease.** Disease in a person with infection in whom symptoms, signs, or radiographic manifestations caused by *M tuberculosis* or *M bovis* are apparent; disease can be pulmonary, extrapulmonary, or both. Infectious tuberculosis refers to tuberculosis disease of the lungs or larynx in a person who has the potential to transmit *M tuberculosis* to other people.

- **Directly observed therapy (DOT).** An intervention by which medication is provided directly to the patient by a health care professional or trained third party (not a relative or friend), who observes and documents that the patient ingests each dose of medication.

Epidemiology

Case rates of tuberculosis for all ages are higher in urban, low-income areas and in nonwhite ethnic groups; two thirds of reported cases in the United States occur in nonwhite individuals. In recent years, foreign-born children have accounted for more than one quarter of newly diagnosed cases in children 14 years of age or younger. Specific groups with high LTBI and disease rates include immigrants, international adoptees, and refugees from high-prevalence regions (eg, Asia, Africa, Latin America, and countries of the former Soviet Union), travelers to countries with endemic infection, homeless people, and residents of corrections facilities.

Infants and postpubertal adolescents are at increased risk of progression of LTBI to tuberculosis disease. Other predictive factors for development of disease include recent infection (within 2 years); immunodeficiency, including HIV infection; use of immunosuppressive drugs; intravenous drug use; and certain diseases or medical conditions, including Hodgkin disease, lymphoma, diabetes mellitus, chronic renal failure, and malnutrition. There have been reports of tuberculosis disease in adolescents and adults being treated for arthritis with tumor necrosis factor (TNF) antagonists, such as infliximab and etanercept. Before use of TNF antagonists, patients should be screened for risk factors for *M tuberculosis* and have a TST performed.

A diagnosis of LTBI or tuberculosis disease in a young child is a sentinel event usually representing recent transmission of *M tuberculosis.* Transmission of *M tuberculosis* is via inhalation of droplet nuclei usually produced by an adult or adolescent with contagious pulmonary or laryngeal tuberculosis disease. Although contagiousness usually lasts only a few days to weeks after initiation of effective drug therapy, it can last longer, especially when an adult has cavitary disease, does not adhere to medical therapy, or is infected with a drug-resistant strain. If the sputum smear is negative for AFB organisms on 3 separate days and the patient has improved clinically, the treated person can be considered at low risk of disease transmission. Children younger than 10 years with pulmonary tuberculosis rarely are contagious because their pulmonary lesions are small (paucibacillary disease), cough is not productive, and few or no bacilli are expulsed.

Incubation Period

2 to 12 weeks to develop a positive TST; many years can elapse between initial tuberculosis infection and tuberculosis disease.

Diagnostic Tests

Isolation of *M tuberculosis* or *M bovis* by culture from specimens of gastric aspirates, sputum, bronchial washings, pleural fluid, CSF, urine, or other body fluids or a biopsy specimen establishes the diagnosis. Children older than 5 years and adolescents frequently can produce sputum by induction with aerosolized hypertonic saline. The best specimen for diagnosis of pulmonary tuberculosis in any child or adolescent in whom the cough is nonproductive or absent and sputum cannot be induced is an early morning gastric aspirate. Gastric aspirate specimens should be obtained with a nasogastric tube on awakening the child and before ambulation or feeding. Aspirates collected on 3 separate days should be submitted for testing. Results of AFB smears of gastric aspirates usually are negative, and false-positive results caused by the presence of nontuberculous mycobacteria can occur. Gastric aspirates have the highest yield in young children on the first day of collection. The overall diagnostic yield of gastric aspirates is less than 50%. Fluorescent staining methods for gastric aspirate smears are more sensitive and, if available, are preferred. Histologic examination for and demonstration of AFB and granulomas in biopsy specimens from lymph node, pleura, mesentery, liver, bone marrow, or other tissues can be useful, but *M tuberculosis* and *M bovis* cannot reliably be distinguished from other mycobacteria in stained specimens. Regardless of results of the AFB smears, each specimen should be cultured.

Because *M tuberculosis* and *M bovis* are slow growing, detection of these organisms can take as long as 10 weeks using solid media; use of liquid media allows detection within 1 to 6 weeks. Even with optimal culture techniques, *M tuberculosis* organisms are isolated from fewer than 50% of children and 75% of infants with pulmonary tuberculosis diagnosed by clinical criteria. Species identification of isolates by culture can be more rapid if a DNA probe is used. Current nucleic acid assays cannot differentiate between *M tuberculosis* and *M bovis*.

Nucleic acid amplification tests for rapid diagnosis are licensed by the FDA only for acid-fast stain positive respiratory tract specimens but have decreased sensitivity for gastric aspirate, CSF, and tissue specimens, with false-negative and false-positive results reported.

Identification of the culture-positive source case supports the child's presumptive diagnosis and provides the likely drug susceptibility of the child's organism. Ingestion of unpasteurized dairy products support a presumptive diagnosis of *M bovis* infection.

Culture material should be collected from children with evidence of tuberculosis disease, especially when (1) an isolate from a source case is not available; (2) the presumed source case has drug-resistant tuberculosis; (3) the child is immunocompromised, including children with HIV infection; or (4) the child has extrapulmonary disease.

Tuberculin Testing. The TST is the most common method for diagnosing LTBI in asymptomatic people. The Mantoux method consists of 5 tuberculin units of purified protein derivative (0.1 mL) injected intradermally using a 27-gauge needle and a 1.0-mL syringe into the volar aspect of the forearm. Creation of a visible wheal 6 to 10 mm in diameter is crucial to accurate testing. Other strengths of TSTs should not be used. Multiple puncture tests are not recommended because they lack adequate sensitivity and specificity.

A TST should be administered to children who are at increased risk of acquiring LTBI and tuberculosis disease (Table 117.2). Routine TST administration, including programs based at schools, child care centers, and camps that include populations at low risk, is to be discouraged because it results in either a low yield of positive results or a large proportion of false-positive results, leading to an inefficient use of health care resources. Simple questionnaires can identify children with risk factors for LTBI who then should be tested with a TST (Table 117.3). Risk assessment for tuberculosis should be performed at first contact with a child and every 6 months thereafter for the first 2 years of life (eg, 2 weeks and 6, 12, 18, and 24 months of age). If at any time risk of

tuberculosis disease is determined, a TST should be performed, although this test is unreliable in infants younger than 3 months. After 2 years of age, risk assessment for tuberculosis should be performed annually, if possible.

A TST can be administered at the same time as immunizations, including live-virus vaccines, except measles vaccine, which temporarily can suppress tuberculin reactivity. If tuberculin testing is indicated, measles immunization should be deferred until testing is complete or the TST should be deferred for 4 to 6 weeks. Previous immunization with bacille Calmette-Guérin (BCG) vaccine is not a contraindication to TST.

Administration of TSTs and interpretation of results should be performed by experienced health care professionals who have been trained in the proper methods because administration and interpretation by unskilled people and family members are unreliable. The recommended time for assessing the TST result is 48 to 72 hours after administration. The diameter of induration in millimeters is measured transversely to the long axis of the forearm. Positive test results can persist for several weeks.

A negative TST result does not exclude LTBI or tuberculosis disease. Approximately 10% to 15% of immunocompetent children with culture-documented disease do not react initially to a TST. Host factors, such as young age, poor nutrition, immunosuppression, other viral infections (especially measles, varicella, and influenza), recent tuberculosis infection, and disseminated tuberculosis disease can decrease TST reactivity. Many children and adults coinfected with HIV and *M tuberculosis* do not react to a TST. Control skin tests to assess cutaneous anergy are not recommended routinely.

Interpretation of TST Results (Table 117.1). Classification of TST results is based on epidemiologic and clinical factors. The size of induration (millimeters) for a positive result varies with the person's risk of LTBI and progression to tuberculosis disease.

Interpretation of TST Results in Previous Recipients of BCG Vaccine. Generally, interpretation of TST results in BCG recipients is the same as for people who have not received BCG vaccine. After BCG immunization, distinguishing between a positive TST result caused by *M tuberculosis* or *M bovis* infection and that caused by BCG can be difficult. Reactivity of the TST after receipt of BCG vaccine does not occur in some patients. The size of the TST reaction (ie, millimeters of induration) attributable to BCG immunization depends on many factors, including age at BCG immunization, quality and strain of BCG vaccine used, number of doses of BCG received, nutritional and immunologic status of the vaccine recipient, and frequency of TST administration.

Tuberculosis disease should be strongly suspected in any symptomatic person with a positive TST result regardless of history of BCG immunization. When evaluating an asymptomatic child who has a positive TST result and who possibly received BCG, the result should not be attributed to BCG vaccine. Certain factors, such as documented receipt of multiple BCG immunizations (as evidenced by multiple BCG scars), decrease the likelihood that the positive TST result is attributable to LTBI. Evidence that increases the probability that a positive TST result is attributable to LTBI includes known contact with a person with contagious tuberculosis, a family history of tuberculosis disease, emigration from a country with a high prevalence of tuberculosis, a long interval (>5 years) since neonatal BCG immunization, and a TST reaction of 15 mm or larger.

Prompt clinical and radiographic evaluation of all children with a positive TST reaction is recommended. In most circumstances, a history of BCG will not account for the positive result. Chest radiographic findings of a granuloma, calcification, or adenopathy can be caused by *M tuberculosis* but not by BCG immunization. For the child with signs and symptoms consistent with abdominal tuberculosis and a history of ingestion of unpasteurized dairy products, a positive TST and a negative chest radiograph, abdominal imaging by CT with contrast should be considered.

Recommendations for TST Usage. The most reliable strategies for preventing LTBI and tuberculosis disease in children are thorough and expedient contact investigations rather than nonselective skin testing of large populations. All children need routine health care evaluations that include an assessment of their risk of exposure to tuberculosis. Only children deemed to have increased risk of contact with people with contagious tuberculosis or children with suspected tuberculosis disease should be considered for a TST. Household investigation is indicated whenever a TST result of a household member converts from negative to positive (indicating recent infection).

HIV Testing. Children with HIV are considered at high risk of tuberculosis, and an annual TST beginning at 3 to 12 months of age is recommended.

Treatment (Table 117.3)

Specific Drugs. Antituberculosis drugs kill *M tuberculosis* and *M bovis* or inhibit multiplication of the organism, thereby arresting progression of LTBI and preventing most complications of early tuberculosis disease. Chemotherapy does not cause rapid disappearance of already caseous or granulomatous lesions (eg, mediastinal lymphadenitis). For treatment of tuberculosis disease, these drugs must always be used in combination to minimize emergence of drug-resistant strains.

Isoniazid is bactericidal, rapidly absorbed, well tolerated, and penetrates into body fluids, including CSF. Isoniazid is metabolized in the liver and excreted primarily through the kidneys. Hepatotoxic effects are rare in children but can be life threatening. In children and adolescents given recommended doses, peripheral neuritis or seizures caused by inhibition of pyridoxine metabolism are rare, and most do not need pyridoxine supplements. Pyridoxine is recommended for exclusively breastfed infants and for children and adolescents on meat- and milk-deficient diets; children with nutritional deficiencies, including all symptomatic HIV-infected children; and pregnant adolescents and women. For infants and young children, isoniazid tablets can be pulverized.

Rifampin is a bactericidal agent that is absorbed rapidly and penetrates into body fluids, including CSF. Rifampin is metabolized by the liver and can alter the pharmacokinetics and serum concentrations of many other drugs. Hepatotoxic effects, influenza-like symptoms, and pruritus can occur rarely. Rifampin is excreted in bile and urine and can cause an orange color in urine, sweat, and tears and discoloration of soft contact lenses. Rifampin can make oral contraceptives ineffective, so other birth control methods should be adopted when rifampin is administered to sexually active adolescents. For infants and young children, the contents of the capsules can be suspended in wild cherry–flavored syrup or sprinkled on semisoft foods (eg, applesauce). *M tuberculosis* resistant to rifampin is uncommon in the United States. Rifabutin is a suitable alternative to rifampin in children with HIV on highly active antiretroviral therapy that proscribes the use of rifampin; however, experience in children is limited.

Pyrazinamide attains therapeutic CSF concentrations, is detectable in macrophages, is administered orally, and is metabolized by the liver. Administration of pyrazinamide with isoniazid and rifampin allows for 6-month regimens in patients with drug-susceptible tuberculosis. *M bovis* intrinsically is resistant to pyrazinamide, precluding 6-month therapy for this pathogen. Some adolescents and many adults develop arthralgia and hyperuricemia because of inhibition of uric acid excretion. Pyrazinamide must be used with caution in people with underlying liver disease.

Ethambutol is well absorbed after oral administration, diffuses well into tissues, and is excreted in urine. However, concentrations in the CSF are low. Ethambutol is bacteriostatic only, and its primary therapeutic role is to prevent emergence of drug resistance. Because ethambutol can cause reversible or irreversible optic neuritis, recipients should be monitored monthly for visual acuity and red-green color discrimination.

Streptomycin is administered intramuscularly but is available only on a limited basis. When streptomycin is not available, kanamycin, amikacin, or capreomycin are alternatives that can be prescribed for the initial 4 to 8 weeks of therapy.

The less commonly used (ie, second-line) antituberculosis drugs have limited usefulness because of decreased effectiveness and greater toxicity and should be used only in consultation with a specialist.

Therapy for LTBI. Isoniazid given to adults who have LTBI (ie, no clinical or radiographic abnormalities suggesting tuberculosis disease) provides substantial protection (54%–88%) against development of tuberculosis disease for at least 20 years. Among children, efficacy approaches 100% with appropriate adherence to therapy. All infants, children, and adolescents who have a positive TST result but no evidence of tuberculosis disease and who never have received antituberculosis therapy should receive isoniazid unless resistance to isoniazid is suspected (ie, known exposure to a person with isoniazid-resistant tuberculosis) or a specific contraindication exists. Isoniazid in this circumstance is therapeutic and prevents development of disease. A physical examination and chest radiograph should be obtained at the time isoniazid therapy is initiated to exclude tuberculosis disease; if the radiograph is normal, the child remains asymptomatic, and treatment is completed, radiography should not be repeated.

Treatment of Tuberculosis Disease. The goal of treatment is to achieve sterilization of the tuberculous lesion in the shortest possible time. Achievement of this goal minimizes the possibility of development of resistant organisms. The major problem limiting successful treatment is poor adherence to prescribed treatment regimens. The use of DOT decreases the rates of relapse, treatment failures, and drug resistance; therefore DOT is recommended strongly for treatment of children and adolescents with tuberculosis disease in the United States.

For *M tuberculosis* disease, a 6-month regimen consisting of isoniazid, rifampin, and pyrazinamide for the first 2 months and isoniazid and rifampin for the remaining 4 months is recommended for treatment of **drug-susceptible** pulmonary disease, pulmonary disease with hilar adenopathy, and hilar adenopathy disease in infants, children, and adolescents. If the chest radiograph shows a cavitary lesion or lesions and sputum remains culture positive after 2 months of therapy, the duration of therapy should be extended to 9 months.

When **drug resistance** is possible (Table 117.4), initial therapy should include a fourth drug, either ethambutol or an aminoglycoside, until drug susceptibility results are available. Data may not be available for foreign-born children or in circumstances of international travel. If this information is not available, a 4-drug initial regimen is recommended.

Therapy for **M bovis** *disease.* Treatment recommendations for *M bovis* disease in adults and children are based on results from treatment trials for *M tuberculosis* disease. Although all strains of *M bovis* are pyrazinamide resistant, multidrug-resistant strains are rare. As knowledge of culture and susceptibility results rarely are available for children with *M bovis* disease, initial therapy should include 3 or 4 drugs appropriate for *M tuberculosis* disease.

Therapy for Drug-Resistant Tuberculosis Disease. Drug resistance is most common in the following: (1) people born in areas such as Russia and the former Soviet Union, Asia, Africa, and Latin America; (2) people previously treated for tuberculosis disease; and (3) contacts, especially children, with tuberculosis disease whose source case is a person from one of these groups. Most cases of pulmonary tuberculosis in children that are caused by an isoniazid-resistant but rifampin-susceptible strain of *M tuberculosis* can be treated with a 6-month regimen of rifampin, pyrazinamide, and ethambutol. For cases of multidrug-resistant tuberculosis disease, the treatment regimen should include at least 4 antituberculosis drugs to which the organism is susceptible. In cases of tuberculosis

with isoniazid- and rifampin-resistant strains, 12 to 24 months of therapy usually is necessary for cure.

Extrapulmonary **M tuberculosis.** In general, extrapulmonary tuberculosis—with the exception of meningitis—can be treated with the same regimens as used for pulmonary tuberculosis. For suspected drug-susceptible tuberculous meningitis, daily treatment with isoniazid, rifampin, pyrazinamide, and streptomycin or another aminoglycoside or ethionamide should be initiated. When susceptibility to all drugs is established, the aminoglycoside or ethionamide can be discontinued. For life-threatening tuberculosis, 4 drugs are given initially because of the possibility of drug resistance and the severe consequences of treatment failure.

Corticosteroids. The evidence supporting adjuvant treatment with corticosteroids for children with tuberculosis disease is incomplete. Corticosteroids are indicated for children with tuberculous meningitis because they decrease rates of mortality and long-term neurologic impairment. Corticosteroids can be considered for children with pleural and pericardial effusions (to hasten reabsorption of fluid), severe miliary disease (to mitigate alveolocapillary block), endobronchial disease (to relieve obstruction and atelectasis), and abdominal tuberculosis (to decrease the risk of strictures). Corticosteroids should be given only when accompanied by appropriate antituberculosis therapy.

Tuberculosis Disease and HIV Infection. Adults and children with HIV infection have an increased incidence of tuberculosis disease. Hence, *HIV testing is indicated for all people with tuberculosis disease.* The clinical manifestations and radiographic appearance of tuberculosis disease in children with HIV infection tend to be similar to those in immunocompetent children, but manifestations in these children can be more severe and unusual and can include extrapulmonary involvement of multiple organs. In HIV-infected patients, a TST result of 5-mm induration or more is considered positive.

Most HIV-infected adults with drug-susceptible tuberculosis respond well to antituberculosis drugs when appropriate therapy is given early. However, optimal therapy for tuberculosis in children with HIV infection has not been established. Consultation with a specialist who has experience in managing HIV-infected patients with tuberculosis is strongly advised .

Tuberculosis During Pregnancy and Breast-feeding. Asymptomatic pregnant women with a positive TST result, normal chest radiographic findings, and recent contact with a contagious person should receive isoniazid therapy. Therapy in these circumstances should begin after the first trimester. Pyridoxine is indicated for all pregnant and breast-feeding women receiving isoniazid. Isoniazid, ethambutol, and rifampin are relatively safe for the fetus. The benefit of ethambutol and rifampin for therapy of tuberculosis disease in the mother outweighs the risk to the infant. Although isoniazid is secreted in human milk, no adverse effects of isoniazid on nursing infants have been demonstrated.

Congenital Tuberculosis. Women who have only pulmonary tuberculosis are not likely to infect the fetus but can infect their infant after delivery. Congenital tuberculosis is rare, but in utero infections can occur after maternal *M tuberculosis* bacillemia.

- *Management of the Newborn Infant Whose Mother (or Other Household Contact) Has LTBI or Tuberculosis Disease.* Management of the newborn infant is based on categorization of the maternal (or household contact) infection.
- *Mother (or household contact) has a positive TST result and normal chest radiographic findings.* The newborn needs no special evaluation or therapy. Because the positive TST result could be a marker of an unrecognized case of contagious tuberculosis within the household, other household members should have a TST and further evaluation, but this should not delay the infant's discharge from the hospital.

- *Mother (or household contact) has clinical signs and symptoms or abnormal findings on chest radiograph consistent with tuberculosis disease.* If the mother has tuberculosis disease, the infant should be evaluated for congenital tuberculosis and the mother should be tested for HIV infection. The mother (or household contact) and the infant should be separated until the mother (or household contact) has been evaluated and, if tuberculosis disease is suspected, until the mother (or household contact) and infant are receiving appropriate antituberculosis therapy, the mother wears a mask, and the mother understands and is willing to adhere to infection control measures. Once the infant is receiving isoniazid, separation is not necessary unless the mother (or household contact) has possible multidrug-resistant *M tuberculosis* disease or has poor adherence to treatment and DOT is not possible.

If the TST result is positive at 3- to 4-month retesting, the infant should be reassessed for tuberculosis disease. If tuberculosis disease is excluded, isoniazid should be continued. If the TST result is negative and the mother (or household contact) has good adherence and response to treatment and no longer is contagious, isoniazid is discontinued.

Table 117.1

Definitions of Positive Tuberculin Skin Test (TST) Results in Infants, Children, and Adolescents[1,2]

Induration ≥5 mm

Children in close contact with known or suspected contagious people with tuberculosis disease
Children suspected to have tuberculosis disease
• Findings on chest radiograph consistent with active or previous tuberculosis disease
• Clinical evidence of tuberculosis disease[3]
Children receiving immunosuppressive therapy[4] or with immunosuppressive conditions, including HIV infection

Induration ≥10 mm

Children at increased risk of disseminated tuberculosis disease
• Children younger than 4 years
• Children with other medical conditions, including Hodgkin disease, lymphoma, diabetes mellitus, chronic renal failure, or malnutrition (See Table 117.2.)
Children with increased exposure to tuberculosis disease
• Children born in high-prevalence regions of the world
• Children frequently exposed to adults who are HIV infected, homeless, users of illicit drugs, residents of nursing homes, incarcerated or institutionalized, or migrant farmworkers
• Children who travel to high-prevalence regions of the world

Induration ≥15 mm

Children 4 years of age or older without any risk factors

[1] HIV indicates human immunodeficiency virus.
[2] These definitions apply regardless of previous bacille Calmette-Guérin immunization; erythema at TST site does not indicate a positive test result. Tests should be read at 48 to 72 hours after placement.
[3] Evidence by physical examination or laboratory assessment that would include tuberculosis in the working differential diagnosis (eg, meningitis).
[4] Including immunosuppressive doses of corticosteroids.

Table 117.2

Tuberculin Skin Test (TST) Recommendations for Infants, Children, and Adolescents[1,2]

Children for whom immediate TST is indicated[3]
• Contacts of people with confirmed or suspected contagious tuberculosis (contact investigation)
• Children with radiographic or clinical findings suggesting tuberculosis disease
• Children emigrating from countries with endemic infection (eg, Asia, Middle East, Africa, Latin America, countries of the former Soviet Union) including international adoptees
• Children with travel histories to countries with endemic infection and substantial contact with indigenous people from such countries[4]
Children who should have annual TST
• Children infected with HIV
• Incarcerated adolescents
Children at increased risk of progression of LTBI to tuberculosis disease: Children with other medical conditions, including diabetes mellitus, chronic renal failure, malnutrition, and congenital or acquired immunodeficiencies deserve special consideration. Without recent exposure, these people are not at increased risk of acquiring tuberculosis infection. Underlying immune deficiencies associated with these conditions theoretically would enhance the possibility for progression to severe disease. Initial histories of potential exposure to tuberculosis should be included for all of these patients. If these histories or local epidemiologic factors suggest a possibility of exposure, immediate and periodic TST should be considered. **An initial TST should be performed before initiation of immunosuppressive therapy, including prolonged steroid administration, use of tumor necrosis factor-alpha antagonists, or immunosuppressive therapy in any child requiring these treatments.**

[1] HIV indicates human immunodeficiency virus; LTBI, latent tuberculosis infection.
[2] Bacille Calmette-Guérin immunization is not a contraindication to a TST.
[3] Beginning as early as 3 months of age.
[4] If the child is well, the TST should be delayed for up to 10 weeks after return.

Table 117.3

Recommended Treatment Regimens for Drug-Susceptible Tuberculosis in Infants, Children, and Adolescents[1]

Infection or Disease Category	Regimen	Remarks
Latent tuberculosis infection (positive TST result, no disease)		
• Isoniazid susceptible	9 mo of isoniazid, once a day	If daily therapy is not possible, DOT twice a week can be used for 9 mo.
• Isoniazid resistant	6 mo of rifampin, once a day	If daily therapy is not possible, DOT twice a week can be used for 6 mo.
• Isoniazid-rifampin resistant[2]	Consult a tuberculosis specialist	
Pulmonary and extrapulmonary (except meningitis)	2 mo of isoniazid, rifampin, and pyrazinamide daily, followed by 4 mo of isoniazid and rifampin[3] by DOT[4] for drug-susceptible *Mycobacterium tuberculosis* 9–12 mo of isoniazid and rifampin for drug susceptible *Mycobacterium bovis*	If possible drug resistance is a concern (see text), another drug (ethambutol or an aminoglycoside) is added to the initial 3-drug therapy until drug susceptibilities are determined. DOT is highly desirable. If hilar adenopathy only, a 6-mo course of isoniazid and rifampin is sufficient. Drugs can be given 2 or 3 times/wk under DOT in the initial phase if nonadherence is likely.
Meningitis	2 mo of isoniazid, rifampin, pyrazinamide, and an aminoglycoside or ethionamide, once a day, followed by 7–10 mo of isoniazid and rifampin, once a day or twice a week (9–12 mo total) for drug-susceptible *M tuberculosis* At least 12 mo of therapy without pyrazinamide for drug-susceptible *M bovis*	A fourth drug, such as an aminoglycoside, is given with initial therapy until drug susceptibility is known. For patients who may have acquired tuberculosis in geographic areas where resistance to streptomycin is common, kanamycin, amikacin, or capreomycin can be used instead of streptomycin.

[1] TST indicates tuberculin skin test; DOT, directly observed therapy.
[2] Duration of therapy is longer for human immunodeficiency virus–infected people, and additional drugs may be indicated.
[3] Medications should be administered daily for the first 2 weeks to 2 months of treatment and then can be administered 2 to 3 times per week by DOT.
[4] If initial chest radiograph shows cavitary lesions and sputum after 2 months of therapy remains positive, duration of therapy is extended to 9 months.

Table 117.4

People at Increased Risk of Drug-Resistant Tuberculosis Infection or Disease

- People with a history of treatment for tuberculosis disease (or whose source case for the contact received such treatment)
- Contacts of a patient with drug-resistant contagious tuberculosis disease
- People born in countries with high prevalence of drug-resistant tuberculosis
- Infected people whose source case has positive smears for acid-fast bacilli or cultures after 2 months of appropriate antituberculosis therapy

Image 117.1

This photomicrograph reveals *Mycobacterium tuberculosis* using acid-fast Ziehl-Neelsen stain (1000x). The acid-fast stains depend on the ability of mycobacteria to retain dye when treated with mineral acid or an acid-alcohol solution such as the Ziehl-Neelsen or the Kinyoun stains that are carbolfuchsin methods specific for *M tuberculosis*.

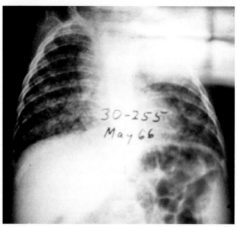

Image 117.2

Tuberculosis, congenital. Miliary lung lesions and striking hepatosplenomegaly. The left upper lobe density is artifactual.

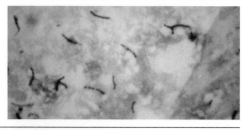

Image 117.3

Tuberculosis, miliary, in a 29-year-old woman 4 months after delivery. Tuberculosis may exacerbate during pregnancy.

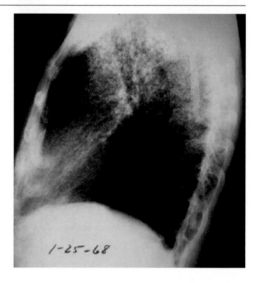

Image 117.4

A: Interpreting the tuberculin skin test by the Sokol ballpoint pen method involves slowly approaching the site of induration using a ball-point or felt-tip pen in the direction perpendicular to the axis on which the test was placed until resistance is felt. The procedure is repeated on the opposite side. B: The distance between the lines where resistance was noted is measured in millimeters. This measures the degree of induration found 48 to 72 hours after application of the test.

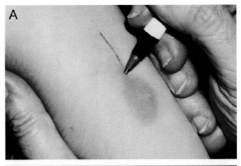

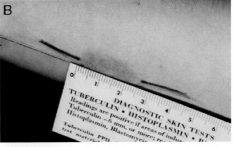

Image 117.5

Young woman with *Mycobacterium tuberculosis* scrofula.

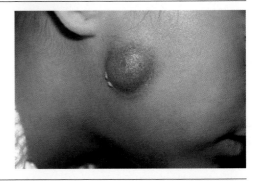

Image 117.6

A 3-month-old infant with tuberculosis. The child had a fever when first examined. Chest radio-graph revealed right upper lobe consolidation. A tuberculin skin test was placed and was positive. *Mycobacterium tuberculosis* grew from gastric aspirate culture.

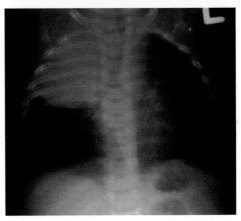

Image 117.7

A 13-year-old male with tuberculosis. The patient had a 1-week history of shortness of breath and sharp pain on his right side while riding his bicycle. A tuberculin skin test revealed 20 by 25 mm of induration at 72 hours. The chest CT scan revealed right hilar adenopathy and a primary complex in the right peripheral lung field.

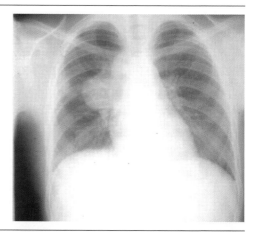

Image 117.8

Miliary tuberculosis with pulmonary cavitation (right lung).

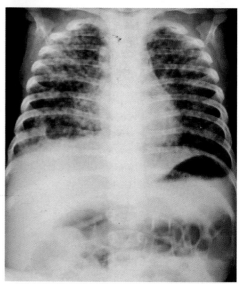

Image 117.9

Tuberculosis of the spine with paravertebral abscess (Pott disease).

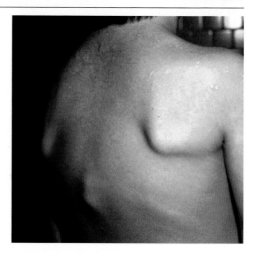

118

Diseases Caused by Nontuberculous Mycobacteria

(Atypical Mycobacteria, Mycobacteria Other Than *Mycobacterium tuberculosis*)

Clinical Manifestations

Several syndromes are caused by nontuberculous mycobacteria (NTM) but in children, the most common is cervical lymphadenitis. Less common infections include cutaneous infection, osteomyelitis, otitis media, central catheter infections, and pulmonary disease. Disseminated infections almost always are associated with impaired cell-mediated immunity, as found in congenital immune defects or HIV infection. Manifestations of disseminated NTM infections depend on the species and route of infection but include fever, night sweats, weight loss, abdominal pain, fatigue, diarrhea, and anemia. NTM, especially *Mycobacterium avium* complex (MAC [including *M avium* and *Mycobacterium intracellulare*]) and *Mycobacterium abscessus*, can be recovered from sputum in 10% to 20% of adolescents and young adults with cystic fibrosis and can be associated with fever and declining clinical and pulmonary function status.

Etiology

Of the almost 100 species of NTM that have been identified, only a few account for most human infections. The species most commonly encountered in infected children in the United States are MAC, *Mycobacterium fortuitum, M abscessus,* and *Mycobacterium marinum* (Table 118.1). NTM disease in patients with HIV infection usually is caused by MAC. *M fortuitum, Mycobacterium chelonae,* and *M abscessus* commonly are referred to as "rapidly growing" mycobacteria because sufficient growth and identification can be achieved in the laboratory within 3 to 7 days. Rapidly growing mycobacteria occasionally have been implicated in wound, soft tissue, bone, pulmonary, central catheter, and middle-ear infections. Other mycobacterial species that usually are not pathogenic have caused infections in immunocompromised hosts or have been associated with the presence of a foreign body.

Epidemiology

Many NTM species are ubiquitous in nature and are found in soil, food, water, and animals. The major reservoir for *Mycobacterium kansasii, Mycobacterium simiae,* and health care–associated infections attributable to the rapidly growing mycobacteria is tap water. For *M marinum,* water in a fish tank or aquarium or an injury in a saltwater environment is the major source of infection. Although many people are exposed to NTM, only a few of these exposures result in chronic infection or disease. The usual portals of entry for NTM infection are believed to be abrasions in the skin (eg, cutaneous lesions caused by *M marinum*), surgical incisions (especially for central catheters), oropharyngeal mucosa (the presumed portal of entry for cervical lymphadenitis), gastrointestinal or respiratory tract for disseminated MAC, and respiratory tract (including tympanostomy tubes for otitis media). Pulmonary disease and rare cases of mediastinal adenitis and endobronchial disease occur. Most infections remain localized at the portal of entry or in regional lymph nodes. Dissemination to distal sites primarily occurs in immunocompromised hosts, especially in people with AIDS. No definitive evidence of person-to-person transmission of NTM exists. Outbreaks of otitis media caused by *M abscessus* have been associated with polyethylene ear tubes and use of contaminated equipment or water. A waterborne route of transmission has been implicated for MAC infection in immunodeficient hosts. Buruli ulcer disease primarily is a skin and bone infection caused by *Mycobacterium ulcerans,* an emerging disease causing significant morbidity and disability in tropical areas, such as Africa, Asia, South America, and the western Pacific.

Incubation Period

Variable.

Diagnostic Tests

Definitive diagnosis of NTM disease requires isolation of the organism. Consultation with the laboratory should be obtained to ensure that culture specimens are handled correctly. Because these organisms commonly are found in the environment, contamination of cultures or transient colonization can occur. Caution must be exercised in the interpretation of cultures obtained from nonsterile sites, such as gastric washing specimens, a single expectorated sputum specimen, or a urine specimen, and if the species cultured usually is nonpathogenic (eg, *Mycobacterium gordonae*). An acid-fast bacillus smear-positive sample or repeated isolation of numerous colonies of a single species on culture media is more likely to indicate disease than culture contamination or transient colonization. Unlike other bacteria, NTM isolates from draining sinus tracts almost always are clinically significant. Recovery of NTM from sites that usually are sterile, such as CSF, pleural fluid, bone marrow, blood, lymph node aspirates, middle ear or mastoid aspirates, or surgically excised tissue, is the most reliable diagnostic method. With radiometric or nonradiometric broth techniques, blood cultures are highly sensitive in recovery of disseminated MAC and other bloodborne NTM species. Disseminated MAC disease should prompt a search for underlying immunodeficiency, usually HIV infection or congenital immune deficiency.

Patients with NTM infection can have a positive tuberculin skin test (TST) result because the purified protein derivative preparation, derived from *Mycobacterium tuberculosis,* shares a number of antigens with NTM species. These TST reactions usually measure less than 10 mm of induration but can measure more than 15 mm.

Treatment

Many NTM are relatively resistant in vitro to antituberculosis drugs. In vitro resistance to these agents, however, does not necessarily correlate with clinical response, especially with MAC infections. The approach to therapy should be dictated by the following: (1) the species causing the infection, (2) the results of drug-susceptibility testing, (3) the site(s) of infection, (4) the patient's underlying disease (if any), and (5) the need to treat a patient presumptively for tuberculosis while awaiting culture reports that subsequently reveal NTM.

For NTM lymphadenitis in otherwise healthy children, especially when the disease is caused by MAC, complete surgical excision almost always is curative. Antituberculosis chemotherapy offers no benefit. Therapy with clarithromycin or azithromycin combined with ethambutol or rifabutin may be beneficial for children in whom surgical excision is incomplete or for children with recurrent disease, but these agents have not been studied in clinical trials (Table 118.2).

M fortuitum, M abscessus, and *M chelonae* commonly are susceptible to amikacin, imipenem, sulfamethoxazole or trimethoprim-sulfamethoxazole, cefoxitin, ciprofloxacin, gatifloxacin, clarithromycin, linezolid, and doxycycline. Clarithromycin and at least one other agent commonly are the treatment of choice for cutaneous (disseminated) infections attributable to *M chelonae* or *M abscessus*. Infected foreign bodies should be removed whenever possible, and surgical debridement for serious localized disease should be considered. The choice of drugs, dosages, and duration should be reviewed with a consultant experienced in the management of NTM infections.

In patients with AIDS and in other immunocompromised people with disseminated MAC infection, multidrug therapy is recommended. Clinical isolates of MAC usually are resistant to many of the approved antituberculosis drugs, including isoniazid, but are susceptible to clarithromycin and azithromycin and often are susceptible to combinations of ethambutol, rifabutin or rifampin, and amikacin or streptomycin. The optimal regimen has yet to be determined. Treatment of disseminated MAC infection should be done in consultation with an expert.

Table 118.1
Diseases Caused by Nontuberculous Mycobacterial Species[1]

Clinical Disease	Common Species	Less Common Species in the United States
Cutaneous infection	M chelonae, M fortuitum, M abscessus, M marinum	M ulcerans[2]
Lymphadenitis	MAC	M kansasii, M fortuitum, M malmoense[3]
Otologic infection	M abscessus	M fortuitum
Pulmonary infection	MAC, M kansasii, M abscessus	M xenopi, M malmoense,[3] M szulgai, M fortuitum, M simiae
Catheter-associated infection	M chelonae, M fortuitum	M abscessus
Skeletal infection	MAC, M kansasii, M fortuitum	M chelonae, M marinum, M abscessus, M ulcerans[2]
Disseminated	MAC	M kansasii, M genavense, M haemophilum, M chelonae

[1] MAC indicates *Mycobacterium avium* complex.
[2] Not endemic in the United States.
[3] Found primarily in northern Europe.

Table 118.2
Treatment of Nontuberculous Mycobacteria Infections in Children[1]

Organism	Disease	Treatment
Slowly Growing Species		
Mycobacterium avium complex (MAC)	Lymphadenitis	Excision of major nodes; if excision incomplete or disease recurs, clarithromycin or azithromycin plus ethambutol with rifampin or rifabutin.
	Pulmonary infection	Clarithromycin or azithromycin plus ethambutol with rifampin or rifabutin (pulmonary resection in some patients who fail drug therapy). For severe disease, an initial course of amikacin or streptomycin often is included.
	Disseminated	See text.
Mycobacterium kansasii	Pulmonary infection	Rifampin plus ethambutol with isoniazid.
	Osteomyelitis	Surgical debridement and prolonged antimicrobial therapy using rifampin plus ethambutol with isoniazid.
Mycobacterium marinum	Cutaneous infection	None, if minor; rifampin, trimethoprim-sulfamethoxazole, clarithromycin, or doxycycline[2] for moderate disease; extensive lesions can require surgical debridement. Susceptibility testing not required.
Mycobacterium ulcerans	Cutaneous and bone infections	Excision of tissue; rifampicin plus streptomycin.

continued

Table 118.2, continued
Treatment of Nontuberculous Mycobacteria Infections in Children[1]

Organism	Disease	Treatment
Rapidly Growing Species		
Mycobacterium fortuitum group	Cutaneous infection	Excision of tissue; initial therapy for serious disease is amikacin plus meropenem, IV, followed by clarithromycin, doxycycline,[2] or trimethoprim-sulfamethoxazole or ciprofloxacin orally based on in vitro susceptibility testing.
	Catheter infection	Catheter removal and amikacin plus meropenem, IV; clarithromycin, trimethoprim-sulfamethoxazole, or ciprofloxacin orally based on in vitro susceptibility testing.
Mycobacterium abscessus	Otitis media	Clarithromycin plus initial course of amikacin plus cefoxitin; may require surgical debridement based on in vitro susceptibility testing (50% are amikacin resistant).
	Pulmonary infection (in cystic fibrosis)	Serious disease, clarithromycin, amikacin, and cefoxitin based on susceptibility testing; may require surgical resection; seek expert advice.
Mycobacterium chelonae	Catheter infection	Catheter removal and tobramycin (initially) plus clarithromycin.
	Disseminated cutaneous infection	Tobramycin and meropenem or linezolid (initially) plus clarithromycin.

[1] IV indicates intravenously.

[2] Doxycycline should not be given to children younger than 8 years unless the benefits of therapy are greater than the risks of dental staining. Only 50% of isolates of *M marinum* are susceptible to doxycycline.

Image 118.1
Atypical mycobacterial tuberculosis (lymphadenitis) with ulceration.

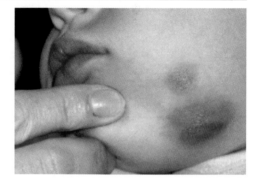

Image 118.2

Disseminated nontuberculous mycobacterial cutaneous lesions in a boy with acute lympho-blastic leukemia.

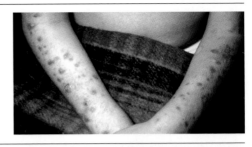

Image 118.3

The same patient as in Image 118.2 with atypical nontuberculous mycobacterial osteomyelitis of the right middle finger.

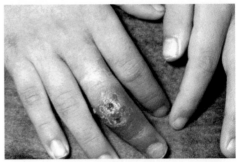

Image 118.4

Mycobacterium avium-intracellulare infection of lymph node in patient with AIDS (Ziehl-Neelsen stain). Histopathology of lymph node shows tremendous numbers of acid-fast bacilli within plump histiocytes.

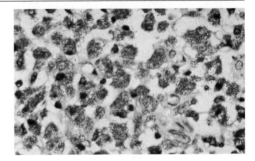

119

Tularemia

Clinical Manifestations

Most patients with tularemia experience abrupt onset of fever, chills, myalgia, and headache. Illness usually conforms to one of the several tularemic syndromes. Most common is the ulceroglandular syndrome, characterized by a painful, maculopapular lesion at the entry site, with subsequent ulceration and slow healing associated with painful, acutely inflamed regional lymph nodes, which can drain spontaneously. The glandular syndrome (regional lymphadenopathy with no ulcer) also is common. Less common disease syndromes are oculoglandular (severe conjunctivitis and preauricular lymphadenopathy), oropharyngeal (severe exudative stomatitis, pharyngitis, or tonsillitis and cervical lymphadenopathy), typhoidal (high fever, hepatomegaly, and splenomegaly), intestinal (intestinal pain, vomiting, and diarrhea), and pneumonic. Pneumonic tularemia, characterized by fever, dry cough, chest pain, and hilar adenopathy, would be the typical syndrome after intentional aerosol release of organisms.

Etiology

Francisella tularensis, the causative agent, is a gram-negative pleomorphic coccobacillus.

Epidemiology

Sources of the organism include approximately 100 species of wild mammals (eg, rabbits, hares, prairie dogs, and muskrats, rats, voles and other rodents), at least 9 species of domestic animals (eg, sheep, cattle, and cats), bloodsucking arthropods that bite these animals (eg, ticks and deerflies), and water and soil contaminated by infected animals. In the United States, ticks and rabbits are major sources of human infection. Infected animals and arthropods, especially ticks, are infective for prolonged periods; frozen rabbits can remain infective for more than 3 years. People at risk are people with occupational or recreational exposure to infected animals or their habitats, such as rabbit hunters and trappers, people exposed to certain ticks or biting insects, and laboratory technicians working with *F tularensis,* which is highly infectious

and easily aerosolized when grown in culture. In the United States, the average annual incidence is highest in males and in people 5 to 9 years of age or older than 54 years. Since 2000, when tularemia became a nationally notifiable disease, there have been 34 to 142 cases reported per year. Ticks are the most important arthropod vectors, and most cases occur during late spring and summer months. Infection also can be acquired by direct contact with infected animals, ingestion of contaminated water or inadequately cooked meat, or inhalation of aerosolized organisms or contaminated particles related to lawn mowing, brush cutting, piling contaminated hay, or bioterrorism. Person-to-person transmission does not occur. Organisms can be present in blood during the first 2 weeks of disease and in cutaneous lesions for as long as 1 month if untreated.

Incubation Period

Usually 3 to 5 days (range, 1–21 days).

Diagnostic Tests

Diagnosis is established most often by serologic testing. A single serum antibody titer of 1:128 or higher determined by microagglutination (MA) or of 1:160 or higher determined by tube agglutination (TA) is consistent with recent or past infection and constitutes a presumptive diagnosis. Confirmation by serologic testing requires a 4-fold or greater titer change between 2 sera obtained at least 2 weeks apart, with one of the specimens having a minimum titer of 1:128 or higher (MA) or 1:160 or higher (TA). Slide agglutination tests are less reliable than TA tests. Nonspecific cross-reactions can occur with specimens containing heterophil antibodies or antibodies to *Brucella* species, *Legionella* species, or other gram-negative bacteria. However, cross-reactions rarely result in MA or TA titers that are diagnostic. Some clinical laboratories identify presumptively *F tularensis* in ulcer exudate or aspirate material by direct fluorescent antibody or PCR assays. Suspect growth on culture can be identified presumptively by direct fluorescent antibody, PCR, or rapid slide agglutination tests. Isolation of *F tularensis* from specimens of blood, skin, ulcers, lymph node drainage, gastric washings, or respiratory tract secretions is best achieved by inoculation of cysteine-enriched media. Because of its propensity for causing laboratory-acquired infections, laboratory personnel should be alerted to the suspicion of *F tularensis*.

Treatment

Streptomycin, gentamicin, or amikacin are recommended for treatment of tularemia. A prolonged course is required for severe illness. Alternative drugs for less severe disease include ciprofloxacin (which is approved only for specific indications in patients younger than 18 years), imipenem-cilastatin, doxycycline (which should not be given to children younger than 8 years unless the benefits of therapy are greater than the risks of dental staining), and chloramphenicol. These drugs are associated with prompt clinical response, but relapses have been reported after treatment with tetracyclines.

Image 119.1
Tularemic ulcer on the thumb. Irregular ulceration occurred at the site of entry of *Francisella tularensis*.

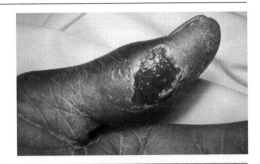

Image 119.2
Tularemic ulcer on the shoulder. Tularemia has been reported in all states except Hawaii.

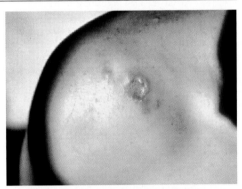

Image 119.3
Tularemia is a relatively rare infection that can manifest with painful adenitis.

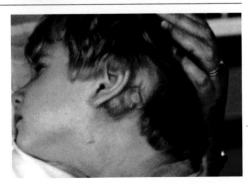

Image 119.4

Tularemia pneumonia. Posterior-anterior chest radiograph shows pleural effusion and pneumonia in the lower lobe of the right lung; the pneumonia was unresponsive to ceftriaxone, azithromycin, and nafcillin. The patient had a history of tick bite and a high fever for 8 days, and his tularemia agglutinin titer was 1:2048. An outbreak of pneumonic tularemia should prompt consideration of bioterrorism.

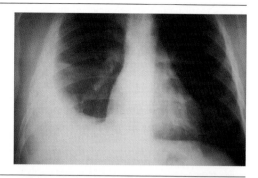

Image 119.5

A tularemic lesion on the dorsal skin of the right hand.

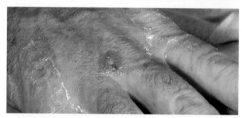

Image 119.6

This is a typical muskrat house camouflaged by reeds in Little Otter Creek, VT. The muskrat is a carrier of the bacterium *Francisella tularensis,* which is considered to be a dangerous potential biological weapon because of its extreme infectivity, ease of dissemination, and substantial capacity to cause illness and death.

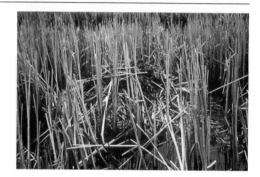

120

Endemic Typhus

(Flea-borne Typhus or Murine Typhus)

Clinical Manifestations

Flea-borne typhus resembles epidemic (louse-borne) typhus but usually has a less abrupt onset with less severe systemic symptoms. In young children, the disease can be mild. Fever can be accompanied by persistent headache and myalgias. A rash typically appears on day 4 to 7 of illness, is macular or maculopapular, lasts 4 to 8 days, and tends to remain discrete, with sparse lesions and no hemorrhage. Illness seldom lasts longer than 2 weeks; visceral involvement is uncommon, but untreated severe disease can be fatal.

Etiology

Flea-borne typhus is caused by *Rickettsia typhi*.

Epidemiology

Rats, in which infection is inapparent, are the natural reservoirs. Opossums and domestic cats and dogs also can be infected and serve as hosts. The vector for transmission among rats and to humans is a rat flea (usually *Xenopsylla cheopis*). Infected flea feces are rubbed into broken skin or mucous membranes or inhaled. The disease is worldwide in distribution and tends to occur most commonly in adults, in males, and during the months of April to October. Endemic typhus is rare in the United States, with most cases occurring in southern California, southern Texas, the southeastern Gulf Coast, and Hawaii. Since 2002 an increased number of cases have been reported from Hawaii. Exposure to rats and their fleas is the major risk factor for infection, although a history of such exposure often is absent. In some regions, peridomestic cycles involving cats, dogs, opossums, and their fleas may exist.

Incubation Period

6 to 14 days.

Diagnostic Tests

Antibody titers determined by an indirect fluorescent antibody test, enzyme immunoassay, latex agglutination test, or complement fixation test peak around 4 weeks after infection. A 4-fold titer change between acute and convalescent serum specimens taken 2 to 3 weeks apart is diagnostic, and immunoassays specific for IgM antibody may aid in confirmation of clinical diagnoses. However, some serologic tests may not reliably differentiate murine typhus from epidemic (louse-borne) typhus without antibody cross-absorption tests, which are not available routinely. Isolation of the organism in culture potentially is hazardous and requires use of specialized laboratories. Molecular diagnostic assays on infected whole blood and skin biopsies can distinguish murine and epidemic typhus reliably and are performed at the CDC.

Treatment

Doxycycline administered intravenously or orally is the treatment of choice. Despite concerns regarding dental staining after the use of tetracyclines in young children, doxycycline provides superior therapy for this potentially severe or life-threatening disease.

Image 120.1
A Norway rat *(Rattus norvegicus)* in a Kansas City, MO, corn storage bin. *R norvegicus* is known to be a reservoir of bubonic plague, endemic typhus fever, and rat-bite fever.

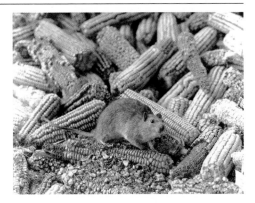

121

Epidemic Typhus
(Louse-borne Typhus)

Clinical Manifestations

Epidemic (louse-borne) typhus is characterized by abrupt onset of high fever, chills, and myalgias accompanied by severe headache and malaise. Influenza illness commonly is suspected. A rash appears 4 to 7 days after illness onset, beginning on the trunk and spreading to the limbs. A concentrated eruption can be present in the axillae. The rash typically is maculopapular, becomes petechial or hemorrhagic, then develops into brownish pigmented areas. The face, palms, and soles usually are not affected. Changes in mental status are common, and delirium or coma can occur. Myocardial and renal failure can occur when the disease is severe. The fatality rate in untreated people is as high as 30%, is less common in children, and increases with advancing age. Untreated patients who recover typically have an illness lasting 2 weeks. Brill-Zinsser disease is a relapse of epidemic typhus that occurs years after the initial episode. Factors that reactivate the rickettsiae are unknown. The recrudescent illness is similar to the primary infection but can be milder and of shorter duration.

Etiology

Epidemic typhus is caused by *Rickettsia prowazekii.*

Epidemiology

Humans are the usual reservoir of the organism, which is transmitted from person-to-person by the human body louse, *Pediculus humanus* subsp *corporis.* Infected louse feces are rubbed into broken skin or mucous membranes or inhaled. All ages are affected. Poverty, crowding, poor sanitary conditions, and poor personal hygiene contribute to the spread of lice and, hence, the disease. Currently cases of epidemic typhus are rare in the United States but have occurred throughout the world, including Asia, Africa, some parts of Europe, and Central and South America. Typhus is most common during winter when conditions favor person-to-person transmission of the vector, the body louse. Rickettsiae are present in the blood and tissues of patients during the early febrile phase but are not found in secretions. Direct person-to-person spread of the disease does not occur in the absence of the louse vector. In the United States, sporadic human cases associated with contact with infected flying squirrels, their nests, or their ectoparasites are occasionally reported. Flying squirrel-related disease typically presents as a milder illness.

Incubation Period

1 to 2 weeks.

Diagnostic Tests

R prowazekii can be isolated from acute blood specimens by animal passage or through tissue culture but these methods can be hazardous. Definitive diagnosis requires immunohistochemical visualization of rickettsiae in tissues, isolation of the organism, detection of the DNA of rickettsiae by PCR assay, or testing of paired serum specimens obtained during the acute and convalescent phases of disease. The indirect fluorescent antibody test is the preferred serologic assay, but enzyme immunoassay, dot immunoassay, and latex agglutination testing also are available. A 4-fold change in antibody titer between acute and convalescent serum specimens taken 2 to 3 weeks apart is diagnostic. Specific molecular assays, isolation, and an immunohistochemical assay for *R prowazekii* in formalin-fixed tissue specimens are available at the CDC.

Treatment

Doxycycline given intravenously or orally is the treatment of choice for epidemic typhus. Children weighing more than 45 kg would receive a standard adult dose of doxycycline. Severe disease can require a longer course of treatment. Despite concerns regarding dental staining after use of a tetracycline-class antimicrobial agent in children 8 years of age or younger, doxycycline provides superior therapy for this potentially life-threatening disease. In people who are intolerant of tetracyclines, intravenous chloramphenicol or fluoroquinolones can be considered. Fluoroquinolones are not approved for this indication in children younger than 18 years, but if illness is life-threatening, the benefit may outweigh potential risks. To halt the spread of disease to other people, louse-infested patients should be treated with cream or gel pediculicides containing pyrethrins (0.16%–0.33%), piperonyl butoxide (2%–4%), crotamiton (10%), or lindane (1%). In epidemic situations in which antimicrobial agents may be limited (eg, refugee camps), a single dose of doxycycline may provide effective treatment. Precautions should be taken to delouse hospitalized patients with louse infestations.

Image 121.1
An adult female body louse *(Pediculus humanus)* and 2 larval young that serve as the vector of epidemic typhus.

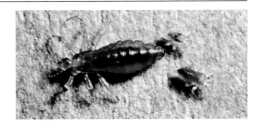

122

Varicella-Zoster Infections

Clinical Manifestations

Primary infection results in varicella (chickenpox), manifesting as a generalized, pruritic, vesicular rash typically consisting of 250 to 500 lesions, mild fever, and other systemic symptoms. Complications include bacterial superinfection of skin lesions, pneumonia, CNS involvement (acute cerebellar ataxia, encephalitis), thrombocytopenia, and other rare complications such as glomerulonephritis, arthritis, and hepatitis. Varicella tends to be more severe in adolescents and adults than in young children. Reye syndrome can follow cases of chickenpox, although the incidence of Reye syndrome has decreased dramatically with decreased use of salicylates during varicella or influenza-like illnesses. In immunocompromised children, progressive severe varicella characterized by continuing eruption of lesions and high fever persisting into the second week of illness as well as encephalitis, hepatitis, and pneumonia can develop. Hemorrhagic varicella is more common among immunocompromised patients than immunocompetent hosts. Pneumonia is relatively less common among immunocompetent children but is the most common complication in adults. In children with HIV infection, recurrent varicella or disseminated herpes zoster can develop. Severe and even fatal varicella has been reported in otherwise healthy children receiving intermittent courses of high-dose corticosteroids for treatment of asthma and other illnesses. The risk is especially high when corticosteroids are given during the incubation period for chickenpox.

The virus establishes latency in the dorsal root ganglia during primary infection. Reactivation results in herpes zoster ("shingles"). Grouped vesicular lesions appear in the distribution of 1 to 3 sensory dermatomes, sometimes accompanied by pain localized to the area. *Postherpetic neuralgia* is defined as pain that persists after resolution of the rash. Zoster occasionally can become disseminated in immunocompromised patients, with lesions appearing outside the primary dermatomes and with visceral complications.

Fetal infection after maternal varicella during the first or early second trimester of pregnancy occasionally results in fetal death or varicella embryopathy, characterized by limb hypoplasia, cutaneous scarring, eye abnormalities, and damage to the CNS (the congenital varicella syndrome). The incidence of congenital varicella syndrome among infants born to mothers with varicella is approximately 1% to 2% when infection occurs before 20 weeks of gestation. Children exposed to varicella-zoster virus (VZV) in utero during the second 20 weeks of pregnancy can develop inapparent varicella and subsequent zoster early in life without having had extrauterine varicella. Varicella infection can be fatal for an infant if the mother develops varicella from 5 days before to 2 days after delivery. When varicella develops in a mother more than 5 days before delivery and gestational age is 28 weeks or more, the severity of disease in the newborn infant is modified by transplacental transfer of VZV-specific maternal IgG antibody.

Etiology

VZV is a member of the herpesvirus family.

Epidemiology

Humans are the only source of infection for this highly contagious virus. Humans are infected when the virus comes in contact with the mucosa of the upper respiratory tract or the conjunctiva. Person-to-person transmission occurs by direct contact with patients with varicella or zoster or by airborne spread from respiratory tract secretions and, rarely, from zoster lesions. In utero infection also can occur as a result of transplacental passage of virus during maternal varicella infection. VZV infection in a household member usually results in infection of almost all susceptible people in that household. Children who acquire their infection at home (secondary family cases) can have more pox lesions than the index case. Health care transmission is well documented in pediatric units, but transmission is rare in newborn nurseries.

In temperate climates, varicella is a childhood disease with a marked seasonal distribution with peak incidence during late winter and early spring. In tropical climates, the epidemiology of varicella is different; acquisition of disease occurs at later ages, resulting in a higher proportion of adults being susceptible to varicella compared with adults in temperate climates. In the prevaccine era, most cases of varicella in the United States occurred in children younger than 10 years. With implementation of universal immunization, a greater number of cases are occurring among adolescents and adults, although the overall incidence in this age group has been greatly reduced. Immunity generally is lifelong. Cellular immunity is more important than humoral immunity for limiting the extent of primary infection with VZV and for preventing reactivation of virus with herpes zoster. Symptomatic reinfection is uncommon in immunocompetent people, although asymptomatic reinfection occurs. Asymptomatic primary infection is unusual, but because some cases are mild, they may not be recognized.

In 2003, 85% of 19- to 35-month-old children in the United States had received 1 dose of varicella vaccine. As vaccine coverage increases and the incidence of wild-type varicella decreases, a greater number of varicella cases are occurring in immunized people as breakthrough disease. This should not be confused as an increasing rate of breakthrough disease or as evidence of increasing vaccine failure. In these surveillance areas with high vaccine coverage, the rate of varicella disease decreased by approximately 85% from 1995 to 2003 with use of varicella vaccine.

Immunocompromised people with primary (varicella) or recurrent (zoster) infection are at increased risk of severe disease. Disseminated varicella and zoster are more likely to develop in children with congenital T-lymphocyte defects or AIDS than in people with B-lymphocyte abnormalities. Other groups of pediatric patients who may experience more severe or complicated disease

include infants, adolescents, patients with chronic cutaneous or pulmonary disorders, and patients receiving systemic corticosteroids or long-term salicylate therapy. Patients are most contagious from 1 to 2 days before to shortly after onset of the rash. Contagiousness persists until crusting of all lesions.

Incubation Period

Usually 14 to 16 days (range, 10–21 days). It can be up to 28 days after receipt of VZIG or IGIV.

Diagnostic Tests

Diagnostic tests for VZV are summarized in Table 122.1. Vesicular fluid or a scab can be used to identify VZV using PCR. VZV also can be isolated from scrapings of a vesicle base during the first 3 to 4 days of the eruption but rarely from other sites, including respiratory tract secretions. Rapid diagnostic tests (PCR, direct fluorescent antibody) are the methods of choice. A significant increase in serum varicella IgG antibody from acute and convalescent samples by any standard serologic assay can confirm a diagnosis retrospectively. These antibody tests are reliable for determining immune status in healthy hosts after natural infection but may not be reliable in immunocompromised people. Commercially available tests are not sufficiently sensitive to demonstrate reliably a vaccine-induced antibody response. IgM tests are not reliable for routine confirmation of acute infection, but positive results indicate current or recent VZV activity.

Treatment

The decision to use antiviral therapy and the route and duration of therapy should be determined by specific host factors, extent of infection, and initial response to therapy. Antiviral drugs have a limited window of opportunity to affect the outcome of varicella-zoster infection. In immunocompetent hosts, most virus replication has stopped by 72 hours after onset of rash; the duration of replication can be extended in immunocompromised hosts. Oral acyclovir is not recommended for routine use in otherwise healthy children with varicella. Administration within 24 hours of onset of rash results in only a modest decrease in symptoms. Oral acyclovir should be consid-

Table 122.1
Diagnostic Tests for Varicella-Zoster Virus (VZV) Infection[1]

Test	Specimen	Comments
Tissue culture	Vesicular fluid, CSF, biopsy tissue	Distinguish VZV from HSV. Cost, limited availability, requires up to a week for result.
PCR	Vesicular swabs or scrapings; scabs from crusted lesions; biopsy tissue, CSF	Very sensitive method. Specific for VZV. Real-time methods (not widely available) have been designed that distinguish vaccine strain from wild-type (rapid, within 3 hours). Requires special equipment.
DFA	Vesicle scraping; swab of lesion base (must include cells)	Specific for VZV. More rapid and more sensitive than culture, less sensitive than PCR.
Tzanck smear	Vesicle scraping; swab of lesion base (must include cells)	Observe multinucleated giant cells with inclusions. Not specific for VZV. Less sensitive and accurate than DFA.
EIA	Acute and convalescent serum specimens for IgG	Specific for VZV. Requires special equipment. May not be sensitive enough to identify vaccine-induced immunity.
LA	Acute and convalescent serum specimens for IgG	Specific for VZV. Rapid (15 min); no special equipment needed. More sensitive but less specific than EIA. Can produce false-positive results. May not be sensitive enough to identify vaccine-induced immunity.
IFA	Acute and convalescent serum specimens for IgG	Specific for VZV. Requires special equipment. Good sensitivity, specificity. May not be sensitive enough to identify vaccine-induced immunity.
gpELISA	Acute and convalescent serum specimens for IgG	Specific for VZV. Highly specific and sensitive but not widely available. Suitable for the evaluation of vaccine seroconversion.
FAMA	Acute and convalescent serum specimens for IgG	Specific for VZV. Highly specific and sensitive but not widely available. Suitable for the evaluation of vaccine seroconversion.
CF	Acute and convalescent serum specimens for IgG	Specific for VZV. Poor sensitivity. Cumbersome to perform.
Capture IgM	Acute serum specimens for IgM	Specific for VZV. IgM consistently detected. Not reliable method for routine confirmation but positive result indicates current/recent VZV activity. Requires special equipment.

[1] CSF indicates cerebrospinal fluid; HSV, herpes simplex virus; PCR, polymerase chain reaction; DFA, direct fluorescent antibody; EIA, enzyme immunoassay; IgG, immunoglobulin G; LA, latex agglutination; IFA, immunofluorescent antibody; gpELISA, glycoprotein-based enzyme-linked immunosorbent assay; FAMA, fluorescent antibody to membrane antigen; CF, complement fixation.

ered for otherwise healthy people at increased risk of moderate to severe varicella, such as people older than 12 years, people with chronic cutaneous or pulmonary disorders, people receiving long-term salicylate therapy, and people receiving short, intermittent, or aerosolized courses of corticosteroids. Some experts also recommend use of oral acyclovir for secondary household cases in which the disease usually is more severe than in the primary case.

Acyclovir is a Category B drug based on FDA drug risk classification in pregnancy. Some experts recommend oral acyclovir for pregnant women with varicella, especially during the second and third trimesters. Intravenous acyclovir is recommended for the pregnant patient with serious complications of varicella. IGIV can be used during pregnancy for susceptible women who are exposed to VZV.

Intravenous antiviral therapy is recommended for immunocompromised patients, including patients being treated with chronic corticosteroids. Therapy initiated early in the course of the illness, especially within 24 hours of rash onset, maximizes efficacy. Oral acyclovir should not be used to treat immunocompromised children with varicella because of poor oral bioavailability. However, some experts have used high-dose oral acyclovir in selected immunocompromised patients perceived to be at lower risk of developing severe varicella, such as HIV-infected patients with relatively normal concentrations of CD4+ T-lymphocytes and children with leukemia in whom careful follow-up is ensured. Although VZIG or, if not available, IGIV given shortly after

exposure can prevent or modify the course of disease, immune globulin preparations are not effective once disease is established.

Famciclovir and valacyclovir have been licensed for treatment of zoster in adults. No pediatric formulation is available for either medication, and insufficient data exist on the use or dose of these drugs in children to support therapeutic recommendations. Children with varicella should not receive salicylates or salicylate-containing products because administration of salicylates to such children increases the risk of Reye syndrome. Acetaminophen can be used for control of fever.

Image 122.1
Congenital varicella with short-limb syndrome and scarring of the skin. The mother had varicella during the first trimester of pregnancy.

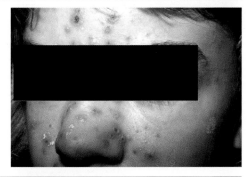

Image 122.2
Adolescent white female with varicella lesions in various stages.

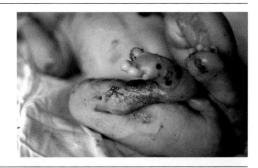

Image 122.3
Varicella with scleral lesions and bulbar conjunctivitis.

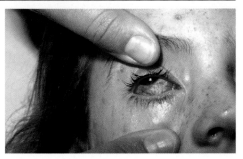

Image 122.4
Adolescent female with varicella lesions in various stages.

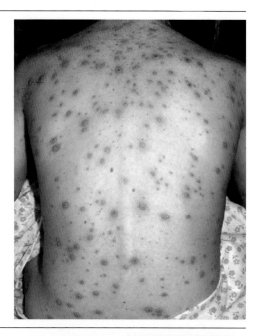

Image 122.5
Hemorrhagic varicella in a 6-year-old white male with eczema.

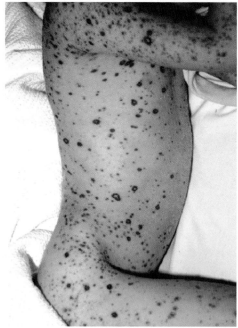

Image 122.6

Diffuse varicella pneumonia bilaterally in the chest radiograph of a patient with Hodgkin disease.

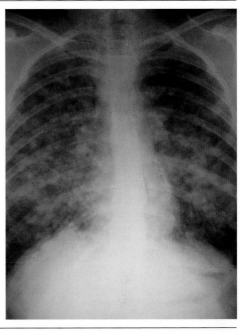

Image 122.7

Varicella and necrotizing fascitis. The blood culture grew group A streptococcus. The disease responded to antibiotics and surgical debridement followed by primary surgical closure.

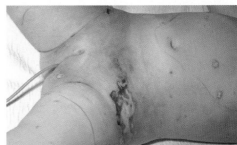

Image 122.8

Bilateral varicella pneumonia in a child with leukemia.

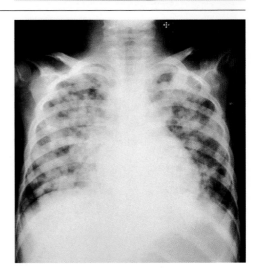

Image 122.9

Herpes zoster in an otherwise healthy child.

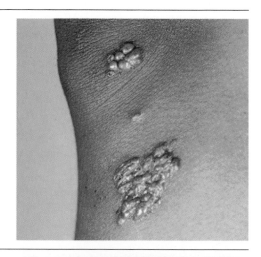

Image 122.10

Varicella-zoster in a 7-year-old girl. The patient had an erythematous vesicular skin rash on the face on first examination. The dermatologic distribution suggested the diagnosis of herpes zoster. This image was taken 3 days after acyclovir therapy was initiated. The lesions are crusting. The child had no prior history of recurring infections and was growing well.

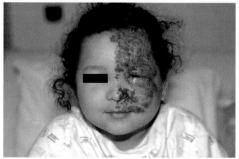

123
Vibrio cholerae Infections

Clinical Manifestations

Cholera is characterized by painless voluminous diarrhea without abdominal cramps or fever. Dehydration, hypokalemia, metabolic acidosis and, occasionally, hypovolemic shock can occur in 4 to 12 hours if fluid losses are not replaced. Coma, seizures, hypoglycemia, and death also can occur, particularly in children. Stools are colorless, with small flecks of mucus ("rice-water"), and contain high concentrations of sodium, potassium, chloride, and bicarbonate. Most infected people with toxigenic *Vibrio cholerae* O1 have no symptoms, and some have only mild to moderate diarrhea lasting 3 to 7 days; fewer than 5% have severe watery diarrhea, vomiting, and dehydration (cholera gravis).

Etiology

V cholerae is a gram-negative, curved, motile bacillus with many serogroups. Only serogroups O1, O139, and O141 cause clinical cholera associated with enterotoxin. There are 3 serotypes of *V cholerae* O1: Inaba, Ogawa, and Hikojima. The 2 biotypes of *V cholerae* are classical and El Tor. El Tor is more commonly observed. Since 1992 toxigenic *V cholerae* serogroup O139 has been recognized as a cause of cholera. Nontoxigenic strains of *V cholerae* O1 and serogroups other than O1 and O139 can cause sporadic diarrheal illness, but they do not cause epidemics.

Epidemiology

During the last 5 decades, *V cholerae* O1 biotype El Tor has spread from India and Southeast Asia to Africa, the Middle East, southern Europe, and the western Pacific Islands (Oceania). In 1991 epidemic cholera caused by toxigenic *V cholerae* O1, serotype Inaba, biotype El Tor, appeared in Peru and spread to most countries in South and North America. In the United States, cases resulting from travel to or ingestion of contaminated food transported from Latin America or Asia have been reported. In addition, the Gulf Coast of Louisiana and Texas has an endemic focus of a

unique strain of toxigenic *V cholerae* O1. Most cases of disease from this strain have resulted from consumption of raw or undercooked shellfish.

Humans are the only documented natural host, but free-living *V cholerae* organisms can exist in the aquatic environment. The usual mode of infection is ingestion of large numbers of organisms from contaminated water or food (particularly raw or undercooked shellfish, raw or partially dried fish, or moist grains or vegetables held at ambient temperature). Direct person-to-person spread has not been documented. People with low gastric acidity are at increased risk of cholera infection.

Incubation Period

Usually 1 to 3 days (range, a few hours–5 days).

Diagnostic Tests

V cholerae can be cultured from fecal specimens or vomitus plated on thiosulfate citrate bile salts sucrose agar. Because most laboratories in the United States do not routinely culture for *V cholerae* or other *Vibrio* organisms, clinicians should request appropriate cultures for clinically suspected cases. Isolates of *V cholerae* should be sent to a state health department laboratory for serogrouping. A 4-fold increase in vibriocidal antibody titers between acute and convalescent serum specimens or a 4-fold decrease in vibriocidal titers available through CDC laboratories between early and late convalescent (more than a 2-month interval) serum specimens can confirm the diagnosis.

Treatment

Oral or parenteral rehydration therapy to correct dehydration and electrolyte abnormalities is the most important modality of therapy and should be initiated as soon as the diagnosis is suspected. Oral rehydration is preferred unless the patient is in shock, is obtunded, or has intestinal ileus. The WHO Oral Rehydration Solution (ORS) has been the standard, but data suggest that rice-based ORS or amylase-resistant starch ORS is more effective.

Antimicrobial therapy results in prompt eradication of vibrios, decreases the duration of diarrhea, and decreases fluid losses. Antimicrobial therapy should be considered for people who are moderately to severely ill. Oral doxycycline or tetracycline is the drug of choice for cholera. Although tetracyclines generally are not recommended for children younger than 8 years, in cases of severe chol-

era, the benefits may outweigh the small risk of staining of developing teeth. If strains are resistant to tetracyclines, ciproflaxin, ofloxacin, or trimethoprim-sulfamethoxazole can be used. Susceptibility of *V cholerae* O139 has changed in recent years; most isolates now are susceptible to trimethoprim-sulfamethoxazole. Antimicrobial susceptibility testing of newly isolated organisms should be determined.

Image 123.1

Typical *Vibrio cholerae*–contaminated water supply. Ingestion of *V cholerae*–contaminated water is a typical mode of pathogen transmission.

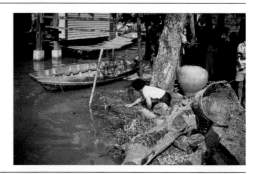

Image 123.2

Adult cholera patient with "washer woman's hand" sign. Due to severe dehydration, cholera manifests itself in decreased skin turgor, which produces the "washer woman's hand" sign.

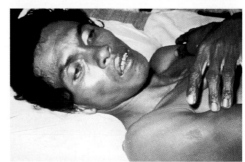

Image 123.3

Here, a cup of typical "rice-water" stool from a cholera patient shows flecks of mucus that have settled to the bottom. These stools are inoffensive, with a faint fishy odor. They are isotonic with plasma and contain high levels of sodium, potassium, and bicarbonate. They also contain extraordinary quantities of *Vibrio cholerae* bacterial organisms.

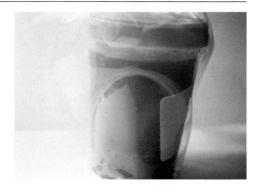

124

West Nile Virus

Clinical Manifestations

Most infections attributable to West Nile virus (WNV) are asymptomatic. Approximately 20% of infected people will develop a self-limited febrile illness called West Nile fever (WNF), and fewer than 1% will develop neuroinvasive disease, such as aseptic meningitis, encephalitis, or flaccid paralysis. The risk of neuroinvasive disease increases with age and is highest among adults older than 60 years. Patients with WNF typically have an abrupt onset of fever, headache, myalgia, weakness and, often, abdominal pain, nausea, vomiting, or diarrhea. Some patients have a transient maculopapular rash. The acute phase of illness usually resolves within several days, but fatigue, malaise, and weakness can linger for weeks. Patients with neuroinvasive disease can present with neck stiffness and headache typical of aseptic meningitis, mental status changes indicating encephalitis, movement disorders such as tremor or Parkinsonism, seizures, or acute flaccid paralysis with or without meningitis or encephalitis. Isolated limb paralysis can occur without fever or apparent viral prodrome. Flaccid paralysis caused by WNV infection is similar clinically and pathologically to poliomyelitis, with damage of anterior horn cells, and can progress to respiratory muscle paralysis requiring mechanical ventilation. Guillain-Barré syndrome also may occur after WNV infection and can be distinguished from anterior horn cell damage by clinical manifestations and electrophysiologic testing. Cardiac dysrhythmias, myocarditis, rhabdomyolysis, optic neuritis, uveitis, chorioretinitis, orchitis, pancreatitis, and hepatitis have been described rarely after WNV infection.

Most women known to have been infected with WNV during pregnancy have delivered infants without evidence of infection or clinical abnormalities. In the single known instance of confirmed congenital WNV infection, the mother developed WNV encephalitis during the 27th week of gestation, and the infant was born with cystic destruction of cerebral tissue and chorioretinitis. One infant who apparently acquired WNV infection from human milk remained asymptomatic.

Etiology

WNV is an RNA flavivirus that is related antigenically to St Louis and Japanese encephalitis viruses.

Epidemiology

WNV is transmitted to humans primarily through the bite of infected mosquitoes. The predominant vectors worldwide are *Culex* mosquitoes, which tend to feed most avidly at dawn and dusk and breed mostly in either peridomestic standing water with high organic content or pools created by irrigation or rainfall. Mosquitoes acquire the virus by feeding on infected birds and then transmit the virus to humans and other mammals during subsequent feeding. Viremia usually lasts fewer than 7 days in immunocompetent people, and viral concentrations in human blood are too low to effectively infect mosquitoes. However, WNV can be transmitted through transfusion of infected blood and through organ transplantation. Percutaneous and aerosol infection has occurred in laboratory workers, and an outbreak of WNV infection among turkey handlers also raised the possibility of aerosol transmission.

The risk of severe WNV disease increases with age and may be slightly higher among males. Organ transplant recipients also are at higher risk of severe illness. Risk of infection is higher during the warmer months, when mosquitoes are more abundant. WNV transmission has been described in Europe and the Middle East, Africa, India, parts of Asia, and Australia (in the form of Kunjin virus, a subtype of WNV). WNV first was detected in North America in 1999 and has spread across the continent, north into Canada, and southward into Mexico, Central America, and the Caribbean. In the United States, WNV transmission has been reported in all states except Alaska and Hawaii.

Most patients who develop WNF or aseptic meningitis recover completely. Patients with encephalitis can have residual neurologic deficits, and patients with flaccid paralysis may not recover full neuromuscular function. The case-fatality rate after neuroinvasive WNV disease is approximately 9% among adult patients and less than 1% in children.

Incubation Period

Usually 2 to 6 days (range, 2–14) up to 21 days in immunocompromised people.

Diagnostic Tests

WNV infection should be considered in the differential diagnosis of any child who presents with a febrile or acute neurologic illness and has had recent exposure to mosquitoes, blood transfusion, or organ transplantation or is born to a mother infected during pregnancy or while breastfeeding. Serum and, if indicated, CSF, should be tested for WNV-specific IgM antibody. Enzyme immunoassays or immunofluorescent assays for WNV-specific IgM currently are available commercially or through state public health laboratories. Positive tests for WNV-specific IgM provide good evidence of recent WNV infection but can cross-react with antibody to other flaviviruses. Because WNV IgM can persist in some patients for more than 1 year, a positive WNV IgM test result occasionally reflects past rather than recent WNV infection. If serum collected within 8 days of illness onset has no detectable IgM, the test should be repeated on a later sample. Plaque-reduction neutralization tests performed in reference laboratories, including some state public health laboratories and the CDC, can help determine the infecting flavivirus and can confirm acute infection by demonstrating a 4-fold change in WNV-specific antibody titer between acute and convalescent serum samples collected 2 to 3 weeks apart.

Viral culture and nucleic acid amplification (NAA) tests for WNV RNA can be performed on serum, CSF, and tissue specimens and, if positive, can confirm WNV infection. Immunohistochemical staining (IHC) can detect WNV antigen in unpreserved or formalin-fixed tissue. Negative results of these tests do not rule out WNV infection. Viral culture, NAA testing, and IHC can be requested through state public health laboratories or the CDC.

Treatment

Treatment of WNV disease is supportive; no specific therapy has been proven effective. IVIG and plasmapheresis should be considered for patients with Guillain-Barré syndrome but not for patients with paralysis because of damage of anterior horn cells. Both ribavirin and interferon have been given to patients with WNV disease with inconclusive results.

Image 124.1

A close-up view of a *Culex tarsalis* mosquito. Note the light-colored band wrapped around its dark-scaled proboscis (A), and the multiple similarly light-colored bands wrapped around its distal appendages (ie, the tibia and femur) of its forelegs and middle pair of legs (B), identifying this as *C tarsalis*.

Other identifying characteristics include the presence of 2 silver dots on its dorsal scutum; however, in this particular image, only 1 of the 2 bilateral silver scutal marks is visible (C), and a blunted distal abdominal tip, which is not visible in this view. *C tarsalis* spreads western equine encephalitis, St Louis encephalitis, and California encephalitis, and is currently the main vector of West Nile virus in the western United States.

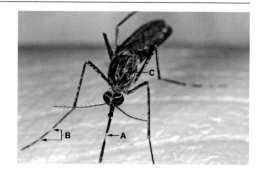

Image 124.2
Photomicrograph of brain tissue from a
West Nile encephalitis patient showing
antigen-positive neurons and neuronal
processes (in red).

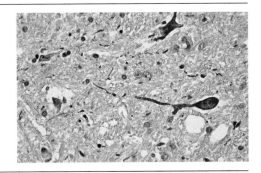

Image 124.3
Staining of West Nile virus antigen in the
cytoplasm of a Purkinje cell in the cerebellum
(40x).

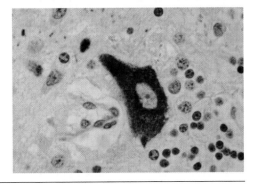

Image 124.4
Histopathologic features of West Nile virus (WNV)
in human tissues. Panels A and B show inflammation, microglial nodules, and variable necrosis
that occur during WNV encephalitis; panel C
shows WNV antigen (red) in neurons and neuronal processes using an immunohistochemical
stain; panel D is an electron micrograph of WNV
in the endoplasmic reticulum of a nerve cell
(arrow). Bar = 100 nm. These 4 images are from
a fatal case of WNV infection in a 39-year-old
African American female.

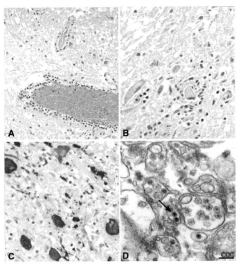

125

Yersinia enterocolitica and *Yersinia pseudotuberculosis* Infections

(Enteritis and Other Illnesses)

Clinical Manifestations

Yersinia enterocolitica causes several age-specific syndromes and a variety of other less common presentations. Infection with *Y enterocolitica* typically manifests as fever and diarrhea in young children; stool often contains leukocytes, blood, and mucus. Relapsing disease and, rarely, necrotizing enterocolitis also have been described. In older children and adults, a pseudoappendicitis syndrome (fever, abdominal pain, tenderness in the right lower quadrant of the abdomen, and leukocytosis) predominates. Bacteremia with *Y enterocolitica* most often occurs in children younger than 1 year and in older children with predisposing conditions, such as excessive iron storage (eg, desferrioxamine use, sickle cell disease, beta-thalassemia) and immunosuppressive states. Focal manifestations of *Y enterocolitica* are uncommon and include pharyngitis, meningitis, osteomyelitis, pyomyositis, conjunctivitis, pneumonia, empyema, endocarditis, acute peritonitis, abscesses of the liver and spleen, and primary cutaneous infection. Postinfectious sequelae with *Y enterocolitica* infection include erythema nodosum, proliferative glomerulonephritis, and reactive arthritis; these sequelae occur most often in older children and adults, particularly people with HLA-B27 antigen.

The major manifestations of *Yersinia pseudotuberculosis* infection are fever, scarlatiniform rash, and abdominal symptoms. Acute pseudoappendiceal abdominal pain is common, resulting from ileocecal mesenteric adenitis or terminal ileitis. Other findings include diarrhea, erythema nodosum, septicemia, and sterile pleural and joint effusions. Clinical features can mimic those of Kawasaki disease.

Etiology

The genus *Yersinia* consists of 11 species of gram-negative bacilli. *Y enterocolitica, Y pseudotuberculosis,* and *Yersinia pestis* are the 3 pathogens most commonly encountered. Fifteen pathogenic O groups of *Y enterocolitica* are recognized. Differences in virulence exist among various O groups of *Y enterocolitica;* serotype O:3 now predominates as the most common type in the United States.

Epidemiology

Y enterocolitica infections are uncommon in the United States. According to the Foodborne Diseases Active Surveillance Network, the annual incidence per 100 000 people is 9.6 for infants, 1.4 for young children, and 0.2 for other age groups. *Y pseudotuberculosis* infections are even more rare. The principal reservoir of *Y enterocolitica* is swine; feral *Y pseudotuberculosis* has been isolated from ungulates (deer, elk, goats, sheep, cattle), rodents (rats, squirrels, beaver), rabbits, and many bird species. Infection with *Y enterocolitica* is believed to be transmitted by ingestion of contaminated food (raw or incompletely cooked pork products and unpasteurized milk), contaminated surface or well water, direct or indirect contact with animals, transfusion with contaminated packed red blood cells and, rarely, person-to-person transmission. Bottle-fed infants can be infected if their caregivers handle raw pork intestines (chitterlings). *Y enterocolitica* is isolated most often during the cool months of temperate climates. The period of communicability is unknown; organisms are excreted for an average of 2 to 3 weeks. Prolonged asymptomatic carriage is possible. Recent outbreaks of *Y pseudotuberculosis* infection in Finland have been associated with eating fresh produce, presumably contaminated by wild animals carrying the organism.

Incubation Period

Typically 4 to 6 days (range, 1–14).

Diagnostic Tests

Y enterocolitica and *Y pseudotuberculosis* can be recovered from stool, throat swabs, mesenteric lymph nodes, peritoneal fluid, and blood. *Y enterocolitica* also has been isolated from synovial fluid, bile, urine, CSF, sputum, and wounds. Stool cultures generally are positive during the first 2 weeks of illness, regardless of the nature of gastrointestinal tract manifestations. Because of the relatively low incidence of *Yersinia* infection in the United States, *Yersinia* is not routinely sought in stool specimens by most laboratories. Consequently, laboratory personnel should be notified when *Yersinia* infection is suspected. Infection can be confirmed by demonstrating increases in serum antibody titer after infection, but these tests generally are available only in reference or research laboratories. Cross-reactions of these antibodies with *Brucella, Vibrio, Salmonella,* and *Rickettsia* species and *Escherichia coli* lead to false-positive *Y enterocolitica* and *Y pseudotuberculosis* titers. In patients with thyroid disease, persistently increased *Y enterocolitica* antibody titers can result from antigenic similarity of the organism with antigens of the thyroid epithelial cell membrane. Characteristic ultrasonographic features demonstrating edema of the wall of the terminal ileum and cecum help to distinguish pseudoappendicitis from appendicitis and can help avoid exploratory surgery.

Treatment

Patients with septicemia or sites of infection other than the gastrointestinal tract and immunocompromised hosts with enterocolitis should receive antimicrobial therapy. Other than decreasing the duration of fecal excretion of *Y enterocolitica* and *Y pseudotuberculosis,* a clinical benefit of antimicrobial therapy for patients with enterocolitis, pseudoappendicitis syndrome, or mesenteric adenitis has not been established. *Y enterocolitica* and *Y pseudotuberculosis* usually are susceptible to trimethoprim-sulfamethoxazole, aminoglycosides, cefotaxime, fluoroquinolones (for patients 18 years of age and older), tetracycline or doxycycline (for children 8 years of age and older), and chloramphenicol. *Y enterocolitica* isolates usually are resistant to first-generation cephalosporins and most penicillins.

Image 125.1

Multiple erythema nodosum lesions over both lower extremities of a 10-year-old female following a *Yersinia enterocolitica* infection. This immunoreactive complication also may occur in association with *Campylobacter jejuni* infections, tuberculosis, leprosy, coccidioidomycocis, histoplasmosis, and other infectious diseases.

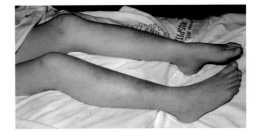

Index

Page numbers followed by *f* indicate a figure.
Page numbers followed by *i* indicate an image.
Page numbers followed by *t* indicate a table.

A

Abdominal abscess
 from *Bacteroides* infection, 24
 from *Prevotella* infection, 24
Abdominal actinomycosis, 1
Abdominal cramps
 from *Clostridium difficile,* 48
 from *Salmonella* infections, 229
 from *Shigella* infections, 239
Abdominal discomfort
 from *Balantidium coli* infection, 26
 from *Clostridium difficile,* 48
 from trichinellosis, 323
 from *Yersinia pseudotuberculosis* infection, 368
Abdominal distention
 from *Escherichia coli,* 72
 from *Giardia intestinalis* infections, 80
Abdominal pain
 from anthrax, 9
 from babesiosis, 21
 from brucellosis, 33
 from *Campylobacter* infections, 35
 from enterovirus infections, 67
 from *Escherichia coli* diarrhea, 75
 from *Giardia intestinalis* infections, 80
 from hookworm infections, 112
 from influenza, 124
 from malaria, 147
 from nontuberculous mycobacteria, 345
 from Rocky Mountain spotted fever, 219
 from schistosomiasis, 236
 from smallpox, 241
 from *Strongyloides,* 275
 from tapeworm infections, 297
 from *Trichomonas vaginalis* infections, 326
 from trichuriasis, 328
 from tuberculosis, 333
 from West Nile virus, 365
Abortion
 lymphocytic choriomeningitis and, 146
 mumps and, 159
 syphilis and, 278
Abscesses
 abdominal
  from *Bacteroides* infection, 24
  from *Prevotella* infection, 24
 from actinomycosis, 1
 actinomycotic, 1*i*
 axillary lymph node, 257*i*
 from *Bacteroides* infection, 24
 from blastomycosis, 29
 brain
  from *Arcanobacterium haemolyticum* infections, 15
  from *Bacteroides* infection, 24
  from *Escherichia coli,* 72
  from *Prevotella* infection, 24

 hepatic, from *Pasteurella* infections, 181
 intra-abdominal, from non–group A or B streptococcal and enterococcal infections, 272
 liver, 5*i*
  from amebiasis, 4
  from *Yersinia enterocolitica,* 368
 lung
  from *Bacteroides* infection, 24
  from *Prevotella* infection, 24
 from nocardiosis, 163
 orbital, 256*i*
 from paracoccidioidomycosis, 172
 paravertebral, 344*i*
 peritonsillar
  from *Arcanobacterium haemolyticum* infections, 15
  from *Bacteroides* infection, 24
  from group A streptococcal infections, 261
  from *Prevotella* infection, 24
 from *Prevotella* infection, 24
 pulmonary, from *Pasteurella* infections, 181
 from rat-bite fever, 213
 retropharyngeal, from group A streptococcal infections, 261
 scalp
  from staphylococcal infections, 248
  from tinea capitis, 302
 spleen, from *Yersinia enterocolitica,* 368
 from toxic shock syndrome, 310
Acanthamoeba species, 6
Acetaminophen
 for influenza, 126
 for varicella-zoster infections, 359
Acid-fast bacillus (AFB), 333
 smear for nontuberculous mycobacteria, 346
Acidosis from rotavirus infections, 223
Acquired immunodeficiency syndrome (AIDS)
 from *Cryptococcus neoformans* infections, 55, 56*i*
Acquired syphilis, 278, 279
 follow-up and management of, 284
 primary stage, 278
 secondary stage, 278
Actinobacillus actinomycetemcomitans, 1*i*
Actinomyces israelii, 1, 1*i,* 163
Actinomycosis, 1–2
 abdominal, 1
 chronic pulmonary, 2*i*
 clinical manifestations of, 1
 diagnostic tests for, 1
 epidemiology of, 1
 etiology of, 1
 incubation period of, 1
 treatment of, 1
Actinomycotic abscesses, 1*i*
Acute follicular adenovirus conjunctivitis, 3*i*
Acute hemorrhagic conjunctivitis from enterovirus infections, 67
Acute hemorrhagic fever from arboviruses, 12
Acute idiopathic polyneuritis, as complication of viral *Campylobacter* infections, 35
Acute myositis from influenza, 124
Acute peritonitis from *Yersinia enterocolitica,* 368

Acute pharyngitis from *Arcanobacterium haemolyticum* infections, 15
Acute polyarthropathy from arboviruses, 12
Acute pulmonary histoplasmosis, 109
Acute respiratory distress syndrome from plague, 195
Acute respiratory tract illness
    from *Mycoplasma pneumoniae* infections, 162
    from respiratory syncytial virus, 215
Acute rheumatic fever, 262
Acute transient pneumonitis from *Ascaris lumbricoides* infections, 17
Acyclovir
    for Epstein-Barr virus, 70
    for herpes simplex virus, 105–106, 106
    for varicella-zoster infections, 357–359
Adamantanes for influenza, 125
Adefovir for hepatitis B virus (HBV), 98–99
Adenitis, 43
    from group B streptococcal infections, 269
Adenopathy
    from leptospirosis, 136
    from rat-bite fever, 213
Adenoviral pneumonia, 3*i*
Adenovirus infections, 3
    clinical manifestations of, 3
    diagnostic tests for, 3
    epidemiology of, 3
    etiology of, 3
    incubation period of, 3
    treatment of, 3
Adolescent, acquisition of human immunodeficiency virus (HIV) during, 117
Aerobic cultures for *Bacteroides* and *Prevotella* infections, 24
Aerosol treatment for respiratory syncytial virus, 216
African trypanosomiasis (African sleeping sickness), 329–330, 330*i*
    clinical manifestations of, 329
    diagnostic tests for, 329
    epidemiology of, 329
    etiology of, 329
    incubation period of, 329
    treatment of, 329
Agranulocytosis from Epstein-Barr virus, 69
Albendazole
    for *Ascaris lumbricoides* infections, 17
    for *Baylisascaris* infections, 27
    for cutaneous larva migrans, 57
    for cysticercosis, 295
    for *Giardia intestinalis* infections, 80
    for hookworm infections, 112
    for hydatid disease, 297, 298
    for pinworm infection, 190
    for strongyloidiasis, 275
    for toxocariasis, 316
    for trichinellosis, 323
    for trichuriasis, 328
Allergic bronchopulmonary aspergillosis, 19
Allergic sinusitis from aspergillosis, 19
Alopecia areata, tinea capitis and, 302
Alveolar disease from *Pneumocystis jiroveci* infections, 204
Amantadine for influenza, 125

Amblyomma americanum, 220*i*
Amebiasis, 4–5
    clinical manifestations of, 4
    diagnostic tests for, 4
    epidemiology of, 4
    etiology of, 4
    incubation period of, 4
    invasive extraintestinal, 5*i*
    treatment of, 4
Amebic meningoencephalitis, 6–8, 7*i*
    clinical manifestations of, 6
    diagnostic tests for, 6
    epidemiology of, 6
    etiology of, 6
    incubation period of, 6
    treatment of, 6
Ameboma from amebiasis, 4
American trypanosomiasis (Chagas disease), 331–332
    clinical manifestations of, 331
    diagnostic tests for, 331
    epidemiology of, 331
    etiology of, 331
    incubation period of, 331
    treatment of, 332
Amikacin
    for nontuberculous mycobacteria, 346
    for tularemia, 351
Aminoglycosides
    for *Arcanobacterium haemolyticum* infections, 15
    for *Campylobacter* infections, 35
    for *Escherichia coli,* 72, 73
    for *Listeria monocytogenes* infections, 138
    for *Yersinia enterocolitica* and *Yersinia pseudo-tuberculosis* infections, 369
Amniocentesis for cytomegalovirus infection, 59
Amnionitis from *Listeria monocytogenes* infections, 138
Amoxicillin
    for actinomycosis, 1
    for Epstein-Barr virus, 70
    for *Haemophilus influenzae* infections, 89
    for Lyme disease, 141
    for *Salmonella* infections, 230
    for *Shigella* infections, 240
Amoxicillin-clavulanate
    for *Haemophilus influenzae* infections, 89
    for nocardiosis, 163
    for otitis media, 201
    for *Pasteurella* infections, 181
Amphotericin B
    for amebic meningoencephalitis, 6
    for aspergillosis, 19
    for blastomycosis, 29
    for coccidioidomycosis, 52
    for *Cryptococcus neoformans* infections, 55
    for histoplasmosis, 110
    for paracoccidioidomycosis, 172
    for sporotrichosis, 246
    in treating candidiasis, 37
Ampicillin
    for actinomycosis, 1
    for Epstein-Barr virus, 70
    for *Escherichia coli,* 72, 73
    for group B streptococcal infections, 270

for *Haemophilus influenzae* infections, 88
for *Listeria monocytogenes* infections, 138–139
for meningococcal infections, 154
for non–group A or B streptococcal and enterococcal
  infections, 273
for *Pasteurella* infections, 181
for *Salmonella* infections, 230
Anaerobic cultures of wound exudate for *Clostridial
  myonecrosis,* 50
Anal infections from granuloma inguinale, 86
Anaplasma infections, 63–66
  clinical manifestations of, 63
  diagnostic tests for, 63
  epidemiology of, 63
  etiology of, 63
  incubation period of, 63
  treatment of, 63
Anaplasma phagocytophilum, 63
Ancylostoma braziliense, 57
Ancylostoma caninum, 57, 113*i*
Anemia
  from African trypanosomiasis, 329
  from *Ehrlichia* and *Anaplasma* infections, 63
  hemolytic
    from Epstein-Barr virus, 69, 70
    from syphilis, 278
  hypochromic microcytic, 112
  from leishmaniasis, 131
  from malaria, 147
  megaloblastic, from tapeworm infections, 297
  from *Mycoplasma pneumoniae* infections, 161
  from nontuberculous mycobacteria, 345
  from parvovirus B19, 178
  from Rocky Mountain spotted fever, 219
  from toxocariasis, 316
Aneurysms from Kawasaki disease, 127–128
Anicteric infection, 97
Anidulafungin for treating candidiasis, 38
Animal feces as cause of *Escherichia coli* diarrhea, 76
Annular erythematous lesions, 306*i*
Anogenital HPV infection, 169, 170
Anogenital warts, 169
Anorectal infection from gonococcal infections, 82
Anorexia
  from anthrax, 9
  from babesiosis, 21
  from brucellosis, 33
  from *Ehrlichia* and *Anaplasma* infections, 63
  from *Escherichia coli,* 72
  from *Giardia intestinalis* infections, 80
  from group A streptococcal infections, 261
  from hepatitis A, 95
  from hepatitis B, 97
  from leishmaniasis, 131
  from lymphocytic choriomeningitis, 146
  from rickettsialpox, 217
  from Rocky Mountain spotted fever, 219
  from *Salmonella* infections, 229
Antemortem diagnosis for rabies, 210
Anterior uveitis from Kawasaki disease, 127
Anthelmintic treatment
  for *Baylisascaris* infections, 27
  for ocular larva migrans, 316
Anthrax, 9–11
  clinical manifestations of, 9
  cutaneous, 9, 10*i*, 11*i*
  diagnostic tests for, 9
  epidemiology of, 9
  etiology of, 9
  incubation period of, 9
  inhalational, 9
  oropharyngeal, 9
  treatment of, 9
Anthrax ulcers, 10*i*
Anticonvulsants for cysticercosis, 295
Antifungal therapy
  for histoplasmosis, 110
  for pityriasis versicolor, 192
Antigen detection tests
  for *Histoplasma capsulatum,* 109
  for malaria, 148
  for respiratory syncytial virus, 215
Antigenic drift from influenza, 124
Antigenic shift from influenza, 124
Anti-HBc for hepatitis B virus (HBV), 99*t*
Anti-HBe for hepatitis B virus (HBV), 99*t*
Anti-HBs for hepatitis B virus (HBV), 99*t*
Anti-inflammatory therapies for *Baylisascaris*
  infections, 27
Antimalarial drugs for malaria, 148–149
Antimicrobial-associated diarrhea from *Clostridium
  difficile,* 48
Antimicrobial susceptibility testing for non–group A
  or B streptococcal and enterococcal
  infections, 272
Antimicrobial therapy
  for brucellosis, 33
  for *Clostridium difficile,* 48
  for diphtheria, 61
  for *Escherichia coli* diarrhea, 77
  for gonococcal infections, 83
  for granuloma inguinale, 86
  for *Haemophilus influenzae* infections, 88
  for Lyme disease, 141
  for meningococcal infections, 154
  for *Mycoplasma pneumoniae* infections, 162
  for pertussis, 187
  for pneumococcal infections, 199, 200*t*
  for respiratory syncytial virus, 216
  for *Salmonella* infections, 230
  for scabies, 234
  for *Shigella* infections, 239
  for toxic shock syndrome, 311
  for *Vibrio cholerae* infections, 364
Antiretroviral therapy for human immunodeficiency
  virus (HIV) infection, 117, 119
Antitoxin
  for *Clostridium botulinum,* 46
  for diphtheria, 61
Antiviral therapy
  for hepatitis B virus, 98
  for herpes simplex virus, 105
  for influenza, 125
  for parainfluenza virus infections, 177
  for varicella-zoster infections, 357–359
Anxiety from rabies, 210

Apnea
  from *Escherichia coli*, 72
  from group B streptococcal infections, 269
  from pertussis, 186
Apneic episodes from respiratory syncytial virus, 215
Appendicitis from *Pasteurella* infections, 181
Aqueous crystalline penicillin G
  for congenital syphilis, 282
  for neurosyphilis, 284
Arboviruses, 12–14
  clinical manifestations of, 12
  diagnostic tests for, 12
  epidemiology of, 12
  etiology of, 12
  incubation period of, 12
  treatment of, 12
Arcanobacterium-associated rash, 16*i*
Arcanobacterium haemolyticum infections, 15–16, 15*i*
  clinical manifestations of, 15
  diagnostic tests for, 15
  epidemiology of, 15
  etiology of, 15
  incubation period of, 15
  treatment of, 15
Arcanobacterium haemolyticum pharyngitis, 16*i*
Areflexia as complication of viral *Campylobacter*
      infections, 35
Arthralgias
  from African trypanosomiasis, 329
  from babesiosis, 21
  from brucellosis, 33
  from coccidioidomycosis, 52
  from *Ehrlichia* and *Anaplasma* infections, 63
  from hepatitis B, 97
  from Kawasaki disease, 127
  from Lyme disease, 140
  from lymphocytic choriomeningitis, 146
  from malaria, 147
  from parvovirus B19, 178
  from rat-bite fever, 213
Arthritis. *See also* Reactive arthritis; Septic arthritis
  from *Bacteroides* infection, 24
  from brucellosis, 33
  group A streptococcal, 267*i*
  from hepatitis B, 97
  from Kawasaki disease, 127
  Lyme, 140, 141–142
  from lymphocytic choriomeningitis, 146
  from meningococcal infections, 153
  migratory, from gonococcal infections, 82
  from mumps, 159
  from *Mycoplasma pneumoniae* infections, 161
  from parvovirus B19, 178
  from *Prevotella* infection, 24
  pyogenic, from pneumococcal infections, 198
  from rat-bite fever, 213
  recurrent, from Lyme disease, 140
  treatment for, 265
  from varicella-zoster infections, 356
  from viral *Campylobacter* infections, 35
Arthritis syndrome from histoplasmosis, 110
Artibeus jamaicensis as carriers of rabies virus, 211*i*

Ascaris lumbricoides infections, 17–18, 17*i*, 18*i*
  clinical manifestations of, 17
  diagnostic tests for, 17
  epidemiology of, 17
  etiology of, 17
  incubation period of, 17
  treatment of, 17
Ascending myelitis from herpes simplex virus, 104
Ascending polyradiculitis from mumps, 159
Ascites from anthrax, 9
Aseptic meningitis
  from arboviruses, 12
  from cat-scratch disease, 40
  from Epstein-Barr virus, 69
  from leptospirosis, 136
  from *Mycoplasma pneumoniae* infections, 161
  from parainfluenza viral infections, 176
  from poliovirus infections, 207
  from West Nile virus, 365
Aspergillomas, 20*i*
  from aspergillosis, 19
Aspergillosis, 19–20, 20*i*
  allergic bronchopulmonary, 19
  clinical manifestations of, 19
  diagnostic tests for, 19
  epidemiology of, 19
  etiology of, 19
  incubation period of, 19
  invasive, 19
  pulmonary, 20*i*
  treatment of, 19
Aspiration pneumonia
  from *Bacteroides* infection, 24
  from *Prevotella* infection, 24
Aspirin therapy for Kawasaki disease, 128–129
Asthma from parainfluenza viral infections, 176
Asymptomatic cyst excreter, 4
Asymptomatic infection, 97
Ataxia as complication of viral *Campylobacter*
      infections, 35
Atelectasis from tuberculosis, 333
Athlete's foot (tinea pedis), 308–309
  clinical manifestations of, 308
  diagnosis of, 308
  epidemiology of, 308
  etiology of, 308
  treatment of, 308–309
Atopic dermatitis, 302
  from tinea capitis, 302
  from tinea pedis, 308
  from tinea unguium, 308
Atovaquone
  for babesiosis, 21
  for *Pneumocystis jiroveci* infections, 205
Atypical lymphocyte, 70*i*
Autoimmune gastritis from *Helicobacter pylori*
      infections, 94
Automated reagin test (ART) for syphilis, 279
Axillary lymph node abscess, 257*i*

Azithromycin
for babesiosis, 21
for *Campylobacter* infections, 35
for cat-scratch disease, 40
for chancroid, 43
for chlamydial pneumonia, 44
for *Chlamydia trachomatis* genital tract infection, 44
for *Escherichia coli* diarrhea, 77
for gonococcal infections, 83
for Lyme disease, 141
for *Mycoplasma pneumoniae* infections, 162
for nontuberculous mycobacteria lymphadenitis, 346
for *Pasteurella* infections, 181
for pertussis, 187
for trachoma, 44

B

Babesia microti, 21, 21*i*
Babesiosis, 21
clinical manifestations of, 21
diagnostic tests for, 21
epidemiology of, 21
etiology of, 21
incubation period of, 21
Lyme disease and, 140
treatment of, 21
Bacille Calmette-Guérin (BCG) vaccine as not recommended for human immunodeficiency virus (HIV) children, 120
Bacillus anthracis, 9
photomicrograph of, 10*i*
Back pain
from *Listeria monocytogenes* infections, 138
from malaria, 147
from smallpox, 241
Bacteremia
from gonococcal infections, 82
from group A streptococcal infections, 261
from group B streptococcal infections, 269
from *Haemophilus influenzae*, 88
from non–group A or B streptococcal and enterococcal infections, 272
from *Pasteurella* infections, 181
from *Shigella* infections, 239
from staphylococcal infections, 248
from toxic shock syndrome, 310
from *Yersinia enterocolitica*, 368
Bacterial antigens in leptospirosis, 137*i*
Bacterial endocarditis, 259*i*
Bacterial infections
from human immunodeficiency virus infection, 116
from pediculosis corporis, 184
Bacterial meningitis, 199–200
Bacterial sepsis from enterovirus infections, 67
Bacterial vaginosis, 22–23
clinical manifestations of, 22
diagnostic tests for, 22
epidemiology of, 22
etiology of, 22
incubation period of, 22
treatment of, 22
Bacteroides fragilis, 24, 25*i*

Bacteroides infections, 24–25, 25*i*
clinical manifestations of, 24
diagnostic tests for, 24
epidemiology of, 24
etiology of, 24
incubation period of, 24
treatment of, 24
Balamuthia mandrillaris, 6, 7*i*
Balantidium coli infections (balantidiasis), 26, 26*i*
clinical manifestations of, 26
diagnostic tests for, 26
epidemiology of, 26
etiology of, 26
incubation period of, 26
treatment of, 26
Bancroftian filariasis, 144–145
from lymphatic filariasis, 144
Bartonella henselae (cat-scratch disease), 40–42
clinical manifestations of, 40
diagnostic tests for, 40
epidemiology of, 40
etiology of, 40
incubation period of, 40
treatment of, 40
Baylisascaris infections, 27–28, 27*i*, 28*i*
clinical manifestations of, 27
diagnostic tests for, 27
epidemiology of, 27
etiology of, 27
treatment of, 27
Baylisascaris procyonis, 27, 27*i*, 28*i*
Beau lines, 268*i*
Beaver direct smear for hookworm infections, 112
Behavioral disturbances
from *Cysticercosis*, 294
from tapeworm diseases, 294
Bell palsy from herpes simplex virus, 104
Benznidazole for American trypanosomiasis, 332
Beta-adrenergic agents for respiratory syncytial virus, 216
Beta-lactam antimicrobial agent for *Escherichia coli*, 73
Beta-lactam penicillin for *Bacteroides* and *Prevotella* infections, 24
Bichloroacetic acid for warts, 170
Bilateral conjunctivitis, as complication of viral *Campylobacter* infections, 35
Bilateral diffuse interstitial disease from *Pneumocystis jiroveci* infections, 204
Bilateral subconjunctival hemorrhages, in infant with pertussis, 188*i*
Bilateral varicella pneumonia, 361*i*
Biliary colic from *Ascaris lumbricoides* infections, 17
Biopsy specimens
for onchocerciasis, 166
for tuberculosis, 334
Bites
cat, 181*i*
human, 1
rat, 214*i*
tick, 142*i*
Bithionol for paragonimiasis, 175
Black Creek Canal virus, 91
Black death, 195
Black-dot ringworm, 302, 303*i*

Black fly larva, 167*i*
Blackwater fever from plague, 195
Bladder cancer from *Schistosoma haematobium,* 236
Bladder incontinence from Rocky Mountain spotted
        fever (RMSF), 219
Blastomyces dermatitidus, 29*i,* 110
    from blastomycosis, 29
Blastomycosis, 29–30, 29*i*
    clinical manifestations of, 29
    cutaneous, 30*i*
    diagnostic tests for, 29
    epidemiology of, 29
    etiology of, 29
    incubation period of, 29
    treatment of, 29
Blindness from onchocerciasis, 166
Blood cultures
    for leishmaniasis, 132
    for pneumococcal infections, 198
    for staphylococcal infections, 251
    for toxic shock syndrome, 311
Blood smears for meningococcal infections, 154
Blood specimen for sporotrichosis, 246
Blueberry muffin lesions from congenital rubella,
        225, 227*i*
Blurred vision from *Toxoplasma gondii* infections, 318
B-lymphocyte count for human immunodeficiency
        virus (HIV), 118
Body infections from staphylococcal infections, 248
Body lice (pediculosis corporis), 184
    clinical manifestations of, 184
    diagnostic tests for, 184
    epidemiology of, 184
    etiology of, 184
    incubation period of, 184
    treatment of, 184
Bone marrow
    for *Histoplasma capsulatum,* 109
    suppression from human herpesvirus 6 and 7, 114
Bordetella pertussis, 186
Borrelia burgdorferi infection (Lyme disease),
        140–141, 140–143
    from babesiosis, 21
    clinical manifestations of, 140
    diagnostic tests for, 141
    epidemiology of, 140–141
    etiology of, 140
    incubation period of, 141
    treatment of, 141–142
Borrelia hermsii, 31
Borrelia infections (relapsing fever), 31–32, 32*i*
    clinical manifestations of, 31
    diagnostic tests for, 31
    epidemiology of, 31
    etiology of, 31
    incubation period of, 31
    treatment of, 31
Borrelia parkeri, 31
Borrelia recurrentis, 31
Borrelia turicatae, 31

Botulism, 46, 47*i*
    food-borne, 46
    infant, 46
        from *Clostridium botulinum,* 46
    intestinal, 46
    ocular muscle paralysis in, 47*i*
    wound, 46, 51*i*
Bowel dilation from *Balantidium coli* infection, 26
Bowel incontinence from Rocky Mountain spotted fever
        (RMSF), 219
Bowel obstruction from tapeworm infections, 297
Brain abscesses
    from *Arcanobacterium haemolyticum* infections, 15
    from *Bacteroides* infection, 24
    from *Escherichia coli,* 72
    from *Prevotella* infection, 24
Brain lesions from candidiasis, 37
Breastfeeding
    postnatal transmission of human immunodeficiency
        virus through, 117
    tuberculosis during, 339
Breath tests for *Helicobacter pylori* infections, 94
Brill-Zinsser disease from epidemic typhus, 354
Bronchiectasis from paragonimiasis, 174
Bronchiolar plugging in infant with pertussis, 188*i*
Bronchiolitis
    from adenovirus infections, 3
    from influenza, 124
    from parainfluenza viral infections, 176
    from respiratory syncytial virus, 215
Bronchopneumonia from measles, 150
Bronchoscopy for *Pneumocystis jiroveci* infections, 204
Brucella abortus, 33
Brucella canis, 33
Brucella granuloma, 34*i*
Brucella melitensis, 33, 34*i*
Brucella suis, 33
Brucellosis, 33–34
    clinical manifestations of, 33
    diagnostic tests for, 33
    epidemiology of, 33
    etiology of, 33
    incubation period of, 33
    treatment of, 33
Brugia malayi, 144
Brugia timori, 144
Bubo aspirate for plague, 195
Bubonic plague, 195
Bulbar conjunctivitis, 359*i*
Bulbar polio, 209*i*
Bullous impetigo, 255*i*
Bunyaviridae, 12
Burkitt lymphoma from Epstein-Barr virus, 69
Butenafine
    for tinea corporis, 305
    for tinea cruris, 307

C

Cachexia from African trypanosomiasis, 329
Calcium alginate swab for pertussis, 186
California serogroup viruses, 13*t*
Calymmatobacterium granulomatis, 86, 87*i*
Campylobacter coli, 35
Campylobacter fetus, 35, 36*i*
Campylobacter infections, 35–36
  clinical manifestations of, 35
  diagnostic tests for, 35
  epidemiology of, 35
  etiology of, 35
  incubation period of, 35
  treatment of, 35
Campylobacter jejuni, 35, 36*i*
Candida albicans, 37, 38*i*
Candida dubliniensis, 37
Candida glabrata, 37
Candida granulomatous lesions, 39*i*
Candida guilliermondii, 37
Candida krusei, 37
Candida lusitaniae, 37
Candida parapsilosis, 37
Candida tropicalis, 37
Candidemia from candidiasis, 37
Candidiasis (moniliasis, thrush), 37–39
  chronic, 39*i*
  clinical manifestations of, 37
  congenital, 38*i*
  cutaneous, 38*i*
  diagnostic tests for, 37
  disseminated, 37, 38
  epidemiology of, 37
  etiology of, 37
  incubation period of, 37
  invasive, 37
  mucocutaneous, 37, 39*i*
  oral, 37
  treatment of, 37–38
  vaginal, 37
Candiduria from candidiasis, 37
Carbuncles from staphylococcal infections, 248
Cardiac care for Kawasaki disease, 129
Cardiac dysrhythmias from West Nile virus, 365
Cardiomyopathy
  from American trypanosomiasis, 331
  from human immunodeficiency virus infection, 116
Carditis
  from Kawasaki disease, 127
  from Lyme disease, 140
Caspofungin for treating candidiasis, 38
Cataracts in congenital rubella, 228*i*
Cat bite, *Pasteurella* infections in, 181*i*
Cat-scratch disease *(Bartonella henselae),* 40–42, 41*i*
  clinical manifestations of, 40
  diagnostic tests for, 40
  epidemiology of, 40
  etiology of, 40
  granuloma of finger of, 42*i*
  incubation period of, 40
  treatment of, 40

Cavitary lesions from tuberculosis, 333
Cefaclor for *Pasteurella* infections, 181
Cefadroxil for *Pasteurella* infections, 181
Cefazolin for staphylococcal infections, 252
Cefixime for gonococcal infections, 83
Cefotaxime
  for *Escherichia coli,* 72, 73
  for gonococcal infections, 83
  for *Haemophilus influenzae* infections, 88
  for meningococcal infections, 154
  for pneumococcal infections, 199
  for *Salmonella* infections, 230
  for *Shigella* infections, 240
  for *Yersinia enterocolitica* and *Yersinia pseudo-tuberculosis* infections, 369
Cefoxitin for nontuberculous mycobacteria, 346
Cefpodoxime
  for gonococcal infections, 83
  for otitis media, 201
  for *Pasteurella* infections, 181
Ceftriaxone
  for gonococcal infections, 83
  for *Haemophilus influenzae* infections, 88
  for leptospirosis, 136
  for meningococcal infections, 154
  for pneumococcal infections, 199
  for *Salmonella* infections, 230
  for *Shigella* infections, 240
  in treating chancroid, 43
Cefuroxime
  for otitis media, 201
  for *Pasteurella* infections, 181
  for staphylococcal infections, 252
Cell cultures
  for adenovirus infections, 3
  for *Clostridium difficile,* 48
  for enterovirus infections, 67
  for herpes simplex virus, 104
  for mumps, 159
  for poliovirus infections, 208
  for rubella, 226
Cellulitis
  from *Arcanobacterium haemolyticum* infections, 15
  from *Bacteroides* infection, 24
  from group A streptococcal infections, 261
  from group B streptococcal infections, 269
  from *Haemophilus influenzae,* 88
  from *Pasteurella* infections, 181
  periorbital, 201*i,* 256*i*
  from *Prevotella* infection, 24
  from staphylococcal infections, 248
  from tinea capitis, 302
Central catheter infections from nontuberculous mycobacteria, 345
Central nervous system (CNS) disease
  from *Baylisascaris* infections, 27
  from human immunodeficiency virus infection, 116
  manifestations from rabies, 210
Cephalexin for *Pasteurella* infections, 181
Cephalic tetanus, 299

Cephalosporins
  for *Campylobacter* infections, 35
  for *Clostridium difficile,* 48
  for *Escherichia coli,* 72, 73
  for gonococcal infections, 83
  for group A streptococcal infections, 264
  for *Listeria monocytogenes* infections, 139
  for *Shigella* infections, 240
Cercarial dermatitis from schistosomiasis, 236
Cerebellar ataxia
  from mumps, 159
  from *Mycoplasma pneumoniae* infections, 161
  from varicella-zoster infections, 356
Cerebral calcifications from *Toxoplasma gondii*
      infections, 318
Cerebral malaria, 147
Cerebral neurocysticercosis, 296*i*
Cerebritis from *Haemophilus influenzae* infections, 90*i*
Cerebrospinal fluid (CSF) specimen for arboviruses, 12
Cervical adenitis, 257*i*
  from *Bacteroides* infection, 24
  from *Prevotella* infection, 24
Cervical lymphadenitis, 266*i*
  from nontuberculous mycobacteria, 345
Cervical lymphadenopathy
  from Kawasaki disease, 127
  from tularemia, 350
Cervical lymph nodes, 304*i*
  aspiration of, 266*i*
Cervicitis from *Chlamydia trachomatis,* 44
Cervicofacial infections from actinomycosis, 1
Cesarean section, in reducing risk of human immuno-
      deficiency virus (HIV) transmission, 117
Chagas disease (American trypanosomiasis), 331–332
  clinical manifestations of, 331
  diagnostic tests for, 331
  epidemiology of, 331
  etiology of, 331
  incubation period of, 331
  treatment of, 332
Chagoma from American trypanosomiasis, 331
Chancroid, 43, 43*i*
  clinical manifestations of, 43
  diagnostic tests for, 43
  epidemiology of, 43
  etiology of, 43
  incubation period of, 43
  treatment of, 43
Chancroidal ulcer, 43
Chemical gastritis from *Helicobacter pylori* infections, 94
Chemoprophylaxis for *Pneumocystis jiroveci*
      infections, 205
Chemotherapy for tuberculosis, 336
Chest pain
  from *Cryptococcus neoformans* infections, 55
  from histoplasmosis, 109
  from tularemia, 350
Chest radiographs
  for anthrax, 9
  for influenza, 126*i*
  for paragonimiasis, 175
Chickenpox. *See* Varicella-zoster virus (VZV) infections

Chikungunya viruses, 12
Chills
  from babesiosis, 21
  from *Ehrlichia* and *Anaplasma* infections, 63
  from epidemic typhus, 354
  from hantavirus pulmonary syndrome, 91
  from influenza, 124
  from leptospirosis, 136
  from malaria, 147
  from meningococcal infections, 153
  from *Pasteurella* infections, 181
  from plague, 195
  from rat-bite fever, 213
  from rickettsialpox, 217
  from tuberculosis, 333
  from tularemia, 350
Chlamydia trachomatis, 44–45, 45*i*, 82, 83, 185, 326
  from bacterial vaginosis, 22
  clinical manifestations of, 44
  diagnostic tests for, 44
  epidemiology of, 44
  etiology of, 44
  genital tract infection, 44
  incubation period of, 44
  treatment of, 44
Chloramphenicol
  for epidemic typhus, 354
  for *Haemophilus influenzae* infections, 88
  for meningococcal infections, 154
  for plague, 196
  for rickettsialpox, 217
  for Rocky Mountain spotted fever, 220
  for tularemia, 351
  for *Yersinia enterocolitica* and *Yersinia pseudo-
      tuberculosis* infections, 369
Chloroquine-resistant *Plasmodium falciparum,* 148
Chloroquine-resistant *Plasmodium vivax,* 148
Choclo virus, 91
Cholangitis from *Ascaris lumbricoides* infections, 17
Cholera *(Vibrio cholerae),* 363–364
  clinical manifestations of, 363
  diagnostic tests for, 363
  epidemiology of, 363
  etiology of, 363
  incubation period of, 363
  treatment of, 363–364
Chorioamnionitis
  from group B streptococcal infections, 269
  from *Haemophilus influenzae,* 88
Chorioretinitis
  from lymphocytic choriomeningitis, 146
  from *Toxoplasma gondii* infections, 318
  from West Nile virus, 365
Chromoblastomycosis, 30*i*
Chronic asymptomatic parasitemia, 147
  Plasmodium malariae infection and, 147
Chronic cardiorespiratory disease, *Mycoplasma pneu-
      moniae* infections and, 161
Chronic meningococcemia from meningococcal infec-
      tions, 153
Chronic onchocerciasis, 168*i*
Chronic pulmonary actinomycosis, 2*i*

Chronic sinusitis
 from *Bacteroides* infection, 24
 from *Prevotella* infection, 24
Ciclopirox
 for candidiasis, 37
 for tinea corporis, 305
 for tinea cruris, 307
Cidofovir
 for molluscum contagiosum, 157
 for smallpox, 242
Ciprofloxacin
 for anthrax, 9
 for cat-scratch disease, 40
 for *Escherichia coli* diarrhea, 77
 for gonococcal infections, 83
 for granuloma inguinale, 86
 for nontuberculous mycobacteria, 346
 for plague, 196
 for *Salmonella* infections, 231
 for *Shigella* infections, 240
 for tularemia, 351
 for *Vibrio cholerae* infections, 364
Cirrhosis from hepatitis C virus (HBV), 101
Citrobacter koseri, 72
Clarithromycin
 for *Mycoplasma pneumoniae* infections, 162
 for nocardiosis, 163
 for nontuberculous mycobacteria, 346
 for nontuberculous mycobacteria lymphadenitis, 346
 for pertussis, 187
Clindamycin
 for actinomycosis, 1
 for babesiosis, 21
 for bacterial vaginosis, 22
 for *Bacteroides* and *Prevotella* infections, 24
 for *Clostridial myonecrosis,* 50
 for *Clostridium difficile,* 48
 for *Pasteurella* infections, 181
 for toxic shock syndrome, 311
 for *Toxoplasma gondii* infections, 320
Clofazimine for leprosy, 134
Clostridial myonecrosis (gas gangrene), 50–51
 clinical manifestations of, 50
 diagnostic tests for, 50
 epidemiology of, 50
 etiology of, 50
 incubation period of, 50
 treatment of, 50
Clostridial omphalitis, 50*i*, 51*i*
Clostridium botulinum, 46–47
 clinical manifestations of, 46
 diagnostic tests for, 46
 epidemiology of, 46
 etiology of, 46
 incubation period of, 46
 treatment of, 46
Clostridium difficile, 48–49, 49*i*
 clinical manifestations of, 48
 diagnostic tests for, 48
 epidemiology of, 48
 etiology of, 48
 incubation period of, 48
 treatment of, 48–49

Clostridium perfringens, 50
Clostridium tetani, 299, 301*i*
Clotrimazole
 for amebic meningoencephalitis and keratitis, 6
 for candidiasis, 37
 for tinea corporis, 305
 for tinea cruris, 307
 for tinea pedis, 308
 for tinea unguium, 308
Clue cells, 23*i*
Clutton joints, 278
 from syphilis, 278
Coagglutination for group A streptococcal infections, 262
Coagulase-negative staphylococci, 248, 250–251
Coagulopathy from histoplasmosis, 109
Coccidioides immitis infection, 52, 53*i*, 54*i*, 110
Coccidioidomycosis, 52–54, 53*i*
 clinical manifestations of, 52
 diagnostic tests for, 52
 epidemiology of, 52
 etiology of, 52
 incubation period of, 52
 pulmonary, 54*i*
 treatment of, 52
Colitis
 from cytomegalovirus infection, 58
 from *Salmonella* infections, 229
 from *Trichuriasis trichiura,* 328
Colorado tick fever, disease caused by arboviruses in
  Western hemisphere, 13*t*
Coma
 from epidemic typhus, 354
 from meningococcal infections, 153
 from *Vibrio cholerae* infections, 363
Common cold
 from adenovirus infections, 3
 from enterovirus infections, 67
 from pertussis, 186
Community-acquired pneumonia from pneumococcal
  infections, 198
Complement fixation assays
 for endemic typhus, 353
 for mumps, 159
 for *Mycoplasma pneumoniae* infections, 161
 for paracoccidioidomycosis, 172
 for Rocky Mountain spotted fever, 220
Complex decongestive physiotherapy for lymphatic
  filariasis, 144
Computed tomography (CT) scan for tapeworm
  diseases, 294
Concentration techniques for trichuriasis, 328
Condylomata acuminata, 169, 171*i*
Condylomata lata, 292*i*
Confusion
 from amebic keratitis, 6
 from amebic meningoencephalitis, 6
Congenital disease from American trypanosomiasis, 331
Congenital heart disease from respiratory syncytial
  virus, 215
Congenital hepatosplenomegaly, 320*i*
Congenital immunodeficiency from *Cryptococcus
  neoformans* infections, 55

Congenital infection from cytomegalovirus infection, 58
Congenital lymphocytic choriomeningitis, 146
Congenital malaria, 147
Congenital rubella syndrome (CRS), 225, 227*i*, 228*i*
Congenital syphilis, 278, 288*i*, 289*i*, 290*i*
  evaluation of newborn infants for, 280–281
  follow-up and management of, 284
  treatment for, 282–283, 286–287*t*
Congenital toxoplasmosis, 318, 319, 320*i*
Congenital tuberculosis, 339, 342*i*
Congenital varicella syndrome, 356, 359*i*
Conidia, inhalation of, in aspergillosis, 19
Conjunctival hemorrhage, 71*i*
  from trichinellosis, 323
Conjunctival injection
  from babesiosis, 21
  from influenza, 124
  from toxic shock syndrome, 310
Conjunctival suffusion from leptospirosis, 136
Conjunctivitis, 45*i*, 151*i*
  from acute follicular adenovirus, 3*i*
  acute hemorrhagic, 67
  from adenovirus infections, 3
  from enterovirus infections, 67
  from gonococcal infections, 82
  from *Haemophilus influenzae*, 88
  from herpes simplex virus, 103, 106
  from measles, 150
  from meningococcal infections, 153
  from *Pasteurella* infections, 181
  from pneumococcal infections, 198
  from rubella, 225
  from tularemia, 350
  from *Yersinia enterocolitica*, 368
Constipation
  from *Clostridium botulinum*, 46
  from *Salmonella* infections, 229
Contact dermatitis
  from tinea pedis, 308
  from tinea unguium, 308
Convalescent serum specimens
  for *Ehrlichia* and *Anaplasma* infections, 63
  for lymphocytic choriomeningitis, 146
  for rickettsialpox, 217
  for Rocky Mountain spotted fever, 219–220
Corneal inflammation
  from amebic keratitis, 6
  from amebic meningoencephalitis, 6
Corneal ulcer endophthalmitis from *Pasteurella*
    infections, 181
Coronary aneurysms from Kawasaki disease, 128
Coronary artery occlusion from Kawasaki disease, 128
Coronary artery thrombosis from Kawasaki disease, 128
Corticosteroid therapy
  for *Baylisascaris* infections, 27
  for cysticercosis, 295
  for Epstein-Barr virus, 70
  for extrapulmonary M tuberculosis, 338
  for hepatitis B virus, 98
  for herpes simplex virus, 106
  for kerion, 303
  for parainfluenza virus infections, 177
  for pediculosis capitis, 183

  for *Pneumocystis jiroveci* infections, 205
  for respiratory syncytial virus, 216
  for *Salmonella* infections, 231
  for toxocariasis, 316
  for trichinellosis, 323
Corynebacterium diphtheriae, 61
Corynebacterium minutissimum, 307, 308
Corynebacterium ulcerans, 61
Coryza
  from measles, 150
  from *Mycoplasma pneumoniae* infections, 161
Cotton rat, 92*i*
Cough
  from babesiosis, 21
  from *Borrelia* infections, 31
  from *Cryptococcus neoformans* infections, 55
  from hantavirus pulmonary syndrome, 91
  from influenza, 124
  from lymphatic filariasis, 144
  from malaria, 147
  from measles, 150
  from paragonimiasis, 174
  from pertussis, 186
  from *Pneumocystis jiroveci* infections, 204
  from schistosomiasis, 236
  from toxocariasis, 316
  from tuberculosis, 333
  from tularemia, 350
Covert toxocariasis, 316
Cowpox, 242
Coxsackievirus lesions, 68*i*
Cranial nerve palsies
  from *Clostridium botulinum*, 46
  from Epstein-Barr virus, 69
Creeping eruption from cutaneous larva migrans, 57
Crepitus from *Clostridial myonecrosis*, 50
Cross-reacting antibodies for *Histoplasma*
    capsulatum, 110
Crotamiton
  for pediculosis capitis, 183
  for scabies, 234
Croup
  from adenovirus infections, 3
  fatal, 177*i*
  from influenza, 124
  from measles, 150
  from parainfluenza viral infections, 176
Cryotherapy for warts, 170, 171
Cryptococcus neoformans infections (*Cryptococcosis*),
    55–56, 56*i*
  clinical manifestations of, 55
  diagnostic tests for, 55
  epidemiology of, 55
  etiology of, 55
  incubation period of, 55
  treatment of, 55
Cryptosporidium from human immunodeficiency
    virus (HIV) infection, 116
CSF pleocytosis, 142
  mumps and, 159
Culex tarsalis mosquito, 366*i*
Cutaneous anthrax, 9, 10*i*, 11*i*
Cutaneous blastomycosis, 30*i*

Cutaneous candidiasis, 38*i*
Cutaneous chancre from African trypanosomiasis, 329
Cutaneous diphtheria, 61
Cutaneous gonococcal lesion, 84*i*
Cutaneous infection from nontuberculous
    mycobacteria, 345
Cutaneous larva migrans, 57, 57*i*
    clinical manifestations of, 57
    diagnostic tests for, 57
    epidemiology of, 57
    etiology of, 57
    treatment of, 57
Cutaneous leishmaniasis, 131, 132*i*
Cutaneous *Nocardia braziliensis,* 165*i*
Cutaneous nocardiosis, 164*i,* 165*i*
Cutaneous nongenital warts, 169
Cutaneous sporotrichosis, 247*i*
Cutaneous syphilis, 288*i*
Cutaneous warts (human papillomavirus infection),
    122*i,* 169
Cyanosis from *Escherichia coli,* 72
Cyanotic from respiratory syncytial virus, 215
Cyclosporin for Epstein-Barr virus, 70
Cysticercal encephalitis, treatment for, 295
Cysticercosis (tapeworm diseases), 294–296
    clinical manifestations of, 294
    diagnosis of, 294
    epidemiology of, 294
    etiology of, 294
    incubation period of, 294
    ocular, 295
    for tapeworm diseases, 295
    treatment of, 294–295
Cysticercus cellulosae, 294
Cysts
    echinococcus, 298*i*
    hydatid, 298*i*
    from tapeworm diseases, 294, 297
Cytomegalovirus (CMV) infections, 58–60, 60*i*
    clinical manifestations of, 58
    diagnostic tests for, 59
    epidemiology of, 58
    etiology of, 58
    from human immunodeficiency virus infection, 116
    incubation period of, 58
    infant with, 59*i*
    treatment of, 59
    white perivascular infiltrates in retina, 60*i*
Cytomegalovirus (CMV) retinitis, 122*i*

D

Dacron alginate swab for pertussis, 186
Dandruff from tinea capitis, 302
Dapsone
    for leprosy, 134
    for paucibacillary leprosy, 134
Darkfield examination for syphilis, 279
Darkfield microscopy in wet mounts for rat-bite fever, 213
Deafness from *Toxoplasma gondii* infections, 318
DEC-albendazole for lymphatic filariasis, 144

Dehydration
    from *Escherichia coli* diarrhea, 75
    from rotavirus infections, 223
    from *Vibrio cholerae* infections, 363
Delirium from epidemic typhus, 354
Delusions from African trypanosomiasis, 329
Demyelinating disease from *Mycoplasma pneumoniae*
    infections, 161
Dengue hemorrhagic fever, 12
    disease caused by arboviruses in Western
        hemisphere, 13*t*
Dental infection
    from *Bacteroides* infection, 24
    from *Prevotella* infection, 24
Dermacentor variabilis, 219
Dermal erythropoiesis from congenital rubella, 225
Dermal infiltration from leprosy, 133
Dermatitis
    atopic, 302
    from onchocerciasis, 166
    seborrheic, 302
    from tinea corporis, 305
Dermatophyte test
    for tinea cruris, 307
    for tinea pedis, 308
    for tinea unguium, 308
Dexamethasone
    for *Haemophilus influenzae* infections, 89
    for parainfluenza virus infections, 177
Diabetes mellitus from group B streptococcal
        infections, 269
Diaphoresis from *Clostridial myonecrosis,* 50
Diaphyseal cortical thickening, 291*i*
Diarrhea
    from anthrax, 9
    from *Balantidium coli* infection, 26
    from *Campylobacter* infections, 35
    from *Clostridium difficile,* 48
    from enterovirus infections, 67
    from *Escherichia coli,* 72, 75
    from *Giardia intestinalis* infections, 80
    from hantavirus pulmonary syndrome, 91
    from hookworm infections, 112
    from influenza, 124
    from malaria, 147
    from measles, 150
    from nontuberculous mycobacteria, 345
    from Rocky Mountain spotted fever, 219
    from rotavirus infections, 223
    from *Salmonella* infections, 229
    from schistosomiasis, 236
    from *Shigella* infections, 239
    from *Strongyloides,* 275
    from tapeworm diseases, 294
    from tapeworm infections, 297
    from toxic shock syndrome, 310
    from trichinellosis, 323
    from trichuriasis, 328
    from tularemia, 350
    from *Vibrio cholerae* infections, 363
    from West Nile virus, 365
    from *Yersinia enterocolitica,* 368
    from *Yersinia pseudotuberculosis* infection, 368

Dicloxacillin for *Pasteurella* infections, 181
Diethylcarbamazine citrate (DEC) for lymphatic
        filariasis, 144
Diffuse adenopathy from histoplasmosis, 109
Diffuse erythematous maculopapular rash from
        coccidioidomycosis, 52
Diffuse intravascular coagulation from plague, 195
Diffuse myalgia from influenza, 124
Diffuse pneumonitis from histoplasmosis, 109
Diloxanide for amebiasis, 4
Diphtheria, 61–62
    clinical manifestations of, 61
    cutaneous, 61
    diagnostic tests for, 61
    epidemiology of, 61
    etiology of, 61
    incubation period of, 61
    pharyngeal, 62*i*
    treatment of, 61
Diphtheria pneumonia, 62*i*
Diphtheritic cervical lymphadenopathy, 62*i*
Diphyllobothrium latum, 297
Dipylidium caninum, 297
Direct aspirate through endoscope for
        strongyloidiasis, 275
Direct fluorescent antibody (DFA) tests
    for pertussis, 187
    for syphilis, 279
    for tularemia, 350
    for varicella-zoster infections, 357
Disseminated candidiasis, 37
    treatment of, 38
Disseminated intravascular coagulation
    from African trypanosomiasis, 329
    from *Ehrlichia* and *Anaplasma* infections, 63
    from histoplasmosis, 109
    from meningococcal infections, 153
    from Rocky Mountain spotted fever, 219
Disseminated *Mycobacterium avium* complex from
        human immunodeficiency virus (HIV)
        infection, 116
Disseminated nontuberculous mycobacterial cutaneous
        lesions, 349*i*
Disseminated sporotrichosis, 246
Dizziness from hantavirus pulmonary syndrome, 91
DNA probes for malaria, 148
Donovanosis, 86
Dot immunoassay for epidemic typhus, 354
Double-centrifugation technique for African trypanoso-
        miasis, 329
Down syndrome, *Mycoplasma pneumoniae* infections
        and, 161
Doxycycline
    for actinomycosis, 1
    for anthrax, 9
    for *Borrelia* infections, 31
    for *Chlamydia trachomatis* genital tract infection, 44
    for *Ehrlichia* and *Anaplasma* infections, 63
    for endemic typhus, 353
    for epidemic typhus, 354
    for gonococcal infections, 83
    for granuloma inguinale, 86
    for leptospirosis, 136
    for Lyme disease, 141
    for *Mycoplasma pneumoniae* infections, 162
    for nontuberculous mycobacteria, 346
    for onchocerciasis, 166
    for *Pasteurella* infections, 181
    for plague, 195–196, 196
    for rat-bite fever, 213
    for rickettsialpox, 217
    for Rocky Mountain spotted fever, 220
    for syphilis, 283
    for trachoma, 44
    for tularemia, 351
    for *Vibrio cholerae* infections, 364
    for *Yersinia enterocolitica* and *Yersinia pseudo-*
        tuberculosis infections, 369
Drug-resistant tuberculosis disease, therapy for, 338
Dumb paralytic rabies, 212*i*
Duodenale, 112
Duodenal ulcers from *Helicobacter pylori* infections, 94
Dwarf tapeworm, 297
Dyshidrotic eczema
    from tinea pedis, 308
    from tinea unguium, 308
Dyspareunia from chancroid, 43
Dysphagia from rabies, 210
Dyspnea
    from hantavirus pulmonary syndrome, 91
    from paragonimiasis, 174
    from *Pneumocystis jiroveci* infections, 204
Dysuria
    from chancroid, 43
    from *Schistosoma haematobium,* 236
    from *Trichomonas vaginalis* infections, 326

E

East African infection, 329
Eastern equine encephalitis virus, disease caused by
        arboviruses in Western hemisphere, 13*t*
Echinococcus cyst, 298*f*
Echinococcus granulosus, 297–298, 298*i*
Echinococcus multilocularis, 297–298, 298, 298*i*
Econazole
    for candidiasis, 37
    for tinea corporis, 305
    for tinea cruris, 307
    for tinea pedis, 308
    for tinea unguium, 308
Ecthyma from staphylococcal infections, 248
Eczema
    from molluscum contagiosum, 157
    from smallpox vaccination, 244*i*
Eczema herpeticum, 107*i*
    from herpes simplex, 103
Eczema vaccinatum lesions, 245*i*
Edema
    from African trypanosomiasis, 329
    from American trypanosomiasis, 331
    from hookworms, 113*i*
    from syphilis, 278
Ehrlichia chaffeensis, 63, 65*i*
Ehrlichia ewingii, 63

Ehrlichia ewingii ehrlichiosis, 64*t*
Ehrlichia infections, 63–66
    clinical manifestations of, 63
    diagnostic tests for, 63
    epidemiology of, 63
    etiology of, 63
    incubation period of, 63
    treatment of, 63
Ehrlichia phagocytophila, 65*i*
Electrocautery for warts, 170, 171
Electrolyte abnormalities from rotavirus infections, 223
Electron micrograph for hepatitis B virus (HBV), 99*i*
Electron microscopic examination
    for molluscum contagiosum, 157
    for smallpox, 242
Elephantiasis, 145*i*
    from lymphatic filariasis, 144
Empirical therapy for *Shigella* infections, 239
Empyema
    from actinomycosis, 1
    from *Bacteroides* infection, 24
    from *Prevotella* infection, 24
    from *Yersinia enterocolitica,* 368
Enanthemas, 242
    from smallpox, 241
Encephalitis
    from adenovirus infections, 3
    from arboviruses, 12
    from enterovirus infections, 67
    from Epstein-Barr virus, 69
    from herpes simplex virus, 103–104, 106
    from human herpesvirus 6 and 7, 114
    from influenza, 124
    from *Mycoplasma pneumoniae* infections, 161
    from parainfluenza viral infections, 176
    from rubella, 225
    from toxocariasis, 316
    from *Toxoplasma gondii* infections, 318
    from varicella-zoster infections, 356
    from West Nile virus, 365
Encephalopathy
    from cat-scratch disease, 40
    from *Ehrlichia* and *Anaplasma* infections, 63
    from human herpesvirus 6 and 7, 114
    from influenza, 124
    from pertussis, 186
Endemic typhus (flea-borne typhus or murine
        typhus), 353
    clinical manifestations of, 353
    diagnostic tests for, 353
    epidemiology of, 353
    etiology of, 353
    incubation period of, 353
    treatment of, 353
Endocardial fibroelastosis from mumps, 159
Endocarditis, 19
    from *Arcanobacterium haemolyticum* infections, 15
    from *Bacteroides* infection, 24
    from brucellosis, 33
    from cat-scratch disease, 40
    from group A streptococcal infections, 261

from *Haemophilus influenzae,* 88
from non–group A or B streptococcal and
        enterococcal infections, 272
from pneumococcal infections, 198
from *Prevotella* infection, 24
from rat-bite fever, 213
from toxic shock syndrome, 310
treatment for, 265
from *Yersinia enterocolitica,* 368
Endocervical swab for gonococcal infections, 82
Endocervicitis from gonococcal infections, 82
Endocrinologic diseases from candidiasis, 37
Endometritis
    from *Chlamydia trachomatis,* 44
    from group B streptococcal infections, 269
Endophthalmitis
    from *Haemophilus influenzae,* 88
    from meningococcal infections, 153
    from staphylococcal infections, 248
    from toxocariasis, 316
Endoscopy
    for amebiasis, 4
    for candidiasis, 37
    for *Helicobacter pylori* infections, 94
Endotracheal aspiration for *Pneumocystis jiroveci*
        infections, 204
Enlarged lymph nodes from paracoccidioidomycosis, 172
Enlarged lymphocyte, 93*i*
Entamoeba dispar, 4
Entamoeba histolytica infections, 4, 4*i*
Entecavir for hepatitis B virus (HBV), 98–99
Enteritis (*Yersinia enterocolitica* and *Yersinia pseudo-
        tuberculosis* infections), 368–369
    clinical manifestations of, 368
    diagnostic tests for, 368–369
    epidemiology of, 368
    etiology of, 368
    incubation period of, 368
    treatment of, 369
Enterobacter sakazakii, 72
Enterobius vermicularis (pinworm infection), 190–191,
        191*i*
    clinical manifestations of, 190
    diagnostic tests for, 190
    epidemiology of, 190
    etiology of, 190
    incubation period of, 190
    treatment of, 190
Enterococcal endocarditis, 273*i*
Enterococcal infections, non–group A or B, 272–274
    clinical manifestations of, 272
    diagnostic tests for, 272
    epidemiology of, 272
    etiology of, 272
    incubation period of, 272
    treatment of, 272–273
Enterocolitis, necrotizing, 248
Entero-Test
    for *Giardia intestinalis* infections, 80
    for strongyloidiasis, 275
Enteroviral exanthem, newborn with, 68*i*

Enterovirus (nonpoliovirus) infections, 67–68, 67*i*, 68*i*
    clinical manifestations of, 67
    diagnostic tests for, 67
    epidemiology of, 67
    etiology of, 67
    incubation period of, 67
    treatment of, 67
Enzyme immunoassay (EIA) tests
    for American trypanosomiasis, 331
    for *Borrelia* infections, 31
    for *Clostridium difficile,* 48
    for *Cryptococcus neoformans* infections, 55
    for cytomegalovirus infection, 59
    for endemic typhus, 353
    for epidemic typhus, 354
    for *Giardia intestinalis* infections, 80
    for hantavirus pulmonary syndrome, 92
    for hepatitis C virus, 101
    for herpes simplex virus, 105
    for *Histoplasma capsulatum,* 109
    for human immunodeficiency virus, 118
    for Lyme disease, 141
    for mumps, 159
    for paracoccidioidomycosis, 172
    for parainfluenza virus infections, 176
    for parvovirus B19, 179
    for Rocky Mountain spotted fever, 220
    for rotavirus infections, 220
    for rubella, 226
    for Shiga toxin for *Shigella* infections, 239
    for strongyloidiasis, 275
    for syphilis, 280
    for toxocariasis, 316
    for *Trichomonas vaginalis* infection, 326
    for West Nile virus, 366
Enzyme-linked DNA probe for *Shigella* infections, 239
Eosinophilia
    from hookworm infections, 112
    from lymphatic filariasis, 144
    from schistosomiasis, 236
    from toxocariasis, 316
    for trichinellosis, 323
Eosinophilic enteritis from cutaneous larva migrans, 57
Eosinophilic meningoencephalitis from *Baylisascaris*
        infections, 27
Epidemic keratoconjunctivitis, 3
Epidemic typhus (louse-borne typhus), 354–355
    clinical manifestations of, 354
    diagnostic tests for, 354
    epidemiology of, 354
    etiology of, 354
    incubation period of, 354
    treatment of, 354–355
Epidermodysplasia verruciformis, 169
Epidermolytic exotoxin, 259*i*
Epidermophyton floccosum, 305, 307, 308
Epididymitis
    acute, 84
    from gonococcal infections, 82
    from lymphatic filariasis, 144
    from *Trichomonas vaginalis* infections, 326
Epigastric pain from *Helicobacter pylori* infections, 94
Epiglottis, swelling of, 89*i*

Epiglottitis from *Haemophilus influenzae,* 88
Epilepsy from tapeworm diseases, 294
Epinephrine for parainfluenza virus infections, 177
Epitrochlear suppurative adenitis, 42*i*
Epstein-Barr virus (EBV) (infectious mononucleosis),
        69–71, 70*t,* 71*i*
    clinical manifestations of, 69
    diagnostic tests for, 69
    epidemiology of, 69
    etiology of, 69
    incubation period of, 69
    treatment of, 70
Equine tetanus antitoxin, 299
Erysipelas, 267*i*
    from group A streptococcal infections, 261
    treatment for, 265
Erythema from tinea corporis, 305
Erythema infectiosum (Fifth disease, parvovirus B19),
        44, 178–180
    clinical manifestations of, 178
    diagnostic tests for, 179
    epidemiology of, 178–179
    etiology of, 178
    incubation period of, 179
    treatment of, 179
Erythema marginatum, 268*i*
Erythema migrans lesions from Lyme disease, 140,
        142*i,* 143*i*
Erythema multiforme from coccidioidomycosis, 52
Erythema nodosum, 53*i,* 369*i*
    from *Campylobacter* infections, 35
    from cat-scratch disease, 40
    from coccidioidomycosis, 52
    from histoplasmosis, 109, 110
    from *Yersinia enterocolitica,* 368
    from *Yersinia pseudotuberculosis* infection, 368
Erythema nodosum leprosum, 134*i,* 135*i*
Erythematous lips, with Kawasaki disease, 129*i*
Erythematous maculopapular rash from measles, 150
Erythematous papules, 235*i*
Erythematous papulovesicular eruptions from
        rickettsialpox, 217
Erythematous rash
    from Kawasaki disease, 127
    from *Listeria monocytogenes* infections, 138
Erythematous tonsils, 266*i*
Erythematous vesicular eruptions
    from tinea pedis, 308
    from tinea unguium, 308
Erythrasma
    from tinea pedis, 308
    from tinea unguium, 308
Erythroderma, 314*i*
    from toxic shock syndrome, 310
Erythroid hypoplasia from parvovirus B19, 178
Erythromycin
    for actinomycosis, 1
    for *Arcanobacterium haemolyticum* infections, 15
    for *Borrelia* infections, 31
    for *Campylobacter* infections, 35
    for chlamydial conjunctivitis, 44
    for chlamydial pneumonia, 44
    for *Chlamydia trachomatis* genital tract infection, 44

for granuloma inguinale, 86
for group A streptococcal infections, 264
for Lyme disease, 141
for *Mycoplasma pneumoniae* infections, 162
for *Pasteurella* infections, 181
for pertussis, 187
for trachoma, 44
in treating cat-scratch disease, 40
Escherichia coli, 73*i*
Escherichia coli diarrhea, 75–79
 classification of, 77*t*
 clinical manifestations of, 75
 diagnostic tests for, 76
 enterohemorrhagic, 78*f*
 epidemiology of, 76
 etiology of, 75–76
 incubation period of, 76
 treatment of, 77
Escherichia coli (nondiarrheal), 72–74
 clinical manifestations of, 72
 diagnostic tests for, 72
 epidemiology of, 72
 etiology of, 72
 incubation period of, 72
 treatment of, 72–73
Esomeprazole for *Helicobacter pylori* infections, 94
Esophagitis, 19
Ethambutol
 for nontuberculous mycobacteria lymphadenitis, 346
 for tuberculosis, 337
Ethmoid sinusitis, 255*i*
 from *Haemophilus influenzae* infections, 90*i*
Ethylsuccinate
 for chlamydial conjunctivitis, 44
 for chlamydial pneumonia, 44
Exanthem subitum from human herpesvirus 6 and 7, 114
Exchange blood transfusions for babesiosis, 21
Extracutaneous sporotrichosis, 246
Extrapulmonary manifestations from paragonimiasis, 174
Extrapulmonary paragonimiasis, 174
Exudative pharyngitis
 from adenovirus infections, 3
 from Epstein-Barr virus, 69
Exudative stomatitis from tularemia, 350

F

Facial nerve palsy in Lyme disease, 143*i*
Failure to thrive from human immunodeficiency virus
   (HIV) infection, 116
Famciclovir
 for herpes simplex virus, 105
  mucocutaneous, 106
 for varicella-zoster infections, 359
Fatigue
 from babesiosis, 21
 from histoplasmosis, 109
 from Lyme disease, 140
 from nontuberculous mycobacteria, 345
 from West Nile virus, 365
Febrile occult bacteremia from meningococcal
   infections, 153

Febrile seizures
 from human herpesvirus 6 and 7, 114
 from influenza, 124
Fecal cultures
 for *Campylobacter* infections, 35
 for *Vibrio cholerae* infections, 363
Fever
 from African trypanosomiasis, 329
 from amebic keratitis, 6
 from amebic meningoencephalitis, 6
 from anthrax, 9
 from *Arcanobacterium haemolyticum* infections, 15
 from *Borrelia* infections, 31
 from brucellosis, 33
 from *Campylobacter* infections, 35
 from cat-scratch disease, 40
 from *Clostridial myonecrosis,* 50
 from *Clostridium difficile,* 48
 from endemic typhus, 353
 from epidemic typhus, 354
 from Epstein-Barr virus, 69
 from *Escherichia coli,* 72
 from *Escherichia coli* diarrhea, 75
 from group A streptococcal infections, 261
 from hantavirus pulmonary syndrome, 91
 from hepatitis A, 95
 from histoplasmosis, 109
 from human herpesvirus 6 and 7, 114
 from influenza, 124
 from Kawasaki disease, 127
 from leishmaniasis, 131
 from leptospirosis, 136
 from *Listeria monocytogenes* infections, 138
 from Lyme disease, 140
 from lymphatic filariasis, 144
 from lymphocytic choriomeningitis, 146
 from malaria, 147
 from measles, 150
 from meningococcal infections, 153
 from *Mycoplasma pneumoniae* infections, 161
 from nontuberculous mycobacteria, 345
 from paracoccidioidomycosis, 172
 from parvovirus B19, 178
 from *Pasteurella* infections, 181
 from pertussis, 186
 from plague, 195
 from *Pneumocystis jiroveci* infections, 204
 from poliovirus infections, 207
 from rat-bite fever, 213
 from rickettsialpox, 217
 from Rocky Mountain spotted fever, 219
 from rotavirus infections, 223
 from *Salmonella* infections, 229
 from schistosomiasis, 236
 from *Shigella* infections, 239
 from smallpox, 241
 from tinea capitis, 302
 from toxic shock syndrome, 310
 from toxocariasis, 316
 from *Toxoplasma gondii* infections, 318
 from trichinellosis, 323
 from tuberculosis, 333
 from tularemia, 350

Fever, continued
  from varicella-zoster infections, 356
  from West Nile virus, 365
  from *Yersinia enterocolitica,* 368
  from *Yersinia pseudotuberculosis* infection, 368
Fifth disease (parvovirus B19, Erythema infectiosum),
        178–180
  clinical manifestations of, 178
  diagnostic tests for, 179
  epidemiology of, 178–179
  etiology of, 178
  incubation period of, 179
  treatment of, 179
Filarial nematodes, 166
Filariasis
  Bancroftian, 144–145
  Malayan, 144–145
  onchocerciasis, 166–168
  Timorian, 144–145
Filiform warts, 169
Fish tapeworm, 297
Fistulas from paracoccidioidomycosis, 172
Fitz-Hugh-Curtis syndrome from gonococcal
        infections, 82
Fixed cutaneous sporotrichosis, 246
Flaccid paralysis from arboviruses, 12
Flatulence from *Giardia intestinalis* infections, 80
Flat warts, 169
Flaviviridae, 12
Flea-borne typhus (endemic typhus, murine typhus), 353
  clinical manifestations of, 353
  diagnostic tests for, 353
  epidemiology of, 353
  etiology of, 353
  incubation period of, 353
  treatment of, 353
Flow-directed pulmonary catheter for hantavirus
        pulmonary syndrome, 92
Fluconazole
  for amebic meningoencephalitis and keratitis, 6
  for blastomycosis, 29
  for coccidioidomycosis, 52
  for *Cryptococcus neoformans* infections, 55
  for histoplasmosis, 110
  for pityriasis versicolor, 192
  for sporotrichosis, 246
  for tinea capitis, 303
  for tinea corporis, 305
  for tinea cruris, 307
  for tinea pedis and tinea unguium, 308
  for treating candidiasis, 38
  in treating candidiasis, 37
Flucytosine
  for *Cryptococcus neoformans* infections, 55
  for treating candidiasis, 38
Flukes, 236
Fluorescein-conjugated monoclonal antibody stain for
        Pneumocystis jiroveci infections, 205
Fluorescent antibody test
  for group A streptococcal infections, 262
  for herpes simplex virus, 105
  for plague, 195
  for *Shigella* infections, 239

Fluorescent microscopy of skin biopsy for rabies, 210
Fluorescent staining for tuberculosis, 334
Fluorescent treponemal antibody absorption (FTA-ABS)
        for syphilis, 279
Fluoroimmunoassays for parainfluenza virus
        infections, 176
Fluoroquinolones
  for *Clostridium difficile,* 48
  for epidemic typhus, 354
  for gonococcal infections, 83
  for *Mycoplasma pneumoniae* infections, 162
  for *Pasteurella* infections, 181
  for plague, 196
  for rickettsialpox, 217
  for Rocky Mountain spotted fever, 220
  for *Salmonella* infections, 230
  for *Yersinia enterocolitica* and *Yersinia pseudo-
        tuberculosis* infections, 369
Folliculitis, tinea capitis and, 302
Fomites, 184
Food-borne botulism, 46
Food poisoning from staphylococcal infections, 248
Francisella tularensis, 350, 352i
Frontal bossing from syphilis, 278
Fulguration for lymphatic filariasis, 144
Fulminant colitis from amebiasis, 4
Fulminant fatal hepatitis, 97
Fungal culture for tinea pedis and tinea unguium, 308
Fungal infection from tinea capitis, 302
Fungal stain for sporotrichosis, 246
Funiculitis from lymphatic filariasis, 144
Furazolidone for *Giardia intestinalis* infections, 80
Furuncles from staphylococcal infections, 248

G

Gagging from pertussis, 186
Gag reflex from *Clostridium botulinum,* 46
Gait disturbance from tapeworm diseases, 294
Gallbladder hydrops from Kawasaki disease, 127
Ganciclovir
  for cytomegalovirus infection, 59
  for human herpesvirus 6 and 7, 115
Gardnerella vaginalis, in bacterial vaginosis, 22
Gas gangrene *(Clostridial myonecrosis),* 50–51
  clinical manifestations of, 50
  diagnostic tests for, 50
  epidemiology of, 50
  etiology of, 50
  incubation period of, 50
  treatment of, 50
Gasping from pertussis, 186
Gastric aspirate specimen for tuberculosis, 334
Gastric biopsy for *Helicobacter pylori* infections, 94
Gastric cancer from *Helicobacter pylori* infections, 94
Gastric ulcers from *Helicobacter pylori* infections, 94
Gastric washings for *Listeria monocytogenes*
        infections, 138
Gastritis from *Helicobacter pylori* infections, 94
Gastroenteritis
  from adenovirus infections, 3
  from *Salmonella* infections, 229
Gastrointestinal tract bleeding from histoplasmosis, 109

Gastrointestinal tract disease from anthrax, 9
Gastrointestinal tract symptoms
    from *Listeria monocytogenes* infections, 138
    from plague, 195
Gatifloxacin for nontuberculous mycobacteria, 346
Gene amplification for hepatitis B virus (HBV), 98
Generalized tetanus, 299
Genital herpes from herpes simplex virus (HSV), 103, 104
Genital tract infection from *Chlamydia trachomatis*, 44
Genital ulcer from chancroid, 43
Genotyping
    for measles, 151
    for staphylococcal infections, 251
Gentamicin
    for brucellosis, 33
    for *Escherichia coli*, 72
    for granuloma inguinale, 86
    for *Listeria monocytogenes* infections, 138
    for non–group A or B streptococcal and enterococcal
        infections, 272, 273
    for tularemia, 351
Geophagia/pica from *Baylisascaris* infections, 27
German measles, rash of, 226*i*
Gianotti-Crosti syndrome from hepatitis B, 97
Giardia intestinalis infections, 80–81
    clinical manifestations of, 80
    diagnostic tests for, 80
    epidemiology of, 80
    etiology of, 80
    incubation period of, 80
    reported cases, 81*f*
    treatment of, 80
Giemsa-stained smear
    for African trypanosomiasis, 329
    for American trypanosomiasis, 331
    identification of intracellular leishmanial
        organism, 132
    for molluscum contagiosum, 157
    for *Plasmodium malariae*, 149*i*
    for *Plasmodium ovale*, 149*i*
    for *Plasmodium vivax*, 149*i*
    for *Pneumocystis jiroveci* infections, 204–205
    in *Yersinia pestis*, 196*i*
Gingivostomatitis, 104
    from herpes simplex virus, 103, 104
Glandular syndrome from tularemia, 350
Glomerulonephritis
    from mumps, 159
    from varicella-zoster infections, 356
Gonococcal infections, 82–85
    clinical manifestations of, 82
    diagnostic tests for, 82–83
    epidemiology of, 82
    etiology of, 82
    incubation period of, 82
    treatment of, 83–84
Gonococcal ophthalmia, 83, 84*i*
Gonococcal urethritis from gonococcal infections, 82
Gonorrhea from gonococcal infections, 82
Gram-negative bacilli, 72–74, 229
    clinical manifestations of, 72
    diagnostic tests for, 72
    epidemiology of, 72

etiology of, 72
    incubation period of, 72
    treatment of, 72–73
Gram stain
    for actinomycosis, 1
    for anthrax, 9
    for *Clostridial myonecrosis*, 50
    for gonococcal infections, 82
    for *Haemophilus influenzae* infections, 88
    for *Listeria monocytogenes* infections, 138
    for meningococcal infections, 154
    for plague, 195
    for staphylococcal infections, 251
    of vaginal secretions in bacterial vaginosis, 22
Granuloma inguinale, 86–87
    clinical manifestations of, 86
    diagnostic tests for, 86
    epidemiology of, 86
    etiology of, 86
    Giemsa-stained Donovan bodies of, 87*i*
    incubation period of, 86
    perianal lesion, 87*i*
    treatment of, 86
Granulomata from cat-scratch disease, 40
Granulomatosis infantisepticum from *Listeria mono-
        cytogenes* infections, 138
Granulomatous adenitis, 110
Granulomatous amebic encephalitis, 6
Granulomatous inflammation of lymph nodes from
        tuberculosis, 333
Granulomatous lesions from paracoccidioidomycosis, 172
Griseofulvin
    for kerion, 303
    for tinea capitis, 303
    for tinea corporis, 305
    for tinea cruris, 307
Gross hematuria from *Schistosoma haematobium*, 236
Group A streptococcal arthritis, 267*i*
Group A streptococcal cellulitis, 267*i*
Group A streptococcal infections, 261–268
    from bacterial vaginosis, 22
    clinical manifestations of, 261
    diagnostic tests for, 262–264
    epidemiology of, 261–262
    etiology of, 261
    incubation period of, 262
    indications for testing, 263–264
    treatment of, 264–265
Group A streptococcal necrotizing fasciitis, 267*i*
Group A streptococcus from influenza, 124
Group B streptococcal infections, 269–271
    clinical manifestations of, 269
    diagnostic tests for, 270
    epidemiology of, 269
    etiology of, 269
    incubation period of, 269
    treatment of, 270
Group B streptococcal meningitis, 270*i*
Group B streptococcal osteomyelitis, 271*i*
Group B streptococcal pneumonia, 270*i*
Group-specific antisera for non–group A or B streptococ-
        cal and enterococcal infections, 272
Growth delay from tuberculosis, 333

Growth retardation
    from congenital rubella, 225
    from trichuriasis, 328
Grunting respirations from *Escherichia coli,* 72
Guaiac-positive stools from *Helicobacter pylori*
                infections, 94
Guillain-Barré (G-B) syndrome
    as complication of viral *Campylobacter* infections, 35
    treatment for, 366
    from West Nile virus, 365

H

Haemophilus ducreyi, 43, 43*i,* 86
Haemophilus influenzae infections, 72, 88–90, 89*i,* 90*i,* 201
    clinical manifestations of, 88
    diagnostic tests for, 88
    epidemiology of, 88
    etiology of, 88
    incubation period of, 88
    treatment of, 88–89
Hair loss from tinea capitis, 302
Hallucinations from African trypanosomiasis, 329
Hansen disease. *See* Leprosy
Hantavirus pulmonary syndrome, 91–93, 93*i*
    clinical manifestations of, 91
    diagnostic tests for, 91–92
    epidemiology of, 91
    etiology of, 91
    incubation period of, 91
    treatment of, 92
Haverhill fever, 213
HBeAg for hepatitis B virus (HBV), 99*t*
HBsAg for hepatitis B virus (HBV), 99*t*
Headaches
    from African trypanosomiasis, 329
    from amebic keratitis, 6
    from amebic meningoencephalitis, 6
    from arboviruses, 12
    from babesiosis, 21
    from brucellosis, 33
    from *Ehrlichia* and *Anaplasma* infections, 63
    from endemic typhus, 353
    from epidemic typhus, 354
    from hantavirus pulmonary syndrome, 91
    from influenza, 124
    from leptospirosis, 136
    from *Listeria monocytogenes* infections, 138
    from Lyme disease, 140
    from lymphatic filariasis, 144
    from malaria, 147
    from *Mycoplasma pneumoniae* infections, 161
    from parvovirus B19, 178
    from plague, 195
    from rat-bite fever, 213
    from rickettsialpox, 217
    from Rocky Mountain spotted fever, 219
    from *Salmonella* infections, 229
    from smallpox, 241
    from tularemia, 350
    from West Nile virus, 365

Head lice (pediculosis capitis), 182–183
    clinical manifestations of, 182
    diagnostic tests for, 182
    epidemiology of, 182
    etiology of, 182
    incubation period of, 182
    treatment of, 182–183
Hearing impairment from mumps, 159
Heart failure from American trypanosomiasis, 331
Heart rate abnormalities from *Escherichia coli,* 72
Helicobacter pylori infections, 94
    clinical manifestations of, 94
    diagnostic tests for, 94
    epidemiology of, 94
    etiology of, 94
    incubation period of, 94
    treatment of, 94
Hemagglutination assay for amebiasis, 4
Hemagglutination inhibition test for mumps, 159
Hematemesis
    from anthrax, 9
    from *Helicobacter pylori* infections, 94
Hemodynamic instability from plague, 195
Hemolytic anemia
    from Epstein-Barr virus, 69, 70
    from syphilis, 278
Hemolytic-uremic syndrome, 75–79
    clinical manifestations of, 75
    diagnostic tests for, 76
    epidemiology of, 76
    from *Escherichia coli* diarrhea, 75
    etiology of, 75–76
    incubation period of, 76
    reported cases of postdiarrheal, 79*f*
    from *Shigella* infections, 239
    treatment of, 77
Hemophagocytic syndrome from Epstein-Barr virus,
                69, 70
Hemoptysis from paragonimiasis, 174
Hemorrhage
    intraventricular, 11*i*
    from parvovirus B19, 178
Hemorrhagic colitis from *Escherichia coli* diarrhea, 75
Hemorrhagic cystitis from adenovirus infections, 3
Hemorrhagic fever, acute from arboviruses, 12
Hemorrhagic meningitis from anthrax, 9
Hemorrhagic retinitis with Roth spots, 274*i*
Hemorrhagic varicella, 356, 360*i*
Hepatic abscess from *Pasteurella* infections, 181
Hepatitis
    from African trypanosomiasis, 329
    from enterovirus infections, 67
    fulminant, 95
    from human herpesvirus 6 and 7, 114
    from human immunodeficiency virus infection, 116
    from varicella-zoster infections, 356
    viral, 96*t*
    from West Nile virus, 365

Hepatitis A, 95–96
    acute, 96*i*
    clinical manifestations of, 95
    diagnostic tests for, 95
    epidemiology of, 95
    etiology of, 95
    incubation period of, 95
    treatment of, 95
    vaccines for children with human immunodeficiency
        virus, 120
Hepatitis B, 97–100
    clinical manifestations of, 97
    diagnostic tests for, 98
    epidemiology of, 97–98
    etiology of, 97
    incubation period of, 98
    treatment of, 98–99
Hepatitis C, 101–102
    clinical manifestations of, 101
    diagnostic tests for, 101–102
    epidemiology of, 101
    etiology of, 101
    incubation period of, 101
    treatment of, 102
Hepatoma from hepatitis B virus (HBV), 100*i*
Hepatomegaly
    from American trypanosomiasis, 331
    from babesiosis, 21
    from *Escherichia coli,* 72
    from human immunodeficiency virus infection, 116
    from leishmaniasis, 131
    from toxocariasis, 316
    from *Toxoplasma gondii* infections, 318
Hepatosplenomegaly
    from American trypanosomiasis, 331
    from *Borrelia* infections, 31
    from brucellosis, 33
    from congenital rubella, 225
    from cytomegalovirus infection, 58
    from Epstein-Barr virus, 69
    from histoplasmosis, 109
    from malaria, 147
    from schistosomiasis, 236
    from syphilis, 278
Herpangina (coxsackievirus), 68*i*
    from enterovirus infections, 67
Herpes labialis from herpes simplex, 103
Herpes simplex infections, 103–108
    adolescent, 103–104
    children beyond neonatal period, 103–104
    clinical manifestations of, 103–104
    diagnostic tests for, 104–105
    epidemiology of, 104
    etiology of, 104
    genital, 103, 104, 105–106
    incubation period of, 104
    mucocutaneous, 106
    neonatal, 103, 104, 105
    recurrent, 107*i*
    treatment of, 105–106
Herpes simplex lesions, 108*i*
    neonatal, 108*i*
Herpes simplex stomatitis, 107*i*

Herpes simplex virus (HSV)
    acyclovir-resistant strains of, 106
    from bacterial vaginosis, 22
    chancroid and, 43
Herpes simplex virus (HSV) conjunctivitis, 106
Herpes simplex virus (HSV) encephalitis, 103–104, 106
Herpes zoster virus (HZV) infection, 362*i*
    from human immunodeficiency virus infection, 116
Herpetic gingivostomatitis, 107*i*
Herpetic whitlow from herpes simplex, 103
Heterophil antibody tests for Epstein-Barr virus, 69
Hilar adenopathy, 344*i*
    from histoplasmosis, 109
    from tularemia, 350
Hirschsprung disease from *Clostridium difficile,* 48
Histologic examination for herpes simplex virus
        (HSV), 105
Histopathologic examination
    for leprosy, 133
    for sporotrichosis, 246
Histoplasma capsulatum, 109, 110*i*
Histoplasmin skin test for histoplasmosis, 110
Histoplasmosis, 109–111
    acute primary, 111*i*
    acute pulmonary, 109
    calcified hilar lymph nodes bilaterally secondary
        to, 111*i*
    clinical manifestations of, 109
    diagnostic tests for, 109–110
    epidemiology of, 109
    etiology of, 109
    incubation period of, 109
    pulmonary, 110
    snowstorm of acute, 111*i*
    treatment of, 110
Hoarseness from hookworm infections, 112
Hookworm infections, 112–113, 113*i*
    anemia and, 113*i*
    clinical manifestations of, 112
    diagnostic tests for, 112
    edema and, 113*i*
    epidemiology of, 112
    etiology of, 112
    incubation period of, 112
    treatment of, 112
Hordeola from staphylococcal infections, 248
HPV DNA testing, 170
HPV RNA testing for human papillomaviruses, 170
Human bite wounds, 1
Human feces as cause of *Escherichia coli* diarrhea, 76
Human granulocytic ehrlichiosis, Lyme disease and, 140
Human granulocytotrophic anaplasmosis, 64*f,* 64*t*
Human herpesvirus 6 and 7, 114–115
    clinical manifestations of, 114
    diagnostic tests for, 114–115
    epidemiology of, 114
    etiology of, 114
    incubation period of, 114
    rash of human, 115*i*
    treatment of, 115
Human immunodeficiency virus (HIV)–associated
        encephalopathy, 122*i*

Human immunodeficiency virus (HIV) infection, 116–123, 123*i*
  from candidiasis, 37
  chancroid and, 43
  clinical manifestations of, 116
  diagnostic tests for, 117–118
  epidemiology of, 116–117
  etiology of, 116
  incubation period of, 117
  laboratory diagnosis of, 120*t*
  treatment of, 119–120
  tuberculosis disease and, 338–339
  Zidovudine regimen for decreasing rate of perinatal transmission of, 120*t*
Human monocytic ehrlichiosis, 66*i*
Human monocytotrophic ehrlichiosis, 64*t,* 65*f*
Human papillomaviruses, 169–171
  clinical manifestations of, 169
  diagnostic tests for, 170
  epidemiology of, 169–170
  etiology of, 169
  incubation period of, 170
  treatment of, 170–171
Human plague, 195
Human plague pneumonia, 197*f*
Human tetanus immune globulin (TIG), 299
Hutchinson teeth, 278, 291*i*
Hutchinson triad, 278
Hybridization assays for hepatitis B virus (HBV), 98
Hydatid cysts, 298*i*
Hydatid disease (other tapeworm infections), 297–298, 298*i*
  alveolar form of, 298
  clinical manifestations of, 297–298
Hydrocele from lymphatic filariasis, 144
Hydrocephalus
  from lymphocytic choriomeningitis, 146
  from *Toxoplasma gondii* infections, 318
Hymenolepis nana from hydatid disease, 297
Hyperbaric oxygen for *Clostridial myonecrosis,* 50
Hyperesthesia from babesiosis, 21
Hypergammaglobulinemia
  from leishmaniasis, 131
  from toxocariasis, 316
Hyperkeratosis, 169
Hypersplenism from malaria, 147
Hypertrophic pulmonary osteoarthropathy, 2*i*
Hyphae, 307*i*
Hypoalbuminemia from leishmaniasis, 131
Hypochromic microcytic anemia from hookworm infections, 112
Hypoesthesia from leprosy, 133
Hypoglycemia
  from malaria, 147
  from *Vibrio cholerae* infections, 363
Hypokalemia from *Vibrio cholerae* infections, 363
Hyponatremia from *Ehrlichia* and *Anaplasma* infections, 63
Hypoplasia from *Ehrlichia* and *Anaplasma* infections, 63
Hypoproteinemia from hookworm infections, 112

Hypotension
  from *Clostridial myonecrosis,* 50
  from toxic shock syndrome, 310
Hypotonia from *Clostridium botulinum,* 46
Hypovolemic shock from *Vibrio cholerae* infections, 363

I

IgG agglutinins for brucellosis, 33
IgG antibody assays for hepatitis C virus (HCV), 101
IgG avidity test for *toxoplasma gondii,* 319
IgG immunoblot assays for Lyme disease, 141
IGIV therapy
  for human immunodeficiency virus, 119
  for Kawasaki disease, 128–129
  for parvovirus B19, 179
  for tetanus, 299
  for toxic shock syndrome, 311
IgM antibody testing
  for human herpesvirus 6 and 7, 114
  for measles, 150
IgM anti-HBc for hepatitis B virus (HBV), 99*t*
IgM immunoblot assays
  for Lyme disease, 141
  for syphilis, 279
IgM test for *toxoplasma gondii,* 319
Ileocecal mesenteric adenitis from *Yersinia pseudo-tuberculosis* infection, 368
Imipenem
  for *Campylobacter* infections, 35
  for *Clostridial myonecrosis,* 50
  for nocardiosis, 163
  for nontuberculous mycobacteria, 346
Imipenem-cilastatin for tularemia, 351
Imiquimod for warts, 170
Immunizations. *See* Vaccines
Immunoassay for adenovirus infections, 3
Immunodeficiencies, *Mycoplasma pneumoniae* infections and, 161
Immunodeficiency disease from respiratory syncytial virus, 215
Immunodiffusion test
  for histoplasmosis, 110
  for paracoccidioidomycosis, 172
Immunofluorescent antibody testing for *Giardia intestinalis* infections, 80
Immunofluorescent assays
  for cytomegalovirus infection, 59
  for parainfluenza virus infections, 176
  for rubella, 226
  for West Nile virus, 366
Immunofluorescent techniques for *Trichomonas vaginalis* infection, 326
Immunohistochemical assay for epidemic typhus, 354
Immunohistochemical examination of brain for rabies, 210
Immunohistochemical staining (IHC)
  for hantavirus pulmonary syndrome, 91
  for West Nile virus, 366
Immunohistochemical techniques for leptospirosis, 136
Immunohistochemical visualization for epidemic typhus, 354

Immunologic disorders from candidiasis, 37
Impetigo
    from staphylococcal infections, 248
    streptococcal, 262
    from tinea capitis, 302
Inactivated poliovirus (IPV-OPV) immunization, 207
Incision and drainage, in treating cat-scratch disease, 40
Incomplete Kawasaki disease, 127
Incontinence from pertussis, 186
Indirect fluorescent antibody tests
    for endemic typhus, 353
    for epidemic typhus, 354
Indirect hemagglutination assays
    for American trypanosomiasis, 331
    for cytomegalovirus infection, 59
    for Rocky Mountain spotted fever, 220
Indirect immunofluorescence for American trypanoso-
    miasis, 331
Indirect immunofluorescent antibody (IFA) assays
    for cat-scratch disease, 40
    for *Ehrlichia* and *Anaplasma* infections, 63
    for Lyme disease, 141
    for rickettsialpox, 217
    for Rocky Mountain spotted fever, 219–220
Infant botulism, 46, 47*i*
    from *Clostridium botulinum,* 46
Infectious mononucleosis (Epstein-Barr virus), 69–71, 70*i*
    clinical manifestations of, 69
    diagnostic tests for, 69
    epidemiology of, 69
    etiology of, 69
    incubation period of, 69
    treatment of, 70
Infectious tuberculosis, 333
Inflammatory bowel disease
    from *Clostridium difficile,* 48
    from trichuriasis, 328
Influenza, 124–126, 126*i*
    clinical manifestations of, 124
    diagnostic tests for, 125
    from epidemic typhus, 354
    epidemiology of, 124–125
    etiology of, 124
    incubation period of, 125
    treatment of, 125–126
Inguinal plague buboes, 196*i*
Inhalational anthrax, 9
Interferon-alfa
    for hepatitis B virus, 98
    for hepatitis C virus, 102
Interior bowing of shins from syphilis, 278
Interstitial keratitis, 278, 292*i*
Interstitial pneumonitis, 93*i*
Interstitial pneumonitis from congenital rubella, 225
Intestinal botulism, 46
Intestinal perforation from *Shigella* infections, 239
Intestinal roundworms, 17
Intestinal ulcers, 5*i*
Intra-abdominal abscesses from non–group A or B strep-
    tococcal and enterococcal infections, 272
Intra-alveolar edema, 93*i*
Intracellular gram-negative diplococci, 85*i*

Intracerebral calcification from cytomegalovirus infec-
    tion, 58
Intracranial calcifications from lymphocytic chorio-
    meningitis, 146
Intracytoplasmic Donovan bodies on Wright or
    Giemsa staining, dark staining of
    for granuloma inguinale, 86
Intramuscular ceftriaxone for otitis media, 201
Intrauterine blood transfusions for parvovirus B19, 179
Intrauterine growth retardation from cytomegalovirus
    infection, 58
Intravenous fluids for *Ascaris lumbricoides* infections, 17
Intraventricular hemorrhage, 11*i*
Invasive aspergillosis, 19
Invasive candidiasis, 37
Invasive extraintestinal amebiasis, 5*i*
In vitro susceptibility and nonsusceptibility, definition
    of, 199*t*
Iododeoxyuridine for herpes simplex virus (HSV), 106
Iodoquinol
    for amebiasis, 4
    for *Balantidium coli* infection, 26
Ipsilateral inguinal lymph nodes, 43*i*
Ipsilateral preauricular adenopathy, 41*i*
Ipsilateral preauricular lymphadenopathy from cat-
    scratch disease, 40
Iridocyclitis from *Borrelia* infections, 31
Iron lung, 208*i*
Irritability
    from *Escherichia coli,* 72
    from group A streptococcal infections, 261
    from respiratory syncytial virus, 215
Isolated limb paralysis from West Nile virus, 365
Isolated ocular toxoplasmosis from *Toxoplasma gondii*
    infections, 318
Isoniazid for tuberculosis, 336, 337
Isospora from human immunodeficiency virus (HIV)
    infection, 116
Itching
    from pediculosis capitis, 182
    from pediculosis corporis, 184
    from scabies, 233
Itraconazole
    for amebic meningoencephalitis and keratitis, 6
    for blastomycosis, 29
    for coccidioidomycosis, 52
    for *Cryptococcus neoformans* infections, 55
    for histoplasmosis, 110
    for paracoccidioidomycosis, 172
    for pityriasis versicolor, 192
    for sporotrichosis, 246
    for tinea capitis, 303
    for tinea cruris, 307
    for tinea pedis, 308
    for tinea unguium, 308
Ivermectin
    for *Ascaris lumbricoides* infections, 17
    for cutaneous larva migrans, 57
    for lymphatic filariasis, 144
    for onchocerciasis, 166
    for scabies, 234
    for strongyloidiasis, 275

Ivermectin-albendazole for lymphatic filariasis, 144
IVIG for West Nile virus (WNV), 366
Ixodes pacificus, 140
Ixodes scapularis, 21, 140

J

Jarisch-Herxheimer reaction
    in *Borrelia* infections, 31
    in leptospirosis, 136
    in Lyme disease, 142
Jaundice
    from *Borrelia* infections, 31
    from cytomegalovirus infection, 58
    from *Escherichia coli,* 72
    from hepatitis A, 95
    from hepatitis B, 97
    from hepatitis C virus, 101
    from malaria, 147
    from *Toxoplasma gondii* infections, 318
Jock itch (tinea cruris), 307
    clinical manifestations of, 307
    diagnostic tests for, 307
    epidemiology of, 307
    etiology of, 307
    incubation period of, 307
    treatment of, 307
Joint effusions from *Yersinia pseudotuberculosis*
            infection, 368
Juvenile plantar dermatosis
    from tinea pedis, 308
    from tinea unguium, 308

K

Kaposi sarcoma, 123*i*
    from human immunodeficiency virus infection, 116
Karyosome, 7*i*
Katayama fever from schistosomiasis, 236
Kato-Katz for hookworm infections, 112
Kawasaki disease (mucocutaneous lymph node
            syndrome), 127–130, 368
    clinical manifestations of, 127–128
    conjunctivitis and, 129*i*
    desquamation of hands with, 130*i*
    diagnostic tests for, 128
    epidemiology of, 128
    erythroderma of, 130*i*
    erythroderma of palm of hand and, 130*i*
    etiology of, 128
    incomplete, 127
    incubation period of, 128
    treatment of, 128–129
    vasculitis of, 128
Keratitis
    amebic, 6–8
        clinical manifestations of, 6
        diagnostic tests for, 6
        epidemiology of, 6
        etiology of, 6
        incubation period of, 6
        treatment of, 6
    from herpes simplex, 103
    interstitial, 278

Keratoconjunctivitis, epidemic, 3
Keratomycosis in treating candidiasis, 37
Kerion, 302
Kerion secondary to tinea capitis, 304*i*
Ketoconazole
    for candidiasis, 37
    for pityriasis versicolor, 192
    for tinea corporis, 305
    for tinea cruris, 307
Kidney lesions from candidiasis, 37
Klebsiella, 72
Klebsiella pneumoniae, 74*i*
Koplik spots, 152*i*
    from measles, 150
Kunjin virus, 365

L

Laguna Negra virus, 91
Lamivudine for hepatitis B virus (HBV), 98
Lansoprazole for *Helicobacter pylori* infections, 94
Larva currens, 275
Laryngeal papillomas, 171*i*
Laryngotracheitis from diphtheria, 61
Laryngotracheobronchitis from measles, 150
Laser surgery for warts, 170
Latent syphilis, 278, 279
    re-treatment of, 285
Latent tuberculosis infection (LTBI), 333
    diagnosis of, 334
Late-onset disease from group B streptococcal
            infections, 269
Latex agglutination assay test
    for *Clostridium difficile,* 48
    for *Cryptococcus neoformans* infections, 55
    for cytomegalovirus infection, 59
    for endemic typhus, 353
    for epidemic typhus, 354
    for group A streptococcal infections, 262
    for Rocky Mountain spotted fever (RMSF), 220
    for rotavirus infections, 220
    for rubella, 226
    for sporotrichosis, 246
Latex particle agglutination for *Haemophilus*
            influenzae infections, 88
Leiomyosarcomas from human immunodeficiency
            virus (HIV) infection, 116
Leishmania aethopica, 131
Leishmania amazonensis, 131
Leishmania braziliensis, 131
Leishmania chagasi, 131
Leishmania donovani, 131
Leishmania guyanensis, 131
Leishmania infantum, 131
Leishmania major, 131
Leishmania mexicana, 131
Leishmania panamensis, 131
Leishmania peruviana, 131
Leishmaniasis, 131–132
    clinical manifestations of, 131
    cutaneous, 131, 132*i*
    diagnostic tests for, 132
    epidemiology of, 131
    etiology of, 131

incubation period of, 131
mucosal, 131, 132
treatment of, 132
visceral, 131, 132
Leishmania tropica, 131
Lemierre syndrome from *Arcanobacterium haemolyticum*
    infections, 15
Leonine facies from leprosy, 133
Lepromatous leprosy, 134*i*, 135*i*
Leprosy, 133–135
    clinical manifestations of, 133
    diagnostic tests for, 133–134
    epidemiology of, 133
    etiology of, 133
    incubation period of, 133
    lepromatous, 133, 134*i*, 135*i*
    treatment of, 134
    tuberculoid, 133
Leptospira, 136
Leptospirosis, 136–137
    clinical manifestations of, 136
    diagnostic tests for, 136
    epidemiology of, 136
    etiology of, 136
    incubation period of, 136
    rash from, 137*i*
    treatment of, 136
Lesions
    annular erythematous, 306*i*
    blueberry muffin, from congenital rubella, 225, 227*i*
    brain, from candidiasis, 37
    candida granulomatous, 39*i*
    cavitary, from tuberculosis, 333
    coxsackievirus, 68*i*
    cutaneous gonococcal, 84*i*
    disseminated nontuberculous mycobacterial, 349*i*
    eczema vaccinatum, 245*i*
    erythema migrans, from Lyme disease, 140, 142*i*, 143*i*
    granulomatous, from paracoccidioidomycosis, 172
    herpes simplex, 108*i*
    kidney, from candidiasis, 37
    liver, from candidiasis, 37
    lobar, from *Pneumocystis jiroveci* infections, 204
    miliary, from *Pneumocystis jiroveci* infections, 204
    modular, from *Pneumocystis jiroveci* infections, 204
    molluscum contagiosum, 158*i*
    from molluscum contagiosum, 157
    mucocutaneous, from syphilis, 278
    mucocutaneous herpes, 122*i*
    mucosal, from *Candidiasis albicans,* 37
    osteolytic, from cat-scratch disease, 40
    papular skin, 155*i*
    papulovesicular, of rickettsialpox, 218*i*
    penile pyodermal, 85*i*
    perianal, 87*i*
    perianal granuloma inguinale, 87*i*
    from pityriasis versicolor, 192
    pruritic skin, from *Strongyloides,* 275
    retinal, from candidiasis, 37
    scalp, from tinea capitis, 302

scaly
    from tinea pedis, 308
    from tinea unguium, 308
skin, 74*i*
    from blastomycosis, 29
    from histoplasmosis, 109
    from leprosy, 133
    from syphilis, 278
    from tinea cruris, 307
    from varicella-zoster infections, 356
smallpox, 243*i*, 244*i*
spleen, from candidiasis, 37
from sporotrichosis, 246
tinea, 303*i*
from tinea corporis, 305
tularemic, 352*i*
ulcerative chancroid, 43*i*
Lesion scrapings for leishmaniasis, 132
Lethargy
    from amebic keratitis, 6
    from amebic meningoencephalitis, 6
    from *Escherichia coli,* 72
    from respiratory syncytial virus, 215
    from *Salmonella* infections, 229
Leucovorin for *Toxoplasma gondii* infections, 320
Leukemia from *Cryptococcus neoformans* infections, 55
Leukocytosis from toxocariasis, 316
Leukopenia
    from leishmaniasis, 131
    from lymphocytic choriomeningitis, 146
    from Rocky Mountain spotted fever, 219
Levofloxacin
    for *Chlamydia trachomatis* genital tract infection, 44
    for gonococcal infections, 83
Lichen planus, 102*i*
Lindane
    for pediculosis capitis, 182–183
    for scabies, 234
Linezolid
    for nocardiosis, 163
    for nontuberculous mycobacteria, 346
Liponyssoides sanguineus, 217
Listeria monocytogenes infections (Listeriosis), 138–139
    clinical manifestations of, 138
    diagnostic tests for, 138
    epidemiology of, 138
    etiology of, 138
    incubation period of, 138
    treatment of, 138–139
Listeriosis (*Listeria monocytogenes* infections),
    138–139, 139*i*
    clinical manifestations of, 138
    diagnostic tests for, 138
    epidemiology of, 138
    etiology of, 138
    incubation period of, 138
    treatment of, 138–139
Liver abscesses
    from amebiasis, 4
    from *Yersinia enterocolitica,* 368
Liver biopsy for toxocariasis, 316

Liver disease
from group B streptococcal infections, 269
from hepatitis C virus, 101
from *Pasteurella* infections, 181
Liver lesions from candidiasis, 37
Lobar lesions from *Pneumocystis jiroveci* infections, 204
Localized tetanus, 299
Lockjaw (tetanus), 299–301. *See also* Tetanus (lockjaw)
clinical manifestations of, 299
diagnostic tests for, 299
epidemiology of, 299
etiology of, 299
incubation period of, 299
treatment of, 299
Löffler-like syndrome from *Strongyloides,* 275
Löffler syndrome
from *Ascaris lumbricoides* infections, 17
from cutaneous larva migrans, 57
Long-term sequelae from Rocky Mountain spotted fever (RMSF), 219
Louse-borne typhus (epidemic typhus), 354–355
clinical manifestations of, 354
diagnostic tests for, 354
epidemiology of, 354
etiology of, 354
incubation period of, 354
treatment of, 354–355
Low birth weight from American trypanosomiasis, 331
Lumbar puncture for *Cryptococcus neoformans* infections, 55
Lung abscess
from *Bacteroides* infection, 24
from *Prevotella* infection, 24
Lung disease
from parainfluenza viral infections, 176
from respiratory syncytial virus, 215
Lung infection from sporotrichosis, 246
Lung tissue secretion specimens for *Pneumocystis jiroveci* infections, 204
Lupus erythematosus, tinea capitis and, 302
Lyme arthritis, 140, 141–142
Lyme disease (*Borrelia burgdorferi* infection), 140–143
clinical manifestations of, 140
diagnostic tests for, 141
epidemiology of, 140–141
etiology of, 140
incubation period of, 141
treatment of, 141–142
Lymphadenitis
cervical, 345
from coccidioidomycosis, 52
from plague, 195
from staphylococcal infections, 248
Lymphadenopathy, 41*i,* 144
from *Arcanobacterium haemolyticum* infections, 15
bilateral cervical, 70*i*
from brucellosis, 33
from Epstein-Barr virus, 69
from group A streptococcal infections, 261
of hilar nodes from tuberculosis, 333
from histoplasmosis, 109
from human immunodeficiency virus infection, 116
from leishmaniasis, 131

from *Pasteurella* infections, 181
from rat-bite fever, 213
from rubella, 225
from schistosomiasis, 236
from syphilis, 278
from tinea capitis, 302
from *Toxoplasma gondii* infections, 318
Lymphangitis from rat-bite fever, 213
Lymphatic filariasis, 144–145
clinical manifestations of, 144
diagnostic tests for, 144
epidemiology of, 144
etiology of, 144
incubation period of, 144
treatment of, 144–145
Lymphedema from lymphatic filariasis, 144
Lymph node specimens for cat-scratch disease, 40
Lymphocytic, congenital, 146
Lymphocytic choriomeningitis, 146
clinical manifestations of, 146
diagnostic tests for, 146
epidemiology of, 146
etiology of, 146
incubation period of, 146
treatment of, 146
Lymphocytosis from Epstein-Barr virus, 69
Lymphogranuloma venereum (LGV) from *Chlamydia trachomatis,* 44
Lymphoid interstitial pneumonia from human immunodeficiency virus (HIV) infection, 116
Lymphoid interstitial pneumonitis/pulmonary lymphoid hyperplasia, 121*i*
Lysis-centrifugation culture
for *Cryptococcus neoformans* infections, 55
for *Histoplasma capsulatum,* 109

M

Macrolides for *Mycoplasma pneumoniae* infections, 162
Maculae ceruleae from pediculosis pubis, 185
Macular rashes from hepatitis B, 97
Macules from pediculosis corporis, 184
Maculopapular exanthem from *Arcanobacterium haemolyticum* infections, 15
Maculopapular rash with necrosis from gonococcal infections, 82
Magnetic resonance imaging (MRI) for tapeworm diseases, 294
Malabsorption from *Strongyloides,* 275
Malaise
from African trypanosomiasis, 329
from brucellosis, 33
from *Campylobacter* infections, 35
from *Ehrlichia* and *Anaplasma* infections, 63
from epidemic typhus, 354
from hepatitis A, 95
from hepatitis B, 97
from influenza, 124
from *Listeria monocytogenes* infections, 138
from Lyme disease, 140
from lymphocytic choriomeningitis, 146
from meningococcal infections, 153
from *Mycoplasma pneumoniae* infections, 161

from paracoccidioidomycosis, 172
from parvovirus B19, 178
from plague, 195
from *Salmonella* infections, 229
from schistosomiasis, 236
from toxocariasis, 316
from *Toxoplasma gondii* infections, 318
from West Nile virus, 365
Malaria, 147–149
　cerebral, 147
　clinical manifestations of, 147
　congenital, 147
　diagnostic tests for, 148
　endemic countries, 149*f*
　epidemiology of, 147–148
　etiology of, 147
　treatment of, 148–149
Malarial ribosomal RNA testing, 148
Malassezia species, 192
Malathion for pediculosis capitis, 182
Malayan filariasis, 144–145
Malazzezia furfur, 193*i*
Malnutrition from histoplasmosis, 109
Mastitis from mumps, 159
Maternal rubella, 225
Mayaro fever, disease caused by arboviruses in
　　　Western hemisphere, 13*t*
Measles, 150–152, 151*f*
　clinical manifestations of, 150
　diagnostic tests for, 150–151
　epidemiology of, 150
　etiology of, 150
　incubation period of, 150
　rash in, 152*i*
　treatment of, 151
Measles encephalitis, 152*i*
Measles-mumps-rubella (MMR) vaccine for human
　　　immunodeficiency virus (HIV) in
　　　children, 120
Mebendazole
　for *Ascaris lumbricoides* infections, 17
　for *Giardia intestinalis* infections, 80
　for hookworm infections, 112
　for pinworm infections, 190
　for toxocariasis, 316
　for trichinellosis, 323
　for trichuriasis, 328
Mediastinitis, 248
　Nocardia, 164*i*
Megacolon
　from amebiasis, 4
　from American trypanosomiasis, 331
　from *Shigella* infections, 239
Megaesophagus from American trypanosomiasis, 331
Megaloblastic anemia from tapeworm infections, 297
Melasma, pityriasis versicolor and, 192
Membranous pharyngitis from *Arcanobacterium*
　　　haemolyticum infections, 15
Meningitis, 19
　from adenovirus infections, 3
　from *Arcanobacterium haemolyticum* infections, 15
　aseptic, 207
　bacterial, 199–200

from *Bacteroides* infection, 24
from *Borrelia* infections, 31
from brucellosis, 33
from *Cysticercosis,* 294
from *Ehrlichia* and *Anaplasma* infections, 63
from enterovirus infections, 67
from group B streptococcal infections, 269
from *Haemophilus influenzae,* 88
hemorrhagic, 9
from herpes simplex virus, 104
from histoplasmosis, 109
from *Listeria monocytogenes* infections, 138
meningococcal, 153, 156*i*
from non–group A or B streptococcal and entero-
　　　coccal infections, 272
from *Pasteurella* infections, 181
pneumococcal, 199
from pneumococcal infections, 198
from *Prevotella* infection, 24
from rat-bite fever, 213
from *Salmonella* infections, 229
from *Strongyloides,* 275
from tapeworm diseases, 294
treatment for, 73, 265, 270
from tuberculosis, 333
viral, 207
from West Nile virus, 365
from *Yersinia enterocolitica,* 368
Meningococcal infections, 153–156
　clinical manifestations of, 153
　diagnostic tests for, 153–154
　epidemiology of, 153
　etiology of, 153
　incubation period of, 153
　treatment of, 154
Meningococcal meningitis, 153, 156*i*
Meningococcemia, 153, 154*i*, 155*i*
　adrenal hemorrhage in, 156*i*
　with cutaneous necrosis, 155*i*
　with gangrene, 155*i*
Meningoencephalitis
　from African trypanosomiasis, 329
　from American trypanosomiasis, 331
　from *Toxoplasma gondii* infections, 318
Mental retardation from lymphocytic
　　　choriomeningitis, 146
Meropenem, 73
　for *Campylobacter* infections, 35
　for *Clostridial myonecrosis,* 50
　for *Haemophilus influenzae* infections, 88
　for nocardiosis, 163
Metabolic acidosis
　from malaria, 147
　from *Vibrio cholerae* infections, 363
Methicillin-resistant CoNS, 251
Methicillin-resistant *Staphylococcus aureus* (MRSA)
　community-associated, 250
　epidemic strains of, 250
Metronidazole
　for amebiasis, 4
　for bacterial vaginosis, 22
　for *Bacteroides* and *Prevotella* infections, 24
　for *Balantidium coli* infection, 26

Metronidazole, continued
  for *Clostridial myonecrosis,* 50
  for *Clostridium difficile,* 49
  for *Giardia intestinalis* infections, 80
  for tetanus, 299
  for *Trichomonas vaginalis* infection, 326
Micafungin for treating candidiasis, 38
Miconazole
  for amebic meningoencephalitis and keratitis, 6
  for tinea corporis, 305
  for tinea cruris, 307
  for tinea pedis and tinea unguium, 308
  in treating candidiasis, 37
Microagglutination tests for Rocky Mountain spotted
        fever (RMSF), 220
Microbial surface components recognizing adhesive
        matrix molecule (MSCRAMM), 249
Microcephaly
  from cytomegalovirus infection, 58
  from lymphocytic choriomeningitis, 146
Micrococcus, 257i
Microfilaria of *Wuchereria bancrofti,* 145i
Microscopic agglutination for leptospirosis, 136
Microsporum audouinii, 304i
Microsporum canis, 305
Microsporum persicolor, 305i
Migratory arthritis from gonococcal infections, 82
Migratory polyarthritis from rat-bite fever, 213
Mild neck stiffness from Lyme disease, 140
Miliary disease from tuberculosis, 333
Miliary lesions from *Pneumocystis jiroveci* infections, 204
Miliary tuberculosis, 342i, 344i
Miller Fisher syndrome, as complication of viral
        Campylobacter infections, 35
Molluscipoxvirus, 157
Molluscum contagiosum, 121i, 157–158, 157i, 158i
  clinical manifestations of, 157
  diagnostic tests for, 157
  epidemiology of, 157
  etiology of, 157
  incubation period of, 157
  lesions of, 158i
  treatment of, 157
  white papules and, 158i
Moniliasis, 37–39
  clinical manifestations of, 37
  diagnostic tests for, 37
  epidemiology of, 37
  etiology of, 37
  incubation period of, 37
  treatment of, 37–38
Monkeypox, 242
Monoclonal antibody-based histochemical method
        for plague, 195
Monongahela virus, 91
Mononuclear pleocytosis, 6
Mononucleosis-like syndromes from human herpesvirus
        6 and 7, 114
Moraxella catarrhalis, 201
Morbilliform rash, 71i
Motor dysfunction from Rocky Mountain spotted fever
        (RMSF), 219
Motor neuron disease from poliovirus infections, 207

Mucocutaneous candidiasis, 37, 39i
  treatment for, 37
Mucocutaneous herpes lesions, 122i
Mucocutaneous herpes simplex infections, 106
Mucocutaneous lesions from syphilis, 278
Mucocutaneous lymph node syndrome (Kawasaki
        disease), 127–130
  clinical manifestations of, 127–128
  diagnostic tests for, 128
  epidemiology of, 128
  etiology of, 128
  incubation period of, 128
  treatment of, 128–129
Mucoid stools from *Shigella* infections, 239
Mucosal leishmaniasis, 131, 132
Mucosal lesions from *Candidiasis albicans,* 37
Mucosal ulceration from histoplasmosis, 109
Mulberry molars from syphilis, 278
Multibacillary leprosy, treatment for, 134
Multidrug therapy (MDT) for leprosy, 134
Multiplex reverse transcriptase-PCR assay for para-
        influenza virus infections, 176
Mumps, 159–160
  clinical manifestations of, 159
  diagnostic tests for, 159
  epidemiology of, 159
  etiology of, 159
  incubation period of, 159
  treatment of, 159
Murine typhus (flea-borne typhus, endemic typhus), 353
  clinical manifestations of, 353
  diagnostic tests for, 353
  epidemiology of, 353
  etiology of, 353
  incubation period of, 353
  treatment of, 353
Muscle enzyme increase for trichinellosis, 323
Muscle pain from rat-bite fever, 213
Muscle spasms from tetanus, 299
Muscle tenderness from leptospirosis, 136
Myalgias
  from babesiosis, 21
  from brucellosis, 33
  from *Ehrlichia* and *Anaplasma* infections, 63
  from endemic typhus, 353
  from epidemic typhus, 354
  from Lyme disease, 140
  from lymphocytic choriomeningitis, 146
  from parvovirus B19, 178
  from rickettsialpox, 217
  from Rocky Mountain spotted fever, 219
  from toxic shock syndrome, 310
  from *Toxoplasma gondii* infections, 318
  from trichinellosis, 323
  from tularemia, 350
  from West Nile virus, 365
Mycelial-phase antigens for *Histoplasma capsulatum,* 110
Mycetoma from nocardiosis, 163
Mycobacterial tuberculosis, 348i
Mycobacterium abscessus, 345
Mycobacterium avium, 345
Mycobacterium avium-intracellulare infection, 349i

Mycobacterium bovis, 333
  therapy for, 338
Mycobacterium chelonae, 345
Mycobacterium fortuitum, 345
Mycobacterium intracellulare, 345
Mycobacterium kansasii, 345
Mycobacterium leprae, 133
Mycobacterium marinum, 345
Mycobacterium simiae, 345
Mycobacterium tuberculosis, 333, 342*i*
  from human immunodeficiency virus infection, 116
Mycobacterium tuberculosis scrofula, 343*i*
Mycobacterium ulcerans, 345
Mycoplasma hominis, in bacterial vaginosis, 22
Mycoplasma pneumoniae infections, 161–162, 162*i*
  clinical manifestations of, 161
  diagnostic tests for, 161–162
  epidemiology of, 161
  etiology of, 161
  incubation period of, 161
  treatment of, 162
Mycoplasmas, 161
Myelitis from Epstein-Barr virus, 69
Myocardial dysfunction from hantavirus pulmonary
    syndrome, 91
Myocardial failure from epidemic typhus, 354
Myocardial infarction from Kawasaki disease, 128
Myocarditis
  from African trypanosomiasis, 329
  from American trypanosomiasis, 331
  from *Borrelia* infections, 31
  from Epstein-Barr virus, 69, 70
  from influenza, 124
  from Kawasaki disease, 127
  from meningococcal infections, 153
  from mumps, 159
  from *Mycoplasma pneumoniae* infections, 161
  from rat-bite fever, 213
  from toxocariasis, 316
  from trichinellosis, 323
Myopericarditis from enterovirus infections, 67
Myositis
  from cutaneous larva migrans, 57
  from group A streptococcal infections, 261
  from toxic shock syndrome, 310
Myringitis from *Mycoplasma pneumoniae* infections, 161
Myringotomy for otitis media, 201

N

Naegleria fowleri, 6, 7*i*
Nafcillin for staphylococcal infections, 252
Naftifine
  for tinea corporis, 305
  for tinea cruris, 307
  in treating candidiasis, 37
Nasal congestion from influenza, 124
Nasogastric suction for *Ascaris lumbricoides* infections, 17
Nasopharyngeal carcinoma from Epstein-Barr virus, 69
Nasopharyngeal specimen for pertussis, 186
Nasopharyngitis from diphtheria, 61
National Hansen's Disease Program, 134

Nausea. *See also* Vomiting
  from anthrax, 9
  from babesiosis, 21
  from *Balantidium coli* infection, 26
  from *Ehrlichia* and *Anaplasma* infections, 63
  from hantavirus pulmonary syndrome, 91
  from *Helicobacter pylori* infections, 94
  from hepatitis A, 95
  from hepatitis B, 97
  from hookworm infections, 112
  from influenza, 124
  from leptospirosis, 136
  from lymphocytic choriomeningitis, 146
  from malaria, 147
  from Rocky Mountain spotted fever, 219
  from schistosomiasis, 236
  from tapeworm diseases, 294
  from trichinellosis, 323
  from West Nile virus, 365
Necator americanus, 112, 113*i*
Neck stiffness from West Nile virus, 365
Necrosis of distal extremities from plague, 195
Necrotizing enterocolitis, 248
  from *Yersinia enterocolitica,* 368
Necrotizing fasciitis, 271*i*, 361*i*
  from *Bacteroides* infection, 24
  from group A streptococcal infections, 261
  management of streptococcal toxic shock syndrome
    with, 313*t*
    without, 313*t*
  from *Prevotella* infection, 24
  from toxic shock syndrome, 310
  treatment for, 265
Necrotizing pneumonia
  from *Bacteroides* infection, 24
  from *Prevotella* infection, 24
Needle aspiration, in treating cat-scratch disease, 40
Neisseria gonorrhoeae, 82, 84*i*, 185, 326
  from bacterial vaginosis, 22
Neisseria meningitidis, 153, 154, 154*i*, 156*i*
Nematode, filarial, 166
Neonatal chlamydial conjunctivitis from *Chlamydia
    trachomatis,* 44
Neonatal conjunctivitis from *Chlamydia trachomatis,* 44
Neonatal herpes simplex lesions, 108*i*
Neonatal herpetic infections from herpes simplex, 103
Neonatal omphalitis
  from group A streptococcal infections, 261
  treatment for, 265
Neonatal septicemia
  from *Haemophilus influenzae,* 88
  from pneumococcal infections, 198
Neonatal tetanus, 299, 300*i*
Nephropathy from human immunodeficiency virus
    (HIV) infection, 116
Nephrotic syndrome, 147
Neuraminidase inhibitors for influenza, 125
Neurocysticercosis, 294, 296*i*
  from tapeworm diseases, 294
Neurocysticercosis treatment for tapeworm diseases, 295
Neuromuscular disorders from pertussis, 186

Neuroretinitis
from *Baylisascaris* infections, 27
from cat-scratch disease, 40
Neurosyphilis, 282
re-treatment of, 285
from syphilis, 278
treatment for, 284
Neutralization for mumps, 159
Neutropenia from parvovirus B19, 178
New York virus, 91
Niclosamide for tapeworm diseases, 294
Nifurtimox for American trypanosomiasis, 332
Night sweats
from brucellosis, 33
from nontuberculous mycobacteria, 345
from tuberculosis, 333
Nikolsky sign, 248
Nitazoxanide
for *Giardia intestinalis* infections, 80
for hydatid disease, 297
for tapeworm diseases, 294
Nits from pediculosis capitis, 183*i*
Nocardia abscessus, 163
Nocardia asteroides, 163
Nocardia brasiliensis, 163
Nocardia braziliensis, cutaneous, 165*i*
Nocardia cyriacigeorgica, 163
Nocardia mediastinitis, 164*i*
Nocardia organisms, 164*i*
Nocardia paucivorans, 163
Nocardia pneumonia, 165*i*
Nocardia pseudobrasiliensis, 163
Nocardia transvalensis, 163
Nocardia veterana, 163
Nocardiosis, 163–165
clinical manifestations of, 163
cutaneous, 164*i*, 165*i*
diagnostic tests for, 163
epidemiology of, 163
etiology of, 163
incubation period of, 163
treatment of, 163
Nodular lesions from *Pneumocystis jiroveci* infections, 204
Nomenclature for *Salmonella organisms,* 229*t*
Noncardiogenic pulmonary edema from malaria, 147
Nongenital warts, 170
Non–group A or B streptococcal and enterococcal infections, 272–274
clinical manifestations of, 272
diagnostic tests for, 272
epidemiology of, 272
etiology of, 272
incubation period of, 272
treatment of, 272–273
Non-Hodgkin B-lymphocyte lymphomas from human immunodeficiency virus (HIV) infection, 116
Nonmeningeal invasive pneumococcal infections
in immunocompromised host, 200
requiring hospitalization, 200

Nonpulmonary primary infection from coccidioidomycosis, 52
Nonradiometric broth technique for nontuberculous mycobacteria, 346
Nonsteroidal anti-inflammatory drugs (NSAIDS) for Lyme disease, 142
Nontreponemal tests for syphilis, 279
Nontuberculous mycobacteria, 345–349
clinical manifestations of, 345
diagnostic tests for, 346
diseases caused by, 347*t*
epidemiology of, 345
etiology of, 345
incubation period of, 345
treatment of, 346, 347–348*t*
Nontuberculous mycobacterial osteomyelitis, 349*i*
Nontuberculous mycobacteria lymphadenitis, 346
Norwegian scabies, 233
Nuchal rigidity
from amebic keratitis, 6
from amebic meningoencephalitis, 6
Nucleic acid amplification (NAA) tests
for *Chlamydia trachomatis,* 44
for gonococcal infections, 82
for hepatitis C virus, 101
for tuberculosis, 335
for West Nile virus, 366
Nucleic acid detection
by DNA PCR assay for human immunodeficiency virus, 118
for human immunodeficiency virus, 117
Nucleic acid hybridization for parvovirus B19, 179
Nucleoside analogues for hepatitis B virus (HBV), 99
Nucleoside analogue reverse transcriptase inhibitors for human immunodeficiency virus (HIV), 119
Nystatin in treating candidiasis, 37

O

Obstructive hydrocephalus
from *Cysticercosis,* 294
from tapeworm diseases, 294
Occult febrile bacteremia from *Haemophilus influenzae,* 88
Ocular cysticercosis, 295
Ocular disease from *Toxoplasma gondii* infections, 318
Ocular infections from *Pasteurella* infections, 181
Ocular muscle paralysis, in botulism, 47*i*
Ocular palsies from *Clostridium botulinum,* 46
Oculoglandular lymphadenopathy from tularemia, 350
Ofloxacin
for *Chlamydia trachomatis* genital tract infection, 44
for gonococcal infections, 83
for *Vibrio cholerae* infections, 364
Omeprazole for *Helicobacter pylori* infections, 94
Omphalitis
from staphylococcal infections, 248
Onchocerca nodule, 167*i*
Onchocerca volvulus, 166

Onchocerciasis, 166–168, 167*i*
    chronic, 168*i*
    clinical manifestations of, 166
    diagnostic tests for, 166
    epidemiology of, 166
    etiology of, 166
    incubation period of, 166
    treatment of, 166
Oophoritis from mumps, 159
Open lung biopsy for *Pneumocystis jiroveci* infections, 204
Ophthalmologic examination for candidiasis, 37
Ophthalmoplegia, as complication of viral *Campylobacter*
        infections, 35
Opisthotonos, 301*i*
Optic neuritis from Epstein-Barr virus, 69
Oral antihistamine agents for pediculosis capitis, 183
Oral candidiasis, 37
    from human immunodeficiency virus infection, 116
Oral cefdinir for otitis media, 201
Oral ivermectin for pediculosis capitis, 183
Oral nystatin suspension, in treating oral candidiasis, 37
Oral poliovirus (OPV) vaccine, 207
Oral quinine for babesiosis, 21
Oral rehydration for *Vibrio cholerae* infections, 363–364
Oran virus, 91
Orbital abscess, 256*i*
Orbital cellulitis, 255*i*
    from *Arcanobacterium haemolyticum* infections, 15
Orchitis
    from Epstein-Barr virus, 69
    from lymphatic filariasis, 144
    from lymphocytic choriomeningitis, 146
    mumps and, 159
    from West Nile virus, 365
Ornithodoros hermsii, 32*i*
Oropharyngeal anthrax, 9
Oropharyngeal from tularemia, 350
Oropharynx inflammation, 265*i*
Oropouche viruses, 12
Oropouche virus fever, disease caused by arboviruses
        in Western hemisphere, 13*t*
Oseltamivir for influenza, 125
Osler nodes, 274*i*
Osteochondritis from syphilis, 278
Osteolytic lesions from cat-scratch disease, 40
Osteomyelitis, 19, 258*i*
    from *Arcanobacterium haemolyticum* infections, 15
    from *Bacteroides* infection, 24
    from brucellosis, 33
    from group A streptococcal infections, 261
    from group B streptococcal infections, 269
    from *Haemophilus influenzae,* 88
    from nontuberculous mycobacteria, 345
    from *Pasteurella* infections, 181
    from pneumococcal infections, 198
    from *Prevotella* infection, 24
    from *Salmonella* infections, 229
    from toxic shock syndrome, 310
    treatment for, 265
    vertebral, 258*i*
    from *Yersinia enterocolitica,* 368

Otitis media, 201, 201*i*
    from adenovirus infections, 3
    from *Bacteroides* infection, 24
    from group A streptococcal infections, 261
    from *Haemophilus influenzae,* 88
    from measles, 150
    from *Mycoplasma pneumoniae* infections, 161
    from nontuberculous mycobacteria, 345
    from *Prevotella* infection, 24
    RSV bronchiolitis and, 216
Otomycosis, 19
    from aspergillosis, 19
Oxacillin for staphylococcal infections, 252
Oxamniquine for schistosomiasis, 237
Oxiconazole
    for tinea corporis, 305
    for tinea cruris, 307
Oxygen desaturation from *Pneumocystis jiroveci*
        infections, 204

P

Pain
    abdominal
        from anthrax, 9
        from babesiosis, 21
        from brucellosis, 33
        from *Campylobacter* infections, 35
        from enterovirus infections, 67
        from *Escherichia coli* diarrhea, 75
        from *Giardia intestinalis* infections, 80
        from hookworm infections, 112
        from influenza, 124
        from malaria, 147
        from nontuberculous mycobacteria, 345
        from Rocky Mountain spotted fever, 219
        from schistosomiasis, 236
        from smallpox, 241
        from *Strongyloides,* 275
        from tapeworm infections, 297
        from *Trichomonas vaginalis* infections, 326
        from trichuriasis, 328
        from tuberculosis, 333
        from West Nile virus, 365
    from amebic keratitis, 6
    from amebic meningoencephalitis, 6
    back
        from *Listeria monocytogenes* infections, 138
        from malaria, 147
        from smallpox, 241
    from *Balantidium coli* infection, 26
    chest
        from *Cryptococcus neoformans* infections, 55
        from histoplasmosis, 109
        from tularemia, 350
    on defecation from chancroid, 43
    epigastric, from *Helicobacter pylori* infections, 94
    muscle, from rat-bite fever, 213
    from tapeworm diseases, 294
Pain syndromes from herpes simplex virus, 104
Palatal enanthem from rubella, 225

Pallor
from *Clostridial myonecrosis,* 50
from malaria, 147
Palmar desquamation of Kawasaki disease, 130*i*
Pancreatitis
from *Ascaris lumbricoides* infections, 17
from mumps, 159
from West Nile virus, 365
Pancytopenia from histoplasmosis, 109
Panhypogammaglobulinemia from human immuno-
deficiency virus (HIV), 118
Pantoprazole for *Helicobacter pylori* infections, 94
Papillomas
laryngeal, 171*i*
respiratory, 169
Papillomatosis
respiratory, 170
respiratory tract, 169
Pap test for human papillomaviruses, 170
Papular acrodermatitis from hepatitis B, 97
Papular rash, 293*i*
Papular skin lesions, 155*i*
Papules from pediculosis corporis, 184
Papulopurpuric gloves-and-socks syndrome from
parvovirus B19, 178
Papulopustules, 235*i*
Papulovesicular rash from hookworm infections, 112
Paracoccidioides brasiliensis, 172, 173*i*
Paracoccidioidomycosis (South American blastomycosis),
172–173
clinical manifestations of, 172
diagnostic tests for, 172
epidemiology of, 172
etiology of, 172
incubation period of, 172
treatment of, 172
Paragonimiasis, 174–175
clinical manifestations of, 174
diagnostic tests for, 174–175
epidemiology of, 174
etiology of, 174
extrapulmonary, 174
incubation period of, 174
treatment of, 175
Paragonimus africanus, 174
Paragonimus ecuadoriensis, 174
Paragonimus heterotremus, 174
Paragonimus kellicotti, 174
Paragonimus mexicanus, 174
Paragonimus miyazakii, 174
Paragonimus skrjabini, 174
Paragonimus uterobilateralis, 174
Paragonimus westermani, 174
life cycle of, 175*f*
Parainfluenza viral infections, 176–177, 177*i*
clinical manifestations of, 176
diagnostic tests for, 176–177
epidemiology of, 176
etiology of, 176
incubation period of, 176
treatment of, 177

Paralysis
from enterovirus infections, 67
from rabies, 210
Paralytic poliomyelitis, 207
from poliovirus infections, 207
Paravertebral abscess, 344*i*
Parenchymal brain infection from *Listeria monocytogenes*
infections, 138
Parenteral gentamicin, in treating cat-scratch disease, 40
Parenteral penicillin for *Arcanobacterium haemolyticum*
infections, 15
Parenteral pentamidine for *Pneumocystis jiroveci* infections, 205
Parenteral rehydration for *Vibrio cholerae* infections,
363–364
Paresthesias from poliovirus infections, 207
Parinaud oculoglandular syndrome, 41*i*
from cat-scratch disease, 40
Paromomycin for amebiasis, 4
Paronychia
from *Arcanobacterium haemolyticum* infections, 15
from staphylococcal infections, 248
Parotitis
from human immunodeficiency virus infection, 116
mumps and, 159
from parainfluenza viral infections, 176
from staphylococcal infections, 248
Parvovirus B19 (Erythema infectiosum, Fifth disease),
178–180, 180*i*
clinical manifestations of, 178
clinical manifestations of human, 179*t*
diagnostic tests for, 179
epidemiology of, 178–179
etiology of, 178
incubation period of, 179
treatment of, 179
Pasteurella infections, 181
clinical manifestations of, 181
diagnostic tests for, 181
epidemiology of, 181
etiology of, 181
incubation period of, 181
treatment of, 181
Pasteurella multocida, 181
Pathognomonic enanthema from measles, 150
Paucibacillary leprosy, treatment for, 134
PCP prophylaxis for human immunodeficiency virus
(HIV) children, 119
PCR assay
for arboviruses, 12
for epidemic typhus, 354
for malaria, 148
for meningococcal infections, 154
for *Mycoplasma pneumoniae* infections, 161
for pertussis, 186
for *Shigella* infections, 239
for smallpox, 242
for syphilis, 279
for tularemia, 350
Pediatric autoimmune neuropsychiatric disorders
associated with streptococcal infection
(PANDAS), 261

Pediculicides
    for epidemic typhus, 355
    for pediculosis capitis, 182, 183
    for pediculosis corporis, 184
    for pediculosis pubis, 185
Pediculosis capitis (head lice), 182–183
    clinical manifestations of, 182
    diagnostic tests for, 182
    epidemiology of, 182
    etiology of, 182
    incubation period of, 182
    treatment of, 182–183
Pediculosis corporis (body lice), 184, 184*i*
    clinical manifestations of, 184
    diagnostic tests for, 184
    epidemiology of, 184
    etiology of, 184
    incubation period of, 184
    treatment of, 184
Pediculosis pubis (pubic lice), 185
    clinical manifestations of, 185
    diagnostic tests for, 185
    epidemiology of, 185
    etiology of, 185
    incubation period of, 185
    treatment of, 185
Pediculus humanus, 354, 355*i*
Pediculus humanus capitis, 182
Pediculus humanus corporis, 184
Peginterferon-alfa for hepatitis C virus (HCV), 102
Pelvic inflammatory disease (PID)
    from *Bacteroides* infection, 24
    from gonococcal infections, 82
    from *Prevotella* infection, 24
Pelvic pain from *Schistosoma haematobium,* 236
Pelvic peritonitis from pinworm infection, 190
Penicillin
    for anthrax, 9
    for *Borrelia* infections, 31
    for *Clostridium difficile,* 48
    for leptospirosis, 136
    for *Pasteurella* infections, 181
    for toxic shock syndrome, 311
Penicillin G
    for actinomycosis, 1
    for *Bacteroides* and *Prevotella* infections, 24
    for *Clostridial myonecrosis,* 50
    for diphtheria, 61
    for group B streptococcal infections, 270
    for leptospirosis, 136
    for meningococcal infections, 154
    for non–group A or B streptococcal and enterococcal
        infections, 272
    for pneumococcal infections, 199
    for rat-bite fever, 213
    for syphilis, 282
    for tetanus, 299
Penicillin G benzathine
    for congenital syphilis, 282
    for group A streptococcal infections, 264
    for latent syphilis, 285

Penicillin G procaine
    for congenital syphilis, 282
    plus oral probenecid for neurosyphilis, 284
Penicillin V for group A streptococcal infections, 264
Penile pyodermal lesion, 85*i*
Pentamidine
    for African trypanosomiasis, 329
    for *Pneumocystis jiroveci* infections, 205
Percutaneous aspiration, infusion of scolicidal agents,
        and re-aspiration (PAIR), 297
Perforation from amebiasis, 4
Perianal cellulitis from group A streptococcal infections,
        261
Perianal desquamation of Kawasaki disease, 130*i*
Perianal granuloma inguinale lesion, 87*i*
Perianal infections
    from *Bacteroides* infection, 24
    from *Prevotella* infection, 24
Pericardial effusion from Kawasaki disease, 127
Pericarditis
    from group A streptococcal infections, 261
    from histoplasmosis, 110
    from meningococcal infections, 153
    from *Mycoplasma pneumoniae* infections, 161
    from pneumococcal infections, 198
Perihepatitis
    from *Chlamydia trachomatis,* 44
    from gonococcal infections, 82
Perinatal bacterial infections from group B streptococcal
        infections, 269
Perinatal death from syphilis, 278
Perinatal transmission of hepatitis B virus (HBV), 97
Perionychia, 257*i*
Periorbital cellulitis, 201*i*, 256*i*
    from *Haemophilus influenzae* infections, 89*i*, 90*i*
    from pneumococcal infections, 198
Periorbital edema from trichinellosis, 323
Peripheral neuropathy
    from Lyme disease, 140
    from *Mycoplasma pneumoniae* infections, 161
    from Rocky Mountain spotted fever, 219
Peritonitis
    from *Haemophilus influenzae,* 88
    from *Pasteurella* infections, 181
    from pneumococcal infections, 198
Peritonsillar abscesses
    from *Arcanobacterium haemolyticum* infections, 15
    from *Bacteroides* infection, 24
    from group A streptococcal infections, 261
    from *Prevotella* infection, 24
Periventricular germinolytic cysts, 60*i*
Permethrin
    for pediculosis capitis, 182
    for scabies, 233–234
Peromyscus leucopus, 21
Peromyscus maniculatus, 92*i*
Person-to-person, spread of hepatitis B virus (HBV)
        by, 97
Pertussis pneumonia, 188*i*

Pertussis (whooping cough), 186–189
    clinical manifestations of, 186
    diagnostic tests for, 186–187
    epidemiology of, 186
    etiology of, 186
    incubation period of, 186
    paroxysmal coughing spell of, 187*i*
    treatment of, 187
Petechiae from parvovirus B19, 178
Pharyngeal carriers, treatment for, 265
Pharyngeal diphtheria, 62*i*
Pharyngeal exudate from *Arcanobacterium haemolyticum*
    infections, 15
Pharyngeal itching from hookworm infections, 112
Pharyngeal swab for gonococcal infections, 83
Pharyngitis
    from enterovirus infections, 67
    food-borne outbreaks of, 261–262
    from gonococcal infections, 82
    from group A streptococcal infections, 261
    from *Mycoplasma pneumoniae* infections, 161
    from non–group A or B streptococcal and entero-
        coccal infections, 272
    streptococcal, 262
    treatment for, 264
    from tularemia, 350
    from *Yersinia enterocolitica,* 368
Pharyngoconjunctival fever from adenovirus infections, 3
Pharyngotonsillitis from group A streptococcal
    infections, 261
Pharynx swabbing for group A streptococcal
    infections, 262
Photophobia
    from amebic keratitis, 6
    from amebic meningoencephalitis, 6
    from babesiosis, 21
    from lymphocytic choriomeningitis, 146
    from onchocerciasis, 166
    from rickettsialpox, 217
Phthirius pubis, 185, 185*i*
Pinworm infection *(Enterobius vermicularis),* 190–191
    clinical manifestations of, 190
    diagnostic tests for, 190
    epidemiology of, 190
    etiology of, 190
    incubation period of, 190
    treatment of, 190
Piperazine solution for *Ascaris lumbricoides* infections, 17
Pipestem cirrhosis, 238*i*
Pityriasis alba, pityriasis versicolor and, 192
Pityriasis rosea, 194*i*
    pityriasis versicolor and, 192
Pityriasis versicolor (tinea versicolor), 192–194, 193*i*, 194*i*
    clinical manifestations of, 192
    diagnosis of, 192
    epidemiology of, 192
    etiology of, 192
    incubation period of, 192
    treatment of, 192

Plague, 195–197
    bioterrorism-related, 195
    bubonic, 195
    clinical manifestations of, 195
    diagnostic tests for, 195
    epidemiology of, 195
    etiology of, 195
    human, 195
    incubation period of, 195
    pneumonic, 195
    primary pneumonic, 195
    secondary pneumonic, 195
    septicemic, 195
    spleen in fatal, 197*i*
    treatment of, 195–196
Plague infection
    gangrene of, 197*i*
    hemorrhages on skin of, 197*i*
Plague pneumonia, 195
Plantar warts, 169, 170
Plaque-reduction neutralization tests for West Nile
    virus (WNV), 366
Plasma HIV-1 RNA PCR assay for human immuno-
    deficiency virus (HIV), 118
Plasmapheresis for West Nile virus (WNV), 366
Plasmodium falciparum, 147, 148, 149*i*
Plasmodium malariae, 147, 148
Plasmodium ovale, 147, 148
Plasmodium vivax, 147, 148
Platelet count for Kawasaki disease, 128
Pleocytosis from poliovirus infections, 207
Pleural effusions
    from hantavirus pulmonary syndrome, 91
    from *Mycoplasma pneumoniae* infections, 161
    from paragonimiasis, 174
    from tuberculosis, 333
    from *Yersinia pseudotuberculosis* infection, 368
Pleural empyema from *Pasteurella* infections, 181
Pleuritic pain from *Borrelia* infections, 31
Pleurodermal sinuses from actinomycosis, 1
Pleurodynia from enterovirus infections, 67
Pneumococcal capsular antigen for pneumococcal
    infections, 198
Pneumococcal infections, 198–203
    children at risk of invasive, 199*t*
    clinical manifestations of, 198
    diagnostic tests for, 198
    epidemiology of, 198
    etiology of, 198
    incubation period of, 198
    treatment of, 199–201
Pneumococcal meningitis, 199
Pneumocystis carinii, 204
Pneumocystis jiroveci infections, 204–206, 206*i*
    clinical manifestations of, 204
    diagnostic tests for, 204–205
    epidemiology of, 204
    etiology of, 204
    incubation period of, 204
    treatment of, 205
Pneumocystis jiroveci pneumonia, 206*i*
    from human immunodeficiency virus infection, 116

Pneumonia
    from actinomycosis, 1
    adenoviral, 3*i*
    from adenovirus infections, 3
    from *Arcanobacterium haemolyticum* infections, 15
    aspiration
        from *Bacteroides* infection, 24
        from *Prevotella* infection, 24
    bilateral varicella, 361*i*
    from cat-scratch disease, 40
    from *Chlamydia trachomatis,* 44
    community-acquired, from pneumococcal
        infections, 198
    from cytomegalovirus infection, 58
    diphtheria, 62*i*
    from enterovirus infections, 67
    from Epstein-Barr virus, 69
    from group A streptococcal infections, 261
    group B streptococcal, 270*i*
    from group B streptococcal infections, 269
    Haemophilus influenzae, 90*i*
    from *Haemophilus influenzae,* 88
    from histoplasmosis, 109
    from human herpesvirus 6 and 7, 114
    human plague, 197*i*
    from influenza, 124
    from *Listeria monocytogenes* infections, 138
    lymphoid interstitial, 116
    from meningococcal infections, 153
    from *Mycoplasma pneumoniae* infections, 161
    necrotizing
        from *Bacteroides* infection, 24
        from *Prevotella* infection, 24
    Nocardia, 165*i*
    from parainfluenza viral infections, 176
    from *Pasteurella* infections, 181
    pertussis, 188*i*
    from pertussis, 186
    plague, 195
    Pneumocystis jiroveci, 116, 206*i*
    from rat-bite fever, 213
    from respiratory syncytial virus, 215
    segmental (nodular), 202*i*
    staphylococcal, 260*i*
    from toxic shock syndrome, 310
    from toxocariasis, 316
    treatment for, 265
    tularemia, 352*i*
    varicella, 361*i*
    from varicella-zoster infections, 356
    from *Yersinia enterocolitica,* 368
Pneumonic plague, 195
Pneumonic tularemia, 350
Pneumonitis
    from *Borrelia* infections, 31
    from hookworm infections, 112
    from *Strongyloides,* 275
    from *Toxoplasma gondii* infections, 318
    from trichinellosis, 323
Pneumothorax from paragonimiasis, 174
Podophyllum resin for warts, 170
Poliomyelitis, paralytic, 207

Poliovirus infections, 207–209
    clinical manifestations of, 207
    deformity caused by, 209*i*
    diagnostic tests for, 208
    epidemiology of, 207
    etiology of, 207
    incubation period of, 208
    photomicrograph of, 209*i*
Polyarthralgia from rubella, 225
Polyarthritis from rubella, 225
Polyarthropathy, acute from arboviruses, 12
Polyarthropathy syndrome from parvovirus B19, 178
Polyhexamethylene biguanide for amebic meningo-
    encephalitis and keratitis, 6
Polymorphonuclear pleocytosis, 6
Polymorphous mucocutaneous eruptions from *Myco-*
    plasma pneumoniae infections, 161
Poor feeding from respiratory syncytial virus, 215
Postdiarrheal thrombotic thrombocytopenic purpura
    from *Escherichia coli* diarrhea, 75
Postherpetic neuralgia, 356
Postinfectious encephalomyelitis from herpes simplex
    virus, 104
Postinflammatory hypopigmentation, pityriasis versicolor
    and, 192
Postnatal rubella, 225
Postoccipital lymphadenopathy from human herpesvirus
    6 and 7, 114
Postoperative wound infection
    from *Bacteroides* infection, 24
    from *Prevotella* infection, 24
Postpolio syndrome from poliovirus infections, 207
Posttransplantation lymphoproliferative disorders from
    Epstein-Barr virus, 69
Potassium hydroxide wet mount
    for pityriasis versicolor, 192
    for tinea capitis, 302
    for tinea pedis, 308
    for tinea unguium, 308
Potassium iodide for sporotrichosis, 246
Powassan encephalitis virus, disease caused by arbovi-
    ruses in Western hemisphere, 13*t*
Praziquantel
    for cysticercosis, 295
    for hydatid disease, 297
    for paragonimiasis, 175
    for schistosomiasis, 237
    for tapeworm diseases, 294
Preauricular lymphadenopathy from tularemia, 350
Precipitation techniques for group A streptococcal
    infections, 262
Pregnancy
    lymphocytic choriomeningitis during, 146
    mumps in, 159
    from parvovirus B19, 178
    parvovirus B19 infections in, 180*f*
    rubella in, 225
    syphilis in, 283
    testing for syphilis in, 280
    tuberculosis during, 339
    varicella-zoster infections during, 355, 358
    West Nile virus during, 365

Prematurity from *Listeria monocytogenes* infections, 138
Prevotella infections, 24–25
    clinical manifestations of, 24
    diagnostic tests for, 24
    epidemiology of, 24
    etiology of, 24
    incubation period of, 24
    treatment of, 24
Prevotella melaninogenica, 24, 25*i*
Primary pneumonic plague, 195
Proctitis from gonococcal infections, 82
Proglottids of *Dipylidium caninum*, 298*i*
Progressive disseminated histoplasmosis (PDH), 109
Proliferative glomerulonephritis from *Yersinia entero-*
    colitica, 368
Propamidine isethionate plus neomycin-polymyxin B
    sulfate-gramicidin ophthalmic solution
    for amebic meningoencephalitis and
    keratitis, 6
Prostatitis from *Trichomonas vaginalis* infections, 326
Prostration
    from meningococcal infections, 153
    from smallpox, 241
Proteus, 72
Protracted nasopharyngitis, 266*i*
Pruritic papules from parvovirus B19, 178
Pruritic skin lesions from *Strongyloides*, 275
Pruritus
    from African trypanosomiasis, 329
    from *Arcanobacterium haemolyticum* infections, 15
    from cutaneous larva migrans, 57
    from hookworm infections, 112
    from pediculosis pubis, 185
    from pinworm infection, 190
    from tinea corporis, 305
Pruritus vulvae from pinworm infection, 190
Pseudoappendiceal abdominal pain from *Yersinia*
    pseudotuberculosis infection, 368
Pseudoappendicitis syndrome from *Yersinia*
    enterocolitica, 368
Pseudomembranous colitis from *Clostridium difficile*, 48
Pseudomonas, 72
Pseudomonas aeruginosa, 73*i*, 74*i*
Pseudoparalysis from syphilis, 278
Psoriasis, tinea capitis and, 302
Pubic lice (pediculosis pubis), 185
    clinical manifestations of, 185
    diagnostic tests for, 185
    epidemiology of, 185
    etiology of, 185
    incubation period of, 185
    treatment of, 185
Puerperal sepsis from group A streptococcal
    infections, 261
Pulmonary abscesses from *Pasteurella* infections, 181
Pulmonary coccidioidomycosis, 54*i*
Pulmonary disease from nontuberculous
    mycobacteria, 345
Pulmonary edema from hantavirus pulmonary
    syndrome, 91
Pulmonary fibrosis from paragonimiasis, 174
Pulmonary histoplasmosis, 110

Pulmonary hypertension
    from respiratory syncytial virus, 215
    from *Schistosoma haematobium*, 236
Pulmonary infections from blastomycosis, 29
Pulmonary infiltrates from histoplasmosis, 109
Pulmonary osteoarthropathy, hypertrophic, 2*i*
Pulmonary sporotrichosis, 246
Punch biopsy for leishmaniasis, 132
Purpura
    from cytomegalovirus infection, 58
    of foot, 155*i*
    from meningococcal infections, 153
Purpuric rash from leptospirosis, 136
Purulent discharge, copious, 327*i*
Purulent pericarditis from *Haemophilus influenzae*, 88
Pustules from nocardiosis, 163
Pyarthrosis from toxic shock syndrome, 310
Pyoderma from nocardiosis, 163
Pyogenic arthritis from pneumococcal infections, 198
Pyomyositis from *Yersinia enterocolitica*, 368
Pyrantel pamoate
    for hookworm infections, 112
    for pinworm infection, 190
Pyrazinamide for tuberculosis, 337
Pyrimethamine for *Toxoplasma gondii* infections, 320

Q

Quantification techniques for hookworm infections, 112
Quantitative antimicrobial susceptibility testing for
    staphylococcal infections, 251
Quinacrine for *Giardia intestinalis* infections, 80
Quinupristin-dalfopristin for non–group A or B strepto-
    coccal and enterococcal infections, 273

R

Rabeprazole for *Helicobacter pylori* infections, 94
Rabies, 210–212
    clinical manifestations of, 210
    diagnostic tests for, 210
    epidemiology of, 210
    etiology of, 210
    incubation period of, 210
    treatment of, 211
Rabies encephalitis, 212*i*
Raccoons as carriers of rabies virus, 211*i*
Radiographs for *Clostridial myonecrosis*, 50
Radioimmunoassay immunoassay test
    for *Histoplasma capsulatum*, 109
    for parvovirus B19, 179
Radiolucent bone disease from congenital rubella, 225
Radiometric broth techniques for nontuberculous
    mycobacteria, 346
Rashes
    from African trypanosomiasis, 329
    from arboviruses, 12
    from *Arcanobacterium haemolyticum* infections, 15
    from *Ehrlichia* and *Anaplasma* infections, 63
    from endemic typhus, 353
    from Epstein-Barr virus, 69
    from group A streptococcal infections, 261
    from human herpesvirus 6 and 7, 114
    from leprosy, 133

from leptospirosis, 136
from Lyme disease, 140
from parvovirus B19, 178
from rat-bite fever, 213
from Rocky Mountain spotted fever, 219
from rubella, 225
from schistosomiasis, 236
from smallpox, 241
from syphilis, 278
from tinea corporis, 305
from *Toxoplasma gondii* infections, 318
from varicella-zoster infections, 356
from West Nile virus, 365
Rat-bite fever, 213–214
  clinical manifestations of, 213
  diagnostic tests for, 213
  epidemiology of, 213
  etiology of, 213
  incubation period of, 213
  rash of, 214*i*
  treatment of, 213
Rat bites, 214*i*
Rattus norvegicus, 353*i*
Reactive airway disease from respiratory syncytial
      virus, 215
Reactive arthritis
  as complication of viral *Campylobacter* infections, 35
  from *Yersinia enterocolitica,* 368
Rectal bleeding from chancroid, 43
Rectal prolapse from trichuriasis, 328
Rectal swab
  for enterovirus infections, 67
  for gonococcal infections, 83
  for *Shigella* infections, 239
Recurrent arthritis from Lyme disease, 140
Recurrent diarrhea from human immunodeficiency
      virus (HIV) infection, 116
Recurrent herpes simplex, 107*i*
Red blood cell aplasia from parvovirus B19, 178
Rehydration for *Campylobacter* infections, 35
Reiter syndrome
  from *Campylobacter* infections, 35
  from *Chlamydia trachomatis,* 44
  from *Shigella* infections, 239
Relapsing bacteremia from cat-scratch disease, 40
Relapsing fever (*Borrelia* infections), 31–32
  clinical manifestations of, 31
  diagnostic tests for, 31
  epidemiology of, 31
  etiology of, 31
  incubation period of, 31
  treatment of, 31
Renal disease from group B streptococcal infections, 269
Renal failure
  from *Clostridial myonecrosis,* 50
  from *Ehrlichia* and *Anaplasma* infections, 63
  from epidemic typhus, 354
  from malaria, 147
  from plague, 195
Renal tuberculosis, 333
Residual paralytic disease from poliovirus infections, 207
Respiratory distress from group B streptococcal infec-
      tions, 269

Respiratory failure
  from *Ehrlichia* and *Anaplasma* infections, 63
  in infant with whooping cough, 189*i*
  from malaria, 147
Respiratory muscle paralysis from West Nile virus, 365
Respiratory papillomas, 169
Respiratory papillomatosis, 170
  treatment for, 170–171
Respiratory syncytial virus (RSV), 215–217
  clinical manifestations of, 215
  diagnostic tests for, 215–216
  electron micrograph of, 216*i*
  epidemiology of, 215
  etiology of, 215
  incubation period of, 215
  treatment of, 216
Respiratory syncytial virus (RSV) bronchiolitis,
      pneumonia and, 216*i*
Respiratory tract infections
  from adenovirus infections, 3
  from *Arcanobacterium haemolyticum* infections, 15
  from non–group A or B streptococcal and entero-
      coccal infections, 272
  from parainfluenza viral infections, 176
  from *Pasteurella* infections, 181
  from pertussis, 186
Respiratory tract papillomatosis, 169
Respiratory tract symptoms from lymphocytic chorio-
      meningitis, 146
Retinal granulomas from toxocariasis, 316
Retinal lesions from candidiasis, 37
Retinitis from cytomegalovirus infection, 58
Retro-orbital headache from lymphocytic chorio-
      meningitis, 146
Retropharyngeal abscesses from group A streptococcal
      infections, 261
Retropharyngeal space infection
  from *Bacteroides* infection, 24
  from *Prevotella* infection, 24
Reverse transcriptase-PCR for mumps, 159
Reye syndrome, 129
  from varicella-zoster infections, 356, 359
Rhagades, 278
  from syphilis, 278
Rheumatic fever
  acute, 262
  from group A streptococcal infections, 261
Rhinitis
  from group A streptococcal infections, 261
  from influenza, 124
Rhipicephalus sanguineus, 219
Rhodococcus equi, 163
Ribavirin
  for hantavirus pulmonary syndrome, 92
  for respiratory syncytial virus, 216
Rib fractures from pertussis, 186
Rice-water stool, 364*i*
Rickettsia akari, 217
Rickettsialpox, 217–218
  clinical manifestations of, 217
  diagnostic tests for, 217
  epidemiology of, 217
  etiology of, 217

Rickettsialpox, continued
    incubation period of, 217
    papulovesicular lesions of, 218*i*
    patient with, 217*i*
    treatment of, 217
Rickettsia prowazekii, cause of epidemic typhus, 354
Rickettsia rickettsii, 217, 219
Rifabutin for nontuberculous mycobacteria lympha-
        denitis, 346
Rifampin
    for brucellosis, 33
    for leprosy, 134
    for paucibacillary leprosy, 134
    in treating cat-scratch disease, 40
    for tuberculosis, 337
Rigors
    from *Ehrlichia* and *Anaplasma* infections, 63
    from influenza, 124
    from malaria, 147
Rimantadine for influenza, 125
Ringworm, 309*i*
    black-dot, 302, 303*i*
    of the body (tinea corporis), 305–306
        clinical manifestations of, 305
        diagnosis of, 305
        epidemiology of, 305
        etiology of, 305
        incubation period of, 305
        treatment of, 305
    of the feet (tinea unguium), 308–309
        clinical manifestations of, 308
        diagnosis of, 308
        epidemiology of, 308
        etiology of, 308
        treatment of, 308–309
    of the scalp (tinea capitis), 302–304
        clinical manifestations of, 302
        diagnostic tests for, 302
        epidemiology of, 302
        etiology of, 302
        incubation period of, 302
        treatment of, 303
Risus sardonicus, 300*i*
Ritter disease, 248
River blindness (onchocerciasis), 166–168, 167*i*
    clinical manifestations of, 166
    diagnostic tests for, 166
    epidemiology of, 166
    etiology of, 166
    incubation period of, 166
    treatment of, 166
RNA PCR assay for human immunodeficiency virus
        (HIV), 118
Rocky Mountain spotted fever (RMSF), 217, 219–222,
        220*i*
    clinical manifestations of, 219
    diagnostic tests for, 219–220
    epidemiology of, 219
    etiology of, 219
    incubation period of, 219
    rashes from, 221*i,* 222*i*
    treatment of, 220

Romaña sign from American trypanosomiasis, 331
Roseola, 114–115
    clinical manifestations of, 114
    diagnostic tests for, 114–115
    epidemiology of, 114
    etiology of, 114
    from human herpesvirus 6 and 7, 114
    incubation period of, 114
    treatment of, 115
Roseola infantum, 115*i*
Rotavirus infections, 223–224, 224*i*
    clinical manifestations of, 223
    diagnostic tests for, 223
    epidemiology of, 223
    etiology of, 223
    incubation period of, 223
    treatment of, 223
RSV bronchiolitis, otitis media and, 216
Rubella, 225–228
    clinical manifestations of, 225
    diagnostic tests for, 226
    epidemiology of, 225–226
    etiology of, 225
    incubation period of, 226
    maternal, 225
    postauricular lymphadenopathy in, 227*i*
    postnatal, 225
    treatment of, 226
Rubella rash, 226*i*
Rubulavirus, 159

S

Sabouraud dextrose agar
    for tinea corporis, 305
    for tinea cruris, 307
Saddle nose from syphilis, 278
St Louis encephalitis virus, disease caused by arboviruses
        in Western hemisphere, 13*t*
Salmonella infections, 72, 229–232
    clinical manifestations of, 229
    diagnostic tests for, 230
    epidemiology of, 229–230
    etiology of, 229
    incubation period of, 230
    osteomyelitis from, 232*i*
    treatment of, 230–231
Salmonella meningitis, 232*i*
Salmonella sepsis with dactylitis, 231*i*
Salmonella septicemia, 232*i*
Salmonella typhi, 231*i*
Salpingitis
    from *Chlamydia trachomatis,* 44
    from gonococcal infections, 82
    from pinworm infection, 190
Sanguinopurulent exudate, 41*i*
Sarcoptes scabiei, 233
Scabicide for scabies, 233

Scabies, 233–235
  clinical manifestations of, 233
  diagnostic tests for, 233
  epidemiology of, 233
  etiology of, 233
  incubation period of, 233
  linear papulovesicular burrows of, 234*i*
  Norwegian, 233
  rash from, 234*i*
  treatment of, 233–234
Scalded skin syndrome from staphylococcal
        infections, 248
Scaling from tinea corporis, 305
Scalp, excoriations of from pediculosis capitis, 183*i*
Scalp abscesses
  from staphylococcal infections, 248
  from tinea capitis, 302
Scalp lesions from tinea capitis, 302
Scaly lesions
  from tinea pedis, 308
  from tinea unguium, 308
Scarlatiniform exanthem from *Arcanobacterium*
        haemolyticum infections, 15
Scarlatiniform rash from *Yersinia pseudotuberculosis*
        infection, 368
Scarlet fever, 267*i*
  from group A streptococcal infections, 261
Schistosoma haematobium, 236, 238*i*
Schistosoma intercalatum, 236
Schistosoma japonicum, 236
Schistosoma mansoni, 236
Schistosoma mekongi, 236
Schistosoma species eggs, 237*i*
Schistosome dermatitis from schistosomiasis, 236
Schistosomiasis, 236–238
  clinical manifestations of, 236
  diagnostic tests for, 237
  epidemiology of, 236–237
  etiology of, 236
  with hepatosplenomegaly, 237*i*
  incubation period of, 237
  treatment of, 237
Scrotal lymphangitis, 145*i*
Seborrheic dermatitis, 302
  pityriasis versicolor and, 192
  from tinea capitis, 302
Secondary pneumonic plague, 195
Secondary syphilis, 292*i*, 293*i*
Secondary uveitis
  from amebic keratitis, 6
  from amebic meningoencephalitis, 6
Sedimentation rate, increased for Kawasaki disease, 128
Segmental (nodular) pneumonia, 202*i*
Seizures
  from amebic keratitis, 6
  from amebic meningoencephalitis, 6
  from American trypanosomiasis, 331
  from *Cysticercosis,* 294
  from human herpesvirus 6 and 7, 114
  from pertussis, 186
  from rabies, 210
  from smallpox, 241

from tapeworm diseases, 294
from *Toxoplasma gondii* infections, 318
from *Vibrio cholerae* infections, 363
Selenium sulfide for pityriasis versicolor, 192
Sepsis from plague, 195
Sepsis syndrome from herpes simplex, 103
Septic arthritis
  from group A streptococcal infections, 261
  from group B streptococcal infections, 269
  from *Haemophilus influenzae,* 88
  from *Pasteurella* infections, 181
Septicemia, 74*i*
  from *Arcanobacterium haemolyticum* infections, 15
  clinical signs of, 72
  from *Escherichia coli,* 72
  from *Listeria monocytogenes* infections, 138
  from *Pasteurella* infections, 181
  from *Strongyloides,* 275
  treatment for, 265
  from *Yersinia pseudotuberculosis* infection, 368
Septicemic plague, 195
Serodiagnosis for strongyloidiasis, 275
Serologic antibody tests for Epstein-Barr virus, 69
Serologic assays
  for enterovirus infections, 67
  for mumps, 159
  for *toxoplasma gondii,* 319
Serologic enzyme immunoassay tests for lymphatic
        filariasis, 144
Serologic tests
  for American trypanosomiasis, 331
  for *Helicobacter pylori* infections, 94
  for hepatitis A, 95
  for hepatitis B virus, 98
  for herpes simplex virus, 105
  for leishmaniasis, 132
  for Lyme disease, 141
  for malaria, 148
  for measles, 150
  for nocardiosis, 163
  for pertussis, 187
  for *Salmonella* infections, 230
  for schistosomiasis, 237
  for *toxoplasma gondii,* 319
  for trichinellosis, 323
  for tularemia, 350
Serratia marescens, 72
Serum antibody assay for tapeworm diseases, 294
Serum antibody concentration for human herpesvirus 6
        and 7, 114
Serum concentrations for rubella, 226
Serum C-reactive protein concentration for Kawasaki
        disease, 128
Serum IgG antibody test for parvovirus B19, 179
Serum specimens
  for epidemic typhus, 354
  for plague, 195
  for *Vibrio cholerae* infections, 363
Serum varicella IgG antibody test for varicella-zoster
        infections, 357
Severe muscular spasms from tetanus, 299
Sexual abuse, acquired syphilis, 279

Shigella boydii, 239
Shigella dysenteriae, 239
Shigella flexneri, 239
Shigella infection, 240*i*
Shigella infections, 239–240
    clinical manifestations of, 239
    diagnostic tests for, 239
    epidemiology of, 239
    etiology of, 239
    incubation period of, 239
    treatment of, 239–240
Shigella species from bacterial vaginosis, 22
Shigellosis, bloody mucoid stool of, 240*i*
Shingles from varicella-zoster infections, 356
Shock
    from group B streptococcal infections, 269
    from meningococcal infections, 153
Short-limb syndrome, 359*i*
Shoulder myalgia from hantavirus pulmonary
        syndrome, 91
Sickle cell dactylitis, 231*i*
Sickle cell disease, *Mycoplasma pneumoniae* infections
        and, 161
Sigmodon hispidus, 92*i*
Sigmoidoscopy for *Balantidium coli* infection, 26
Sin Nombre virus (SNV), 91
Sinusitis, 201
    allergic, 19
    from *Arcanobacterium haemolyticum* infections, 15
    from group A streptococcal infections, 261
    from *Haemophilus influenzae,* 88
    from *Mycoplasma pneumoniae* infections, 161
    from pneumococcal infections, 198
Sixth disease from human herpesvirus 6 and 7, 114
Skeletal muscle biopsy specimen for trichinellosis, 323
Skin biopsies for leprosy, 133
Skin lesions, 74*i*
    from blastomycosis, 29
    from histoplasmosis, 109
    from leprosy, 133
    from syphilis, 278
    from tinea cruris, 307
    from varicella-zoster infections, 356
Skin scrapings
    for pityriasis versicolor, 192
    for tinea cruris, 307
    for tinea pedis and tinea unguium, 308
Skin warts, 169
Skunks as carriers of rabies virus, 211*i*
Slant culture of paracoccidioidomycosis, 173*i*
Slapped cheek appearance, in parvovirus B19 infections,
        178, 180*i*
Slate-colored maculae from pediculosis pubis, 185
Sleep disturbance from pertussis, 186
Slide agglutination tests for tularemia, 350
Slit-lamp examination for onchocerciasis, 166
Slit-smears for leprosy, 133
Smallpox (variola), 241–245, 245*i*
    clinical manifestations of, 241–242
    diagnostic tests for, 242
    epidemiology of, 242
    etiology of, 242
    incubation period of, 242

    lesions from, 243*i,* 244*i*
    pustules, 243*i,* 244*i*
    treatment of, 242
Snowstorm of acute histoplasmosis, 111*i*
Snuffles from syphilis, 278
Sodium hyposulfite for pityriasis versicolor, 192
Sodium thiosulfate for pityriasis versicolor, 192
Soft tissue infection from pneumococcal infections, 198
Somnolence from African trypanosomiasis, 329
Sore throat
    from babesiosis, 21
    from influenza, 124
    from poliovirus infections, 207
    from *Toxoplasma gondii* infections, 318
South American blastomycosis (paracoccidioido-
        mycosis), 172–173
    clinical manifestations of, 172
    diagnostic tests for, 172
    epidemiology of, 172
    etiology of, 172
    incubation period of, 172
    treatment of, 172
Specific IgM antibody tests for parvovirus B19, 179
Specific serologic assays for *Baylisascaris* infections, 27
Spectinomycin for gonococcal infections, 83
Spinal fluid specimens for mumps, 159
Spiramycin for *Toxoplasma gondii* infections, 320
Spirillum minus, 213, 214*i*
Spirillum moniliformis infection, 213
Spleen abscesses from *Yersinia enterocolitica,* 368
Spleen lesions from candidiasis, 37
Splenic rupture from Epstein-Barr virus, 69
Splenomegaly
    from babesiosis, 21
    from Epstein-Barr virus, 70
    from human immunodeficiency virus infection, 116
    from leishmaniasis, 131
    from *Toxoplasma gondii* infections, 318
    from tularemia, 350
Splinter hemorrhages, 325*i*
Spontaneous hemorrhage from *Ehrlichia* and *Anaplasma*
        infections, 63
Sporothrix schenckii, 246, 247*i*
Sporotrichosis, 246–247
    clinical manifestations of, 246
    diagnostic tests for, 246
    disseminated, 246
    epidemiology of, 246
    etiology of, 246
    extracutaneous, 246
    fixed cutaneous, 246
    incubation period of, 246
    pulmonary, 246
    treatment of, 246–247
Staphylococcal enterotoxins, 310
Staphylococcal infections, 248–260
    clinical manifestations of, 248
    diagnostic tests for, 251
    epidemiology of, 249–251
    etiology of, 248–249
    incubation period of, 251
    treatment of, 252–253

Staphylococcal pneumonia, 260*i*
Staphylococcal pustules, 315*i*
Staphylococcal scalded skin syndrome (SSSS), 248, 259*i*, 260*i*
Staphylococcal toxic shock syndrome, clinical case definition, 312*t*
Staphylococcus aureus hordeolum, 255*i*
Staphylococcus aureus infections, 159, 233, 248, 310
    abscesses, 256*i*
    chronic osteomyelitis of, 258*i*
    colonization and disease, 249
    health care–associated methicillin-resistant, 249–250
    from influenza, 124
    parenteral antimicrobial agents for treatment of, 253–254*t*
    pyoderma caused by, 255*i*
    transmission of, in hospitals, 249
Staphylococcus epidermidis, 248
Staphylococcus haemolyticus, 248
Staphylococcus lugdunensis, 248
Staphylococcus saprophyticus, 248
Staphylococcus schleiferi, 248
Stillbirth from syphilis, 278
Stoll antigen test for *Helicobacter pylori* infections, 94
Stoll egg counting techniques for hookworm infections, 112
Stomatitis from enterovirus infections, 67
Stool cultures
    for *Balantidium coli* infection, 26
    for *Giardia intestinalis* infections, 80
    for *Salmonella* infections, 230
    for strongyloidiasis, 275
    for *Yersinia enterocolitica* infections, 368–369
    for *Yersinia pseudotuberculosis* infections, 368–369
Stool specimens
    for hookworm infections, 112
    for poliovirus infections, 208
    for schistosomiasis, 237
Strand-displacement assays for gonococcal infections, 83
Strawberry cervix, 327*i*
Strawberry tongue of scarlet fever, 268*i*
Streptobacillary fever, 213
Streptobacillus moniliformis, 213, 214*i*
Streptococcal impetigo, 262
    treatment for, 265
Streptococcal infections, non–group A or B, 272–274
    clinical manifestations of, 272
    diagnostic tests for, 272
    epidemiology of, 272
    etiology of, 272
    incubation period of, 272
    treatment of, 272–273
Streptococcal pharyngitis, 262, 266*i*
Streptococcal skin infections from group A streptococcal infections, 261
Streptococcal toxic shock syndrome
    clinical case definition, 312*t*
    treatment for, 265
Streptococcus agalactiae, 269
Streptococcus aureus–mediated TSS, 310

Streptococcus pneumoniae, 153, 198, 199, 201*i*, 202*i*, 203*i*
    from influenza, 124
    meningeal infection with, 203*i*
    pericarditis due to, 203*i*
Streptococcus pyogenes, 233, 261, 310
Streptococcus pyogenes—mediated TSS, 310
Streptococcus viridans bacterial endocarditis, 273*i*
Streptococcus viridans subacute bacterial endocarditis, 273*i*
Streptomycin
    for brucellosis, 33
    for plague, 195
    for rat-bite fever, 213
    for tuberculosis, 337
    for tularemia, 351
Strongyloides stercoralis (strongyloidiasis), 275–277, 277*i*
    clinical manifestations of, 275
    diagnostic tests for, 275
    epidemiology of, 275
    etiology of, 275
    incubation period of, 275
    larvae, 277*i*
    life cycle for, 276*f*
    treatment of, 275
Strongyloidiasis (*Strongyloides stercoralis*), 275–277
    clinical manifestations of, 275
    diagnostic tests for, 275
    epidemiology of, 275
    etiology of, 275
    incubation period of, 275
    treatment of, 275
Subacute diffuse pneumonitis from *Pneumocystis jiroveci* infections, 204
Subacute sclerosing panencephalitis (SSPE), 150
Subdural bleeding, in whooping cough neonate, 188*i*
Submandibular adenopathy from herpes simplex, 103
Submucosal hemorrhage of human anthrax, 10*i*
Subungual hemorrhage from trichinellosis, 323
Sucking blisters, 108*i*
Sulbactam for *Pasteurella* infections, 181
Sulconazole
    for tinea corporis, 305
    for tinea cruris, 307
Sulfacetamide
    for *Chlamydia trachomatis,* 44
    for trachoma, 44
Sulfadiazine for *Toxoplasma gondii* infections, 320
Sulfamethoxazole
    for nocardiosis, 163
    for nontuberculous mycobacteria, 346
Sulfisoxazole for nocardiosis, 163
Sulfonamide
    for group A streptococcal infections, 264
    for nocardiosis, 163
    for paracoccidioidomycosis, 172
Suppressive therapy for cytomegalovirus infection, 59
Suppurative cervical adenitis from group A streptococcal infections, 261
Suramin for African trypanosomiasis, 329
Surgical excision for warts, 170, 171
Surgical wound infection from group A streptococcal infections, 261

Sweats
    from babesiosis, 21
    from malaria, 147
    from rickettsialpox, 217
Swimmer's itch, 237, 238*i*
    from schistosomiasis, 236
Syncope from pertussis, 186
Synergistic bacterial gangrene
    from *Bacteroides* infection, 24
    from *Prevotella* infection, 24
Syphilis, 278–293
    acquired, 278, 279
    chancroid and, 43
    clinical manifestations of, 278
    congenital, 278, 280–281, 288*i*, 289*i*, 290*i*
    cutaneous, 288*i*
    diagnostic tests for, 279–281
    epidemiology of, 278–279
    etiology of, 278
    incubation period of, 279
    latent, 278, 279
    with penile chancre, 291*i*
    secondary, 292*i*
    tertiary, 279
    treatment of, 282–287
Syphilis serologic test, guide for interpretation of, 285*t*
Systemic lupus erythematosus from *Cryptococcus neo-
    formans* infections, 55
Systemic toxicity from *Clostridium difficile,* 48
Systemic toxoplasmosis from *Toxoplasma gondii
    * infections, 318

T

Tachycardia from *Clostridial myonecrosis,* 50
Tachypnea from *Pneumocystis jiroveci* infections, 204
Taenia asiatica, 294
Taenia saginata, 294, 295*i*
Taeniasis (tapeworm diseases), 294–296
    clinical manifestations of, 294
    diagnosis of, 294
    epidemiology of, 294
    etiology of, 294
    incubation period of, 294
    treatment of, 294–295
Taenia solium, 294, 295*i*
Tapeworm diseases (*taeniasis* and cysticercosis), 294–296
    clinical manifestations of, 294
    diagnosis of, 294
    epidemiology of, 294
    etiology of, 294
    incubation period of, 294
    treatment of, 294–295
Temperature instability from *Escherichia coli,* 72
Tenesmus
    from *Shigella* infections, 239
    from trichuriasis, 328
Tenosynovitis
    from gonococcal infections, 82
    from *Pasteurella* infections, 181

Terbinafine
    for tinea capitis, 303
    for tinea corporis, 305
    for tinea cruris, 307
    for tinea pedis and tinea unguium, 308
Terminal ileitis from *Yersinia pseudotuberculosis*
    infection, 368
Tertiary syphilis, 279
Tetanus (lockjaw), 299–301, 301*i*
    cephalic, 299
    clinical manifestations of, 299
    diagnostic tests for, 299
    epidemiology of, 299
    etiology of, 299
    generalized, 299
    incubation period of, 299
    infant with, 300*i*
    localized, 299
    neonatal, 299, 300*i*
    treatment of, 299
Tetracycline
    for actinomycosis, 1
    for anthrax, 9
    for *Balantidium coli* infection, 26
    for *Borrelia* infections, 31
    for brucellosis, 33
    for *Chlamydia trachomatis,* 44
    for epidemic typhus, 354
    for group A streptococcal infections, 264
    for *Mycoplasma pneumoniae* infections, 162
    for plague, 195, 196
    for Rocky Mountain spotted fever, 220
    for syphilis, 283
    for trachoma, 44
    for tularemia, 351
    for *Vibrio cholerae* infections, 364
    for *Yersinia enterocolitica* and *Yersinia pseudo-
    tuberculosis* infections, 369
Thalassemia from parvovirus B19, 178
Thiabendazole
    for cutaneous larva migrans, 57
    for strongyloidiasis, 275
Thigh myalgia from hantavirus pulmonary syndrome, 91
Thoracic disease from actinomycosis, 1
Thread-like warts, 169
Throat specimens for enterovirus infections, 67
Throat swab specimens for poliovirus infections, 208
Throat washing for mumps, 159
Thrombocytopenia
    from African trypanosomiasis, 329
    from *Borrelia* infections, 31
    from congenital rubella, 225
    from *Ehrlichia* and *Anaplasma* infections, 63
    from Epstein-Barr virus, 69
    from hepatitis B, 97
    from leishmaniasis, 131
    from malaria, 147
    from mumps, 159
    from parvovirus B19, 178
    from Rocky Mountain spotted fever, 219

from rubella, 225
from syphilis, 278
from *Toxoplasma gondii* infections, 318
from varicella-zoster infections, 356
Thrombocytopenic purpura from cat-scratch disease, 40
Thrombosis, 19
Thrush, 37–39
  from candidiasis, 37
  clinical manifestations of, 37
  diagnostic tests for, 37
  epidemiology of, 37
  etiology of, 37
  incubation period of, 37
  treatment of, 37–38
Thyroiditis from mumps, 159
Ticarcillin-clavulanate for *Pasteurella* infections, 181
Tick bite, rash of, in Lyme disease, 142*i*
Timorian filariasis, 144–145
Tinea capitis (ringworm of the scalp), 302–304, 303*i*, 304*i*
  clinical manifestations of, 302
  diagnostic tests for, 302
  epidemiology of, 302
  etiology of, 302
  incubation period of, 302
  treatment of, 303
Tinea corporis (ringworm of the body), 305–306, 306*i*
  clinical manifestations of, 305
  diagnosis of, 305
  epidemiology of, 305
  etiology of, 305
  incubation period of, 305
  treatment of, 305
Tinea cruris (Jock itch), 307
  clinical manifestations of, 307
  diagnostic tests for, 307
  epidemiology of, 307
  etiology of, 307
  incubation period of, 307
  treatment of, 307
Tinea lesion, 303*i*
Tinea pedis (athlete's foot), 308–309, 309*i*
  clinical manifestations of, 308
  diagnosis of, 308
  epidemiology of, 308
  etiology of, 308
  treatment of, 308–309
Tinea unguium (ringworm of the feet), 308–309, 309*i*
  clinical manifestations of, 308
  diagnosis of, 308
  epidemiology of, 308
  etiology of, 308
  treatment of, 308–309
Tinea versicolor (pityriasis versicolor), 192–194, 193*i*
  clinical manifestations of, 192
  diagnosis of, 192
  epidemiology of, 192
  etiology of, 192
  incubation period of, 192
  treatment of, 192

Tinidazole
  for amebiasis, 4
  for *Giardia intestinalis* infections, 80
  for *Trichomonas vaginalis* infection, 326
Tissue biopsy
  for candidiasis, 37
  for paracoccidioidomycosis, 172
Tissue infection from toxic shock syndrome, 310
Togaviridae, 12
Tolnaftate
  for tinea corporis, 305
  for tinea cruris, 307
Tonsillar inflammation from Epstein-Barr virus, 70
Tonsillitis
  from adenovirus infections, 3
  from tularemia, 350
Tonsillopharyngeal infection from gonococcal
      infections, 82
Tonsillopharyngitis, 15
Tonsil swabbing for group A streptococcal infections, 262
Toxic encephalopathy from *Shigella* infections, 239
Toxic shock syndrome, 310–315, 314*i*, 315*i*
  clinical manifestations of, 310
  diagnostic tests for, 311
  epidemiology of, 310
  etiology of, 310
  management of staphylococcal or streptococcal, 313*t*
  management of streptococcal, with necrotizing
      fasciitis, 313*t*
  from staphylococcal infections, 248
  treatment of, 311
Toxocara canis, 316, 317*i*
Toxocara cati, 316
Toxocariasis (visceral larva migrans, ocular larva mi-
      grans), 316–317
  clinical manifestations of, 316
  diagnostic tests for, 316
  epidemiology of, 316
  etiology of, 316
  incubation period of, 316
  treatment of, 316
Toxoplasma gondii encephalitis, 320
Toxoplasma gondii infections (toxoplasmosis),
      318–322, 322*i*
  clinical manifestations of, 318
  diagnostic tests for, 319–320
  epidemiology of, 318
  etiology of, 318
  from human immunodeficiency virus infection, 116
  incubation period of, 318
  treatment of, 320
Toxoplasma gondii-specific IgE antibody test for toxo-
      plasma, 319
Toxoplasmosis, congenital, 318, 319
Toxoplasmosis of myocardium, 322*i*
Trachoma, 44
  from *Chlamydia trachomatis*, 44
Transbronchial biopsy for *Pneumocystis jiroveci* infec-
      tions, 204
Transcription-mediated amplification for gonococcal
      infections, 82
Transient aplastic crisis from parvovirus B19, 178

Transient pneumonitis, acute from *Ascaris lumbricoides* infections, 17
Transverse myelitis
    from Epstein-Barr virus, 69
    from mumps, 159
    from *Mycoplasma pneumoniae* infections, 161
    from tapeworm diseases, 294
Tremors
    from American trypanosomiasis, 331
    from West Nile virus, 365
Treponemal tests for syphilis, 279
Treponema pallidum, 278, 279, 288*i*
Treponema pallidum particle agglutination (TP-PA) for syphilis, 279
Tretinoin for warts, 170
Triatomine bug, 332*i*
Trichinella nativa, 323
Trichinella spiralis, 323
Trichinellosis *(Trichinella spiralis),* 323–325, 325*i*
    clinical manifestations of, 323
    diagnostic tests for, 323
    epidemiology of, 323
    etiology of, 323
    incubation period of, 323
    treatment of, 323
Trichloroacetic acid for warts, 170
Trichomonas vaginalis infections (trichomoniasis), 326–327, 327*i*
    from bacterial vaginosis, 22
    clinical manifestations of, 326
    diagnostic tests for, 326
    epidemiology of, 326
    etiology of, 326
    incubation period of, 326
    treatment of, 326
Trichophyton mentagrophytes, 305, 307, 308
Trichophyton rubrum, 307, 308
Trichophyton tonsurans, 302, 305
Trichotillomania, tinea capitis and, 302
Trichuriasis trichiura, 328
Trichuriasis trichiura colitis, 328
Trichuriasis (whipworm infection), 328
    clinical manifestations of, 328
    diagnostic tests for, 328
    epidemiology of, 328
    etiology of, 328
    incubation period of, 328
    treatment of, 328
Trichuris trichiura, 328, 328*i*
Trichuris trichiura dysentery syndrome, 328
Trifluridine for herpes simplex virus (HSV), 106
Trigeminal neuralgia from herpes simplex virus, 104
Trimethoprim-sulfamethoxazole
    for brucellosis, 33
    for *Escherichia coli* diarrhea, 77
    for granuloma inguinale, 86
    for *Listeria monocytogenes* infections, 139
    for nocardiosis, 163
    for nontuberculous mycobacteria, 346
    for *Pasteurella* infections, 181

    for pediculosis capitis, 183
    for pediculosis pubis, 185
    for pertussis, 187
    for plague, 196
    for *Pneumocystis jiroveci* infections, 205
    for *Salmonella* infections, 230
    for *Shigella* infections, 240
    for *Toxoplasma gondii* infections, 320
    in treating cat-scratch disease, 40
    for *Vibrio cholerae* infections, 364
    for *Yersinia enterocolitica* and *Yersinia pseudotuberculosis* infections, 369
Trismus from tetanus, 299
Tropheryma whippelii, 163
Trypanosoma brucei gambiense infection, 329
Trypanosoma brucei rhodesiense infection, 329
Trypanosoma cruzi, 331, 332*i*
Trypanosomiasis
    African, 329, 330*i*
    American, 331–332, 332*i*
Tube agglutination for tularemia, 350
Tuberculin skin test (TST), 343*i*
    results from, 335
    for tuberculosis, 333, 335
Tuberculosis, 333–344
    clinical manifestations of, 333
    congenital, 339, 342*i*
    definitions of, 333
    definitions of positive tuberculin skin tests, 340*t*
    diagnostic tests for, 334–336
    epidemiology of, 333–334
    etiology of, 333
    incubation period of, 334
    miliary, 342*i*
    mycobacterial, 348*i*
    people at increased risk of drug-resistant, 341*t*
    recommended treatment regimens for drug-susceptible, 341*t*
    renal, 333
    from sporotrichosis, 246
    treatment of, 336–339
    tuberculin skin test recommendations for, 340*t*
Tuberculosis disease, 333
    drug resistance, 338, 341*t*
    human immunodeficiency virus infection and, 338–339
    treatment of, 337–338
Tularemia, 350–352, 351*i*
    clinical manifestations of, 350
    diagnostic tests for, 350–351
    epidemiology of, 350
    etiology of, 350
    incubation period of, 350
    pneumonic, 350
    treatment of, 351
Tularemia pneumonia, 352*i*
Tularemic lesion, 352*i*
Tularemic ulcer, 351*i*
Tympanocentesis for otitis media, 201

Typhus
    endemic, 353
        clinical manifestations of, 353
        diagnostic tests for, 353
        epidemiology of, 353
        etiology of, 353
        incubation period of, 353
        treatment of, 353
    epidemic, 354–355
        clinical manifestations of, 354
        diagnostic tests for, 354
        epidemiology of, 354
        etiology of, 354
        incubation period of, 354
        treatment of, 354–355

U

Ulcerative chancroid lesions, 43*i*
Ulcerative enanthem from herpes simplex, 103
Ulceroglandular syndrome from tularemia, 350
Ulcers
    from amebiasis, 4
    anthrax, 10*i*
    from *Balantidium coli* infection, 26
    chancroidal, 43
    duodenal, from *Helicobacter pylori* infections, 94
    gastric, from *Helicobacter pylori* infections, 94
    genital, from chancroids, 43
    tularemic, 351*i*
Undifferentiated B- or T-lymphocyte lymphomas from
        Epstein-Barr virus, 69
Unilateral inguinal adenitis from chancroid, 43
Upper respiratory tract culture for pneumococcal
        infections, 198
Upper respiratory tract illness from respiratory
        syncytial virus, 215
Urease testing for *Helicobacter pylori* infections, 94
Urethral exudate, 84*i*
Urethral obstruction from granuloma inguinale, 86
Urethritis
    from *Chlamydia trachomatis,* 44
    from *Campylobacter* infections, 35
    from gonococcal infections, 82
    from Kawasaki disease, 127
    from pinworm infection, 190
    from *Trichomonas vaginalis* infections, 326
Urgency from *Schistosoma haematobium,* 236
Urinary tract infections
    from group B streptococcal infections, 269
    from non–group A or B streptococcal and
        enterococcal infections, 272
    from *Pasteurella* infections, 181
    from *Schistosoma haematobium,* 236
    from staphylococcal infections, 248
Urine specimens for gonococcal infections, 82
Urticarial rash from trichinellosis, 323
Uveitis
    from leptospirosis, 136
    from West Nile virus, 365

V

Vaccine-associated paralytic poliomyelitis (VAPP), 207
Vaccines
    for children with human immunodeficiency virus
        infection, 119–120
    for diphtheria, 61
    oral poliovirus, 207
Vaccinia, 242, 243*i*
Vaginal candidiasis, 37
Vaginal discharge
    from chancroid, 43
    from *Trichomonas vaginalis* infections, 326
Vaginal swabs for gonococcal infections, 83
Vaginitis
    from bacterial vaginosis, 22
    from *Chlamydia trachomatis,* 44
    from gonococcal infections, 82
    from group A streptococcal infections, 261
    from pinworm infection, 190
Vaginosis, bacterial, 22–23
    clinical manifestations of, 22
    diagnostic tests for, 22
    epidemiology of, 22
    etiology of, 22
    incubation period of, 22
    treatment of, 22
Valacyclovir
    for Epstein-Barr virus, 70
    for herpes simplex virus, 105
    mucocutaneous, 106
    for varicella-zoster infections, 359
Valvular heart disease from non–group A or B strepto-
        coccal and enterococcal infections, 272
Vancomycin
    for *Clostridium difficile,* 49
    for non–group A or B streptococcal and enterococcal
        infections, 273
    for pneumococcal infections, 199
    for staphylococcal infections, 252
    for toxic shock syndrome, 311
Vancomycin-intermediately susceptible *Staphylococcus*
        aureus (VISA), 250, 252
Vancomycin-resistant *Staphylococcus aureus* (VRSA), 250
Varicella fasciitis, 361*i*
Varicella lesions, 359*i*, 360*i*
Varicella pneumonia, 361*f*
Varicella-zoster virus (VZV) infections, 356–362
    clinical manifestations of, 356
    diagnostic tests for, 357, 358*t*
    epidemiology of, 356–357
    etiology of, 356
    human immunodeficiency virus children and, 120
    incubation period of, 357
    treatment of, 357–359
Variola major, 241–242
Variola minor, 241, 242*i*

Variola (smallpox), 241–245
  clinical manifestations of, 241–242
  diagnostic testing for, 242
  diagnostic tests for, 242
  epidemiology of, 242
  etiology of, 242
  incubation period of, 242
  treatment of, 242
Vascular collapse and shock from malaria, 147
Vasculitis
  from *Haemophilus influenzae* infections, 90*i*
  from Rocky Mountain spotted fever, 221*i*
Venereal Disease Research Laboratory (VDRL) slide test
      for syphilis, 279
Venezuelan equine encephalitis virus, 12
  disease caused by arboviruses in Western
      hemisphere, 13*t*
Venoarterial ECMO for hantavirus pulmonary
      syndrome, 92
Vertebral osteomyelitis, 258*i*
Vesicular fluid for varicella-zoster infections, 357
Vesiculopapular herpes genitalis lesions, 108*i*
Vibrio cholerae (cholera), 363–364, 364*i*
  clinical manifestations of, 363
  diagnostic tests for, 363
  epidemiology of, 363
  etiology of, 363
  incubation period of, 363
  treatment of, 363–364
Vibriocidal antibody titers for *Vibrio cholerae*
      infections, 363
Vibrio cholerae infections, 363–364
  clinical manifestations of, 363
  diagnostic tests for, 363
  epidemiology of, 363
  etiology of, 363
  incubation period of, 363
  treatment of, 363–364
Vidarabine for herpes simplex virus (HSV), 106
Viral antigen
  in nasopharyngeal specimens for respiratory
      syncytial virus, 215
  for parainfluenza virus infections, 176
Viral cultures
  for hantavirus pulmonary syndrome, 92
  for West Nile virus, 366
Viral gastroenteritis from *Campylobacter* infections, 35
Viral meningitis from poliovirus infections, 207
Viral nucleic acid for human papillomaviruses, 170
Viral shedding
  from influenza, 124
  in respiratory syncytial virus, 215
Viremia, 365
Viridans streptococci from non–group A or B streptococ-
      cal and enterococcal infections, 272
Visceral leishmaniasis, 131, 132
Visual impairment from tapeworm diseases, 294
Vitamin A supplementation for measles, 151
Vitamin B$_{12}$ deficiency from tapeworm infections, 297
Vitiligo, pityriasis versicolor and, 192

Vomiting. *See also* Nausea
  from anthrax, 9
  from babesiosis, 21
  from *Balantidium coli* infection, 26
  from *Ehrlichia* and *Anaplasma* infections, 63
  from enterovirus infections, 67
  from *Escherichia coli,* 72
  from hantavirus pulmonary syndrome, 91
  from *Helicobacter pylori* infections, 94
  from hookworm infections, 112
  from influenza, 124
  from leptospirosis, 136
  from malaria, 147
  from pertussis, 186
  from rat-bite fever, 213
  from rickettsialpox, 217
  from Rocky Mountain spotted fever, 219
  from rotavirus infections, 223
  from smallpox, 241
  from *Strongyloides,* 275
  from toxic shock syndrome, 310
  from trichinellosis, 323
  from tularemia, 350
  from *Vibrio cholerae* infections, 363
  from West Nile virus, 365
Voriconazole for aspergillosis, 19
Vulvitis from bacterial vaginosis, 22
Vulvovaginal burning from *Trichomonas vaginalis*
      infections, 326
Vulvovaginal candidiasis, treatment for, 37
Vulvovaginal infections
  from *Bacteroides* infection, 24
  from *Prevotella* infection, 24
Vulvovaginal itching from *Trichomonas vaginalis*
      infections, 326

W

Warts, 169
  anogenital, 169
  cutaneous, 169
  cutaneous nongenital, 169
  filiform, 169
  flat, 169
  nongenital, 170
  plantar, 169, 170
  skin, 169
  thread-like, 169
Washer woman's hand, 364*i*
Water contamination as cause of *Escherichia coli*
      diarrhea, 76
Waterhouse-Friderichsen syndrome from meningococcal
      infections, 153
Wayson stain for plague, 195
Weakness
  from brucellosis, 33
  from West Nile virus, 365

Weight loss
  from African trypanosomiasis, 329
  from babesiosis, 21
  from brucellosis, 33
  from *Ehrlichia* and *Anaplasma* infections, 63
  from histoplasmosis, 109
  from leishmaniasis, 131
  from nontuberculous mycobacteria, 345
  from paracoccidioidomycosis, 172
  from tuberculosis, 333
Weil syndrome from leptospirosis, 136
West African infection, 329
Western blot assays for hantavirus pulmonary
      syndrome, 92
Western blot serologic antibody test for paragonimiasis,
      174–175
Western equine encephalitis virus, disease caused by
      arboviruses in Western hemisphere, 13*t*
West Nile encephalitis virus, 367*f*
  disease caused by arboviruses in Western
      hemisphere, 13*t*
West Nile fever (WNF), 365
West Nile virus (WNV), 14*i*, 365–367
  antigen for, 367*i*
  clinical manifestations of, 365
  diagnostic tests for, 366
  epidemiology of, 365–366
  etiology of, 365
  histopathologic features of, 367*i*
  incubation period of, 366
  treatment of, 366
Wet-mount preparation of vaginal discharge for
      Trichomonas vaginalis infection, 326
Wheezing
  from respiratory syncytial virus, 215
  from toxocariasis, 316
Whipple disease, 163
Whipworm infection (trichuriasis), 328, 328*i*
  clinical manifestations of, 328
  diagnostic tests for, 328
  epidemiology of, 328
  etiology of, 328
  incubation period of, 328
  treatment of, 328
White blood cell count for pertussis, 187
Whooping cough (pertussis), 186–189
  clinical manifestations of, 186
  diagnostic tests for, 186–187
  epidemiology of, 186
  etiology of, 186
  incubation period of, 186
  treatment of, 187
Widal test for *Salmonella* infections, 230
Winterbottom sign, 329
Wood light examination
  for pityriasis versicolor, 192
  for tinea capitis, 302

World Health Organization (WHO), Oral Rehydration
      Solution (ORS), 363–364
Wound botulism, 46, 51*i*
Wound infections
  from *Arcanobacterium haemolyticum* infections, 15
  from staphylococcal infections, 248
Wright-stained smear
  for African trypanosomiasis, 329
  for American trypanosomiasis, 331
  identification of intracellular leishmanial organism,
      132
  for molluscum contagiosum, 157
  for *Plasmodium malariae*, 149*i*
  for *Plasmodium ovale*, 149*i*
  for *Plasmodium vivax*, 149*i*
  for *Pneumocystis jiroveci* infections, 204–205
  in *Yersinia pestis*, 196*i*
Wuchereria bancrofti, 144

X

Xenodiagnosis for American trypanosomiasis, 331
Xenopsylla cheopis, 353
X-linked lymphoproliferative syndrome from Epstein-
      Barr virus, 69

Y

Yeast-phase antigen for *Histoplasma capsulatum*, 110
Yellow fever virus, 12, 14*i*
  disease caused by arboviruses in Western
      hemisphere, 13*t*
Yersinia enterocolitica infections (enteritis and other
      illnesses), 368–369
  clinical manifestations of, 368
  diagnostic tests for, 368–369
  epidemiology of, 368
  etiology of, 368
  incubation period of, 368
  treatment of, 369
Yersinia pestis, 195, 196*i*, 368
Yersinia pseudotuberculosis infections (enteritis and
      other illnesses), 368–369
  clinical manifestations of, 368
  diagnostic tests for, 368–369
  epidemiology of, 368
  etiology of, 368
  incubation period of, 368
  treatment of, 369

Z

Zanamivir for influenza, 125, 126